Freebirth Stories

Edited by Mavis Kirkham and Nadine Edwards

Freebirth Stories

First edition published 2023 by Birth Practice and Politics Forum
Sheffield

© Mavis Kirkham and Nadine Edwards

Mavis Kirkham and Nadine Edwards have asserted their moral right to be named as the authors of this work in accordance with the Copyright, Designs and Patents Act of 1988.

ISBN: 9781916060623

Also available as an e-book

Cover design by Nikki Chhokar

All rights reserved. No part of this book may be reproduced or transmitted in any form by any means for any commercial or non-commercial use without the prior written permission of the authors. This book is sold subject to the condition that it shall not, by way of trade and otherwise, be lent, resold, hired out or otherwise circulated without the publisher's prior consent in any form, or binding, or cover other than that in which it is published and without a similar condition being imposed upon the subsequent purchaser.

This book offers general information for interest only and does not constitute or replace individualised professional midwifery or medical care and advice. The authors accept no liability or responsibility for any loss or damage caused, or thought to be caused, by making decisions based upon the content of this book.

Dedication to Beverley Lawrence Beech

We dedicate this book to the birth activist Beverley Lawrence Beech (1944-2023). Beverley's achievements are legendary: she was renowned both nationally and internationally by those working in the field of birth. Her campaigning led to changes in maternity practice for the benefit of women and their families. Nothing was more important to her than supporting women to make the decisions that they felt were best for them and their babies. Whether she agreed with women's decisions or not, she worked tirelessly to make sure that these were respected and that pregnant, birthing and postnatal women were treated with dignity and kindness.

"The universe, somebody said, and I know now it is true, is made of stories, not particles; they are the wave functions of our existence. If they constitute the event horizon of our particular black hole they are also our only means of escape."

Andre Brink (1996)

Contents

Glossary ix

Introduction 1

Four Freebirth Stories 7

Section 1: Why Freebirth? 17

Chapter 1: Journeying away from trauma and institutionalisation 19

Chapter 2: The journey towards freebirth 35

Chapter 3: "Finding your safe place": safety, trust and fear 51

Section 2: Preparation for Freebirth 57

Chapter 4: Preparation: learning and unlearning 59

Chapter 5: Letting go of fear and control: building confidence and taking responsibility 67

Section 3: Relationships around Freebirth 79

Chapter 6: Partners 81

Chapter 7: Family and freebirth 91

Chapter 8: Friends and the freebirth community: holding safe space 99

Chapter 9: Doulas 107

Chapter 10: Midwives and "the system" 119

Section 4: Labours and births 143

Chapter 11: Labours and births 145

Chapter 12: Three first labours and births 157

Chapter 13: More labours and births 167

Chapter 14: A mother's story and her doula's story ---------------------------------------183

Chapter 15: A twin birth: a mother's story and her doula's story------------------------193

Chapter 16: A premature twin birth and the death of a baby ---------------------------201

Chapter 17: A stillbirth ---205

Section 5: After the Birth and Wider Issues------------------------------------ 209

Chapter 18: After the birth: joy and compliance ---------------------------------------211

Chapter 19: Problems --223

Chapter 20: Referral to Social Services ---237

Chapter 21: The impact of the freebirth on the mother --------------------------------251

Our reflections ---259

References---265

Glossary

ADHD: Attention Deficit Hyperactivity Disorder

AIMS: Association for Improvements in the Maternity Services

Apgar score: A measure of the physical condition of a newborn infant, obtained by giving points (2, 1, or 0) for heart rate, respiratory effort, muscle tone, response to stimulation, and skin coloration. A score of ten represents the best possible condition

BBA: Birth Before Arrival. An NHS term for mothers booked for home birth where the baby is born before the midwife arrives or mothers booked for hospital birth who give birth before they arrive at the hospital

BMI: Body Mass Index

Braxton Hicks contractions: Uterine contractions experienced in pregnancy which prepare the uterine muscle for labour, named after the nineteenth century physician who "discovered" them

CTG: Cardiotocograph, electronic monitoring of the fetal heart rate

EMCS/ECS: Emergency caesarean section

HBAC: Home birth after caesarean section

HCP: Health care professional

IM: Independent midwife, self employed

Inco pad: Incontinence pads which are absorbent and disposable

MSLC: Maternity Services Liaison Committee. A committee made up of those using maternity services and various disciplines of service providers. Replaced in 2019 by Maternity Voices Partnerships in England. Term still sometimes used

NCT: National Childbirth Trust

NHS: National Health Service

NICU: Neonatal intensive care unit

NIPT: Noninvasive prenatal testing, a test of maternal blood for fetal DNA

Pinard: Ear trumpet shaped fetal stethoscope for listening to the unborn baby's heartbeat

PND: Postnatal depression

PPC: Pregnancy and Parents Centre, Edinburgh

PTSD: Post-Traumatic Stress Disorder

Puppy pads: Inco pads sold for training puppies

Rebozo: Traditional Mexican shawl which can be used in pregnancy and labour to encourage optimal fetal positioning

SPD: Symphysis pubis dysfunction, now usually referred to as pelvic girdle pain

Supervisor of Midwives (SoM): This statutory role, independent of employers, provided both supervision for midwives and someone to whom mothers could appeal if they thought their maternity care did not meet their needs. This role was abolished in 2017. There are a few occasions in this book where the term was used for a senior midwifery manager after that date

VBAC: Vaginal birth after caesarean section

VE: Vaginal examination

Ventouse Extraction: Birth helped by traction on a suction cup attached to the baby's head. This is now often preferred to a forceps delivery as it is thought to be less traumatic

WBAC: Water birth after caesarean

Introduction

This is a collection of stories about freebirth by women who have given birth without health professional attendance in the United Kingdom (UK). The stories were woven together by a midwife and a birth activist. We have each spent several decades listening to women and, in different ways, being with them on their journeys of pregnancy, birth and parenting. We have witnessed many types of misogyny and disrespect, as well as a continual decline in the services offered to childbearing women and families in the UK. This has taken place alongside a devaluing of midwifery knowledge, practice and services, and we have both written about this (Kirkham 2010, 2018, Reed and Edwards 2023). The move towards freebirth is not the only result of the cultural changes that have taken place during these years, but it is an important result, and one that we wanted to help document.

We aim to share the stories of women and families so that others may learn from them. We will define and explain how we came to collect these stories, but this book is not about us or our voices. Our aim in undertaking this project has been to raise awareness of the issues, and to help women and families to share their own stories. We have used our experience of research, analysis and writing to collect and weave these stories together in a way that we hope will be meaningful to the reader, but we have sought to add as little of our own voices as possible, and to prioritise those of the women who shared their stories with us. In order to do this, we have italicised our own comments throughout.

Why freebirth matters

Freebirth matters because it tells us about what those concerned want for their births, their babies and themselves and what they seek to avoid. Stories matter because they render our experiences coherent and enable others to understand our experiences (Kirkham 1997). Every story is more than a tale. Stories speak of context and values. The stories in this book can be seen as voicing resistance (McKenzie-Mohr and La France 2014) to the dominant message of maternity services which no longer meets so many women's needs (Wickham 2022, Cohen Shabot 2020). In addition, overburdened staff prioritise tasks and are unable to care for women individually in their own unique circumstances. They therefore no longer provide safe emotional care for women and sometimes are unable to provide care which is safe in any sense of the word.

It is generally agreed that the number of freebirths is growing, though it is not possible to count cases which, by definition, are absent from official birth statistics. Freebirth has been described as the 'Canary in the Coal Mine' (Dahlen et al 2020) because the traumas many of these women have previously experienced within conventional maternity care and their decisions to avoid that system highlight its toxic nature; just as canaries in coal mines succumbed to toxic gases and thereby warned miners who were less sensitive. "They choose to birth outside the system because what we offer is hurting them and we are simply not listening to their concerns" (Dahlen et al 2020 p4). Thus freebirth is important for what it tells us about the system that the women who plan to freebirth wish to avoid. It is also important in showing what these women believe needs to be in place for them to have positive births for their babies and themselves, and why they make the decision to freebirth.

It is important to distinguish between present NHS maternity services and the fundamental concept of the NHS. We wholeheartedly support a health service free at the point of need for all, including pregnant, birthing and postnatal women. We do not wish to further undermine the concept or ideology of the NHS, to which we are committed. But there is clearly a need to criticise the current organisation and delivery of NHS maternity services.

The presence of the NHS gives a particular quality to freebirth in the UK. While planning a freebirth, almost all the women who entrusted us with their stories saw NHS maternity services as a safety net which they were happy to use in an emergency. We did not encounter the kind of opposition to medical services which pervades some online freebirth communities in other countries. Online freebirth communities in this country, whilst supporting maternal choice, usually have a flexible approach.

Definition

For this book we are defining freebirth as birth without a midwife or doctor in attendance, when that attendance is available without charge, and the decision not to be professionally attended is made by the mother and usually the family concerned. Such births are sometimes called "unassisted" or "unattended births" by professionals and we have heard them called "unhindered births" or "wild births" by parents. "Freebirth" is now the term most commonly used.

If the woman received some NHS antenatal care and was booked for an NHS birth, her birth would be recorded in NHS statistics as a BBA, birth before arrival, despite the fact that a midwife was neither summoned nor sought, (or sometimes deliberately called too late) nor did the woman attempt to attend a maternity hospital. Such recording means that freebirths cannot be counted separately from births en route to hospital, precipitate births where the mother wished to be in hospital but could not get there in time, or births where the mother was not aware she was pregnant. Recording freebirths is made more difficult by the many women who have NHS antenatal care and plan to freebirth but do not tell their midwives of their plan. Freebirths, where no NHS care was sought, do not appear in NHS statistics.

A few of the women in this book had no contact with maternity services in pregnancy or in labour. Some booked for NHS home births, had NHS antenatal care to varying extents and omitted to call the midwife to the birth or deliberately called her so she arrived after the birth. Some called the midwife after the birth, some did not. There were different degrees of planning in terms of not calling the midwife: a few even had telephone access to a friendly midwife during labour, but all the mothers whose stories we collected felt they made the right decision not to have a midwife at the birth. One gave birth during the 45 minutes her partner was on the phone trying to call a midwife to their NHS booked home birth. We include her story because after the event she was pleased she gave birth without a midwife and would freebirth if she had another pregnancy.

The women in this book are spread throughout the UK. They differ greatly in age, cultural, educational, social, and economic circumstance and have very different backgrounds, belief systems and lifestyles. We have mainly anonymised geographical locations except on a few occasions to give some idea of the spread of stories across the UK. Almost all of the women had very positive outcomes, but tragically two of the babies died.

How this book came about

We have long been interested in women's experiences of birth and in why some women decide to freebirth and how they experience this. We have both had a career long commitment to helping women achieve the birth they feel is right for them, which becomes more difficult as NHS maternity services become increasingly underfunded, centralised, standardised and run on an industrial model (Kirkham 2018). In their struggles to achieve a birth which is physically and emotionally right for them, women who freebirth appear more frequently in many contexts, from newspapers (e.g. Summers 2020), to academic articles (e.g. Shorey et al 2023), to the popular writings of the Yorkshire Shepherdess (Owen 2016). In all these contexts, women who have freebirthed so often say, "It was wonderful. I simply believe that it was right for our family."

About the Authors

I, Mavis, am long retired after a career in midwifery research and clinical midwifery. I was fortunate to train as a midwife at a time when my training left me with a deep respect for women and their ability to birth their babies with the support of midwives who they often knew well. My central professional concern has been how women are engaged with the process of birth, the enabling effects of active engagement upon mothers, families and midwives and the conditions which foster "normal" birth. The relationships around birth are also important to me. I have long been concerned with how birth stories evolve in the light of changing relationships and experiences. Also the impact of these stories on tellers and hearers.

I, Nadine, have been a birth activist and campaigner for over four decades. Part of my work has been supporting women to negotiate the care they need during pregnancy, labour and birth. As services have become increasingly under-resourced, highly regulated, rule bound and thus inflexible, health practitioners have become less able to support women's agency, especially when they decline previously unchallenged routine practices such as vaginal examinations and fetal heart monitoring. This inflexibility is leading more women to consider freebirthing. Seeking and understanding women's experiences of maternity care systems, their decisions, what facilitates and undermines these and the politics behind these is central to my work.

At one time we naively sought funding in order to research freebirth. But efforts to obtain funding were futile when it was impossible to answer the first question "How many per year in the UK?" On further reflection it became clear that looking at women's decisions to reject the NHS bureaucratic structures around birth could not wisely be contained within the bureaucratic structures of academic health research. We wanted to be led by the women who wanted to tell their stories of freebirth. We wanted to collect more stories than in previous studies and we wanted to present those stories from the woman's perspective.

We were inspired by the work of Svetlana Alexievich, who allowed people to tell their painful and nuanced stories, some of which the authorities concerned did not want to hear. We cannot reach the skill of a winner of the Nobel Prize for literature, but we have learned from Svetlana Alexievich and seek to allow the women to tell their nuanced and difficult stories.

We were also inspired by Reginald Ray (1994), writing in a very different context, that we can best understand a situation "not by arriving at some supposedly balanced and objective viewpoint, but rather by hearing clearly the different voices that have spoken – without being too put off by contrary perspectives or trying too hard to resolve contradictions." We believe, with Elif Shafak, that, "It is mostly through stories that we learn to think, perceive and remember the world in a more nuanced and reflective way." (Shafak 2020 p87).

The stories

We collected stories firstly from women we knew, and then from women they knew. Doulas and freebirth networks led others to offer their stories. As the collection of stories grew, we sought out women with different experiences. There must also be women with other experiences who may have contributed if they had known of our project. We are not claiming a representative sample but we did collect far more freebirthing stories than any of the research studies on this subject.

We were entrusted with 52 stories. Some were written by the mothers soon after the birth and some were written later at our request. One story was written for the baby and specifically addressed to that baby when older. Some of the stories were collected verbally, mostly in person, and by telephone or zoom during times of Covid and when distances were great. All the stories told verbally were recorded and transcribed. Most of the mothers were given their transcript which some chose to amend, but a major computer problem prevented this in some cases. Most of the births were relatively recent, though the baby in one story is now an adult.

Most of these women wanted us to use their own names, and we added an initial where more than one woman had the same first name. Some preferred a pseudonym or initials.

As we collected the stories, the importance of doulas became clear. Many of the women had doulas at their births and a considerable number of them were doulas themselves. Some were doulas to each other. After one gave us her written account of a birth as a doula, we went on to interview 5 doulas who work particularly with women who plan to freebirth. We have referred to doulas and everyone except the mothers in this book by an initial. A number of the doulas in the stories have the same initial. We kept the full names of those who have since died: Mary Cronk and Beverley Beech.

Language

We are respectfully aware of current moves to refer to those giving birth as persons without ascribing gender. We are also grateful for the clarity of Gribble et al (2022) in this regard. Covid restrictions have led pregnant people of differing sexual and gender orientations to consider freebirth (Greenfield et al 2021). However, all those whose stories are included here saw themselves as women and used the words "woman", "mother" and "she." We speak of them as they spoke of themselves.

There is a considerable difference between written and spoken use of language. We wanted all the stories to be equally readable. We have therefore removed from the recorded stories many hesitations, and use of terms such as "you know", "sort of" and "like" where these are used as verbal punctuation rather than contributing to meaning.

Structure of the book

We are very aware that the creation of chapters required the cutting up of stories. Three dots indicate gaps in the original text. We have built the book around the issues which were important to those who shared their stories. We also sought to create an easily readable book which conveyed the diversity of experiences and was not overly repetitive. We start the book with four complete stories.

Thanks

We are most grateful to all the women who gave generously of their time and entrusted us with their stories. We are also grateful to those who put us in touch with other women who had freebirthed, especially Beverley Beech, Daisy Dinwoodie and Samantha Gadsden. We would like to thank Gill Boden, Sarah Davies, Naomi Nygaard, Caroline Weddell and Sara Wickham for their constructive comments on earlier drafts, Becky Reed for her meticulous proofreading, Jane Flint and Janet Lightfoot and her team for their accurate and timely transcripts and Nikki Chhokar for the beautiful book cover.

We are particularly grateful to Sara Wickham. Without her expertise and constant technical support this book would never have been published.

We dedicate this book to Beverley Beech, who died as it approached completion and who suggested another important contributor in one of our last conversations with her. She helped so many women and continues to inspire us.

Four Freebirth Stories

Claire's story

When we decided to have another baby, I already knew that I would freebirth. It had taken me some time and five births, but I truly knew that assuming that all was well during pregnancy I didn't need, in fact actively needed to not have any interruption or interference during the birth. I chose to dip into antenatal care with the local NHS team as and when I needed/wanted. This worked very well for me. One of my grievances with NHS care is the feeling of handing over control and being swept along a conveyor belt of backside-covering, impersonal "care." I simply declined and cancelled where necessary, staying and feeling very much in control of myself and my pregnancy - as it should be! (At what other point in life do we expect grown adults to let you "allow" them to do things to their bodies because, "it's what we do"?!)...

The birth itself was a wonderful, normal, every-day amazing thing. I was exactly 41 weeks pregnant. My contractions started sometime in the late morning, quietly and gently at first, not even enough for me to be sure that they were for real. I carried on as normal with my day, still totally in denial that this was actually real. By lunchtime I was thinking this probably was it. I made my lunch and ate as much as I could, knowing that I can't eat in labour, and played Hearthstone! I also cleaned my kitchen sink, a job I'd been saving to do in labour as it had distracted me well last time! The contractions were short and not particularly regular, but really packed a punch. I didn't manage to clean the sink as much as I'd intended, and the cooker didn't get a look in! This labour was demanding much more of my attention and was way more intense. About 5pm-ish I accepted that yep, these were for real, this baby had decided to come today. But I was sure I had ages! My husband went to collect our son from work and I walked around downstairs, swaying and leaning on things through the contractions now, they were starting to pinch somewhat! While L [husband] was out I messaged my friend to say something was happening (still pretty sure at this point that I had aaaages). Things really picked up while I was alone for that half hour and L came home to find me in the bathroom (a sure sign things are well on the way!) leaning on the sink and swaying through the now pretty intense contractions. My eldest son chatted to us for a few minutes but I was well away and needed privacy, so we shut the door with the children occupied by a film downstairs and I settled somewhat uncomfortably leaning and swaying on our chest of drawers in the bedroom. The contractions were really INTENSE and I felt like I couldn't keep up with them, my breathing was too fast and I was getting a tingly face from almost hyperventilating. It was like being swept out to sea and I was desperately trying to swim with it and not drown! My waters broke and I knew the baby was coming fast, and she did - I squatted down and she was roared out in two almighty contractions/involuntary pushes, only a few hours after I'd decided that yes, I probably was in labour. The best way to describe it is like a freight train! Fast, huge, and bloody uncomfortable! I'd hoped for another easy, relatively pain freebirth with being unobserved, but it seems for me that just meant things happened even faster! I half caught her, half just cushioned her landing onto the inco pads we'd just managed to get down in time. This bit seems like it happened in slow-mo, that weird time-slowing-down-before-your-eyes feeling when something happens that leaves you acting totally on autopilot! I saw that she was wrapped in her cord, remarked that she was, and unwrapped her as I picked her up. She was utterly covered head to toe in meconium which made her really slippy, but I cuddled her to my chest as she started protesting quite vehemently at the annoyance of being born! I said something to L about the meconium meaning we might need the midwives (meaning if she wasn't okay, but I don't think I was very clear in my just-gave-birth-a-moment-ago state and he gave me a surprised, "really?!"). I checked that she was a girl - we hadn't known the sex of the baby but I was already referring to her as a girl as she was born, before I'd even checked! I think we knew we had a girl all along. We had no boy's names; this is always a giveaway for us!

Her tone and colour were perfect at birth and I had no concerns at all - she was perfect. L took some video and the other children came in to say hello to her, our four year-old being most unimpressed at the volume of her crying! She had a little feed and then I was ready to move as I was uncomfortable on the floor and ready to birth the placenta. I knew from previous experience that my placentas can take a while to come, but I was sure that this was simply because they sit at my cervix. I recognised the feeling clearly this time: the placenta had detached within minutes of the birth and was indeed ready to come out. I squatted again over a bowl and half pushed half pulled the placenta and membranes out (I gave it a bit of a pull when one or the other, not sure which (!) was out). My blood loss as I expected was very minimal (my periods are heavier!). We then sat in bed together and baby-gazed for hours, eventually getting a tiny bit of sleep in the early hours. I tied and cut the cord after a few hours, once it became a bit inconvenient to keep it attached, and I felt ready. This was one of my bug-bears about previous births: there's always someone saying, "Right, shall we do this now?", interrupting my instinctive behaviour and interfering with my space. It seems like such a small thing but it sticks out like a sore thumb from my previous births. This time I did everything exactly when the baby and I were ready. When she was eight hours old I had her wrapped on my chest for the first time while I got food and everyone slept! I called the hospital the next morning to let them know that she was here and had a call back from a lovely but slightly confused midwife! She asked what I'd like her to do and so I asked her to come out and check us over, which she did about an hour later. She went through the forms with us and weighed the baby, 8lb 10oz just like most of her siblings!

And that is the story of my sweet A's uneventful, like a freight train, normal, extraordinary birth. Exactly what I'd hoped for – just a normal event fitted into our day. No one in the way, interrupting or bringing me out of my birthing zone. **Claire**

Keri's story

For pregnancy number four, I had already decided before I knew I was pregnant that I really did want a freebirth this time, and that I was going to fight tooth and nail for it. My reasoning was that I had birthed the previous two babies myself, and had healthy pregnancies where I monitored myself and tried to avoid the midwives as much as I could (naughty I know, but I felt like I didn't need them – I wasn't ill, just undergoing a perfectly natural process for which my body had been perfectly designed). I knew my body better than any midwife could ever do, and I knew what pregnancy and labour entailed. I think the deciding argument for my husband was the fact that I refused to take the three boys, now aged one, three and five to the surgery for any appointments that I might have, so I told him that if he wanted me to see a midwife, then he would have to take time off work, roughly every two weeks, and look after the boys while I went. He agreed only with the caveat that I was sensible and went to the midwives at the slightest problem. So, I didn't see a midwife or doctor for the entire duration of my pregnancy. I monitored my own health as I had done during my other pregnancies, and I felt marvellous. I drank "pregnancy tea" (a blend of raspberry leaf, alfalfa, nettle and peppermint) as I had done during my previous pregnancy – a tea dubbed "disgusting tea" by my kids (the kitchen did stink when I was brewing it) and afterwards I took the label on too as during the ninth month I ramped up my intake and also increased the strength of the tea, holding my nose and glugging it down – research had led me to do this and I believed that this was in part responsible for my short and relatively painless third labour.

On the morning of the 11th of March, I woke up and discovered that I had lost my mucus plug; something I had done just before onset of labour with all my previous pregnancies. I carried on as normal, having the odd Braxton Hicks now and then – nothing that I would have called a contraction. Still, they were irritating me that they weren't getting any stronger, just fiddling around. So, at about 11am, with the other three playing happily with their wooden train track in our oldest's bedroom, I had a lie down on our bed. While I relaxed, I was hit out of nowhere with a very strong contraction.

Marvellous, I thought, and waited to see if anything else happened. I had another four very strong contractions, and then boy number three walked in wafting an unmistakable smell with him. So I got up to change his nappy and made it as far as the door, bending over as contraction number six arrived. I then felt like I desperately needed a wee, so asking the little one to wait for me, I went into our shower room, sat down and discovered that I didn't need a wee, but rather that the head was almost crowning. "Right", I thought and decided that the most sensible thing would be to get in the shower and give birth, rather than trying to make it downstairs to get the phone to ring my husband – he was working half an hour away and I figured he was going to miss it anyway, and as we were in a rented house, I don't want to ruin someone else's carpet. So, I stripped off, put my dressing gown on and got in the shower. As nothing was happening, I decided to break my waters as I could feel that bulging out with the head not too far behind. I used my fingernail, and once they broke, a contraction arrived and the head was on its way out. It was during this contraction that I heard footsteps and I looked round to see our second boy looking at me. "What are you doing Mummy," he asked, to which I managed to reply mid-contraction, "I'm having a baby, please go away." He did, but only to tell his brothers the exciting news that Mummy was having a baby, come and see. Just as the head was out and I breathed a sigh of relief (my least favourite part of labour), I turned to see all three of them, lined up against the side of the shower. In the pause in between contractions, they were bent over, looking at the part of their sibling they could see, making comments like, "ahhh, isn't it cute" and so on. Then our oldest asked me where the rest of it was and why wasn't it coming out. "I'm waiting for a contraction to push the rest out," to which he replied, "what's a contraction?" I was just contemplating a) how do I answer that in a way a six year old will understand and b) this is by far the strangest conversation I've ever had in labour. Fortunately I was spared having to make that reply by the eighth and final contraction arriving and the three of them witnessed me birthing their little brother. There was great joy and clapping and their faces were wreathed in awe and wonder, it was fantastic. As I had cuddled the baby close to me, they hadn't actually spotted whether it was a little brother or a sister, so they asked, and more joy when it was revealed – our second child was going through an "I don't like girls" phase and had publicly stated that if this baby was a girl he would put it in the bin! After our oldest had brought me the phone, they stood around, looking at me and the baby for a bit, and then asked if they could go back to their train track! It was a very matter of fact question, as if watching a baby being born was a perfectly normal thing; get up, have breakfast, play with train track, watch little brother being born, more trains, lunch with Daddy and so on – perfectly "normal" day! I birthed the placenta into a washing up bowl, and carried it and baby, still attached, downstairs after I had showered and dressed. My parents arrived and my Mum buried the placenta in the hole in the field next door that my squeamish husband had dug – he said that he'd dig the hole but wouldn't go anywhere near the "goo" as he called it, otherwise he'd probably pass out! This was a beautiful, quiet, intimate, gentle birth, and I am always thankful that I have a supportive family, and that I have been blessed with a healthy body that works perfectly during labour. The presence of midwives at this final birth would have been superfluous and would probably have spoiled its magical quality. We don't plan on having any more children, but if we do, then I know that I would plan and pray for an identical re-run of this one – a perfect, joyful family event. **Keri**

Kendal's story

F's birth story begins 17 days after he was due, on a snowy day in March. And it begins in the days before, when I wondered if that night would be the night. When I saw the first signs of labour, the gelatinous slip of mucous, the strange dreams.

It begins with a surprise pink line on a pregnancy test months before, unplanned but not unwanted.

And the evening just a few days before when I stared through the dense snow fall and saw a fox paused in the middle of the road, and wondered if that was some sign that birth was imminent.

It begins, for sure, the night before, when I had a sense of extreme giddiness, accompanied by a tingling in my lower back. It had to be soon, I told myself, surely I cannot be the first woman ever just not to have her baby.

Hours later, I woke up to waves that were coming and going, but always returning. Not particularly regular, or intense, but I knew that this was the something that would lead to birth, and I woke my husband just before 6am to tell him that I was pretty sure I may be in labour. Maybe it would be a good idea to put the pool up.

Four births in, and yet I am still surprised by birth. By the strange and different sensations that move through your body. Could I be in labour if I felt so calm, if the surges were so easy? Maybe not. I messaged my doula anyway, told her that it might be happening, that she should maybe be prepared, just in case.

Still, they were little more than sensations that came every so often. But when they persisted, stuck in the certainty that when labour really got going, F [baby] would come quickly, I asked H [partner] to call L my doula, and she and my photographer friend, arrived around 8am.

I wish I could remember when my children got up, how much they were around, but I don't. I knew they were in the dining room with my husband, but beyond that, I can't recall if they came in and out of the room. I vaguely remember my daughter's presence, because I knew how much she wanted to be there.

By the time L [photographer] and L [doula] arrived I felt like I was probably in labour, having the first surges that were something close to intense, but really, still quite painless and quite spaced out. I moved a lot, as seems to be my way. Swaying hips and crouching, walking up and down the stairs. I went to the bathroom, felt like throwing up once (but didn't!) and then kept moving some more. I don't remember anything increasing in intensity, and the surges felt quite short.

But the second time I went to the bathroom, I felt a pressure that made me want to stick my fingers inside and feel about, and there was a smooth, round bubble, around the size of an apple, inside my vagina. My waters! I ran down the stairs, somewhat scaring my doula, as I declared I thought I might need to push.

I got into the birth pool and right away, the need to push was there. Squatting by the side of the pool, I still didn't feel any surges that felt particularly strong or intense, and I wondered if I could be mistaken. But there was no resisting the pressure and, with my hand still inside me, I couldn't stop feeling the bulging waters, unyielding even with my prodding fingers. I knew once they broke there would be some relief, and when they did go, the burst gave way to wrinkled skin, hair. Right there.

I asked H [partner] to get A [daughter], who I knew wanted to be there, and she came through and stood close by, her birthing goddess necklace around her neck. I don't recall where L was, and have only a vague sense of L being next to me, stroking my arm. Yet I also recall feeling quite conscious and aware, not really having had the time to immerse myself in that odd, liminal labour-land. I know I spoke to them and told them the head was right there.

And as soon as I felt his head, I wanted to push again, but the pushing was a completely different sensation to having contractions and pushing. It was simply a need to bear down, to urge out, to expel. And with my hand still on his head, squatting, his head came out. I could feel the skin, rippled and soft, and then flicked my fingers over something strange on the side – an ear! I breathed and felt the size of his body in my birth canal, the moment just before I knew he would be earthside and in my arms.

After a small pause, his body popped out, and I brought him up, leaning back in the pool. Laughter shaking me, the quickness of it all somewhat overwhelming. We stayed in the water for a while, and when we got out I still felt quite overcome by the speed with which he came. The after-surges were intense but then seemed to desist, and after a couple of jelly-like clots came out, nothing much seemed to happen.

F fed well, straight away, and I kept feeling inside to see if the placenta was there. We decided to cut the cord and H did it with sterilised scissors. His cord was thin and easier to cut than the others. I went to the bathroom, and managed to wee, but the placenta was still inside. As we neared the two hour mark, my doula asked if she should phone an independent midwife we know to ask what she thought, and she assured us that it was fine for the placenta to take a while, so long as I felt fine, and was not bleeding heavily. She suggested going to the toilet, and also trying to relax.

After a hug and some calming down, I went to the bathroom and felt the placenta lying right there, so I pushed it out whilst holding the cord and it came out, caught in the plastic bowl I had placed in the toilet.

My doula and photographer were doing their thing in the background, helping, tidying, shuffling, organising, and I had tea. We weighed the baby on faulty scales, but managed to determine later he must have been at least 11lbs, and then I had a shower and went to bed and all of it was before noon.

Although I had known this would be a quick birth, I was in active labour for at most an hour, so I wasn't prepared for how much of a shock it can feel to birth a baby so quickly, which I only really acknowledged in the days and weeks after. But it was as normal a thing as anything, and it felt relaxed and informal – a tiny, brilliant moment in time interrupting a regular Sunday, and there I was at the end of it in bed with this big, beautiful, round-cheeked baby and he had shown up after all, albeit later than I'd have guessed, sharing the birthday of my oldest childhood friend. **Kendal**, the birth of F, her fourth child and second freebirth.

Lindsay's story

I had a doula and we employed her quite early on in the pregnancy, maybe after my first scan. We discussed with her our decision to freebirth and she was supportive of that. We also discussed quite carefully the role of the doula.

So I woke up one morning, a Friday morning, about five in the morning, got out of bed quite suddenly and my waters just broke on the floor of the bedroom. I was like, "oh I wasn't expecting that". It was just over 37 weeks. I was supposed to be going to work that day. I had yoga classes that afternoon. I wasn't planning to start my maternity leave until the Saturday, the following day. So I rang one of my colleagues at the yoga studio and said, "I don't think I'll be coming into work today – I think I'm in labour. My waters have broken, and I'll keep you posted as to how things go." So pretty soon, straight after my waters broke, my contractions started, but they weren't regular. They were strong to start with but coming and going, coming and going. I knew that A was in a back-to-back position, but I didn't know how that would affect my labour. I didn't have any sort of understanding really there… what implications that would have… I didn't have any worry about that. I just knew that was the position he was in. We went for a long walk. I had this idea in my head that – we've got a dog – and that when I was in labour I wanted to go for a walk in the park near where we lived. There was a river there and I wanted to be near that river and I wanted to walk by it. So we went for a walk there, but it was quite uncomfortable and it was cold and we didn't last that long, and we came back home. I just spent most of the time pottering around. A, my partner, was with me, and the dog and we just spent the day at home, got everything dark and cosy… And then by about 8.30 in the evening things were just really similar. I was still getting quite strong contractions but there was no pattern to it. It was just sort of coming and going, coming and going. They were really intense. I felt the discomfort of them. I think we called the doula to come that evening when it started getting dark. I got in the pool for a bit. We had a birth pool upstairs but I really didn't like that. I stayed in it for a while and I thought, urgh, this isn't doing it for me. I felt like labour was taking forever. I think in my head I thought by now the baby should have come out! (Laughs). I was expecting it to be a really short labour, for some reason. I had a fantasy that I would go into labour and then six hours later the baby would be born. But obviously that wasn't how it was. I realised that it was just going to take longer. So it was very normal. It was very boring. I was just dealing with the contractions coming and going. I got out of the pool, came downstairs, spent a bit of time lying on the bed, did a bit of up and down stairs movement, just because moving felt better than being still. I spent a bit of time in the kitchen downstairs, decided I didn't want to be in the kitchen – I wanted to be back upstairs in the toilet… and spent quite a long time just sitting on the toilet. I remember me and my partner… I was sitting on the toilet and he was just talking to me and talking to the baby, and encouraging the baby to move down, and we were just repeating this mantra of "move down, move down, move down." Time just didn't seem to be real, in a way. It was just one hour moved into the next. I think it got to about midnight and I had this urge to have a shower, and I just wanted to get in and have this water running on me. I didn't want to get back in the pool. I just wanted to get in the shower. I got in the shower and I felt quite a big movement in my belly. It was a definite shift of position of A, our baby. And then I had a massive bloody show. And then I felt A's head move down really significantly, and I could really feel him in my pelvis, and I don't think before then that he had been in my pelvis. He was obviously just floating about, but I felt this sudden feeling of him really getting down low. I got out of the shower and I remember leaning over the bath thinking I don't want to have my baby in the bathroom. Our bathroom was on the top floor and our bedroom was on the next floor down. I had this really awkward sort of trying to get back downstairs but having to walk down the stairs like a cowboy because I could feel his head really low. It felt like it was taking up the whole of my lower pelvis. Eventually I somehow got back down to the bedroom. I don't even know what time that would have been – maybe like two in the morning or something – then kneeling at the bottom of my bed, looking onto my bed with all the cushions that were on there, thinking, "soon this is going to be over and I can get into that bed, and it's going to be snuggly and I'm going to have a baby and it's going to be OK." And I felt tired but I could tell that the end was coming. I was getting the sensation to push, and I think I must have had a pushing phase which lasted about two hours. It was really intense and I remember squeezing my partner's hands and him afterwards telling me that he felt I was going to break it (laughs). But I didn't, obviously! And then just feeling this head coming down bit by bit. I remember I kept saying to A [partner] "is it out yet? Is it out yet?" And he just kept saying, "I can see it coming, I can see it coming, but it's not out yet." And just thinking, is this head ever going to come out? And then eventually, slowly, slowly, the head did come out and I could fully feel and see the head. And then in the next push, the whole of A's body came out and A caught him, and then passed him through my legs to me. I somehow managed to get out of my kneeling position into a seated position and sat against the bed… just on the floor. We hadn't planned to have him in the bedroom. We'd planned to have him in the pool, so the bedroom was not birth-ready. So I just sat on a rug at the bottom of the bed. He instantly went to the breast. There was a bit of gurgling when he first came out. I put him to the breast and he had a little bit of a suckle and then he started this sort of gurgling noise. I instinctively put my mouth to his nose and sucked. I don't know why I did that. I just felt that was the right thing to do. And then put him back to my… it was my left breast… and he just started feeding properly and then the placenta just came out really quickly. I remember - between giving birth and the placenta coming out - eating jelly babies. I obviously needed sugar and I dropped one. I was just scoffing them like a cake out of the packet, and after the placenta had come out, I dropped one on the floor. I remember it was a green one and it dropped into this bloody mess of the placenta, and I said it was a good job it was a green one, because nobody likes them anyway! And everyone was just looking at me thinking, " – making jokes. She's just given birth after a 25 hour labour!" I just remember thinking, oh that was quite normal. I've just had a baby at home and it was really normal and boring and not exciting. But I felt like in some ways it was the most amazing thing I've ever done. But then in other ways it was just the most normal thing I've ever done.

And it was that real weird mix of those two emotions. I was like "wow, I've just given birth to a baby in my bedroom", but also, "well that was quite normal". It was this really weird combination of the two things. It's quite hard to describe. It was like, "wow, I'm amazing", and then also, "I'm also really normal". It was just a weird sort of, "oh yes, I've just had a baby - look what I just did"! And it was yes, weirdly normal. **Lindsay**, freebirth of her first baby.

Section 1: Why Freebirth?

Women's motivations for freebirth are the obvious way to start this book if we are to understand the rest of their stories. Their motivation can be very difficult to understand for those involved with or committed to existing services. From the professional viewpoint other options can easily be seen as deviant and therefore wrong. But we urge those involved with existing services to read on. The motivations of women who freebirth tell us so much about the shortcomings of existing services and what is unavailable to those who use them, as well as about what freebirthing women want.

The mothers who entrusted us with their stories did not see freebirth as a clear either/or one-off decision. They spoke of their journeys towards freebirth. These journeys were sometimes long journeys over much of their lives or over successive pregnancies. For some the journey was made quite early in their first pregnancy, and for others it was a possibility which they felt was right, only when they were in labour.

People differ and the birth they journeyed towards embodied the different priorities of different women. Some would have been happy with what we know as good evidence-based care but which was not available to them within the NHS. This usually involved continuity of midwifery carer and no routine interventions or distractions. Some prioritised privacy, autonomy or the presence of supporters who would not have been allowed at a birth within the maternity care system.

The journey towards freebirth was a journey to a place and a state of mind where they felt safe to labour and give birth. They wanted to labour in their own home and in their own space, usually with people they trusted and who trusted them to be able to birth their baby. They wanted to be able to focus on the labour and birth with no other demands being made upon them.

Chapter 1: Journeying away from trauma and institutionalisation

The women who entrusted us with their stories had very different paths towards freebirth. They saw it as a journey, rather than a simple decision. Many sought to avoid the trauma that they had previously experienced within maternity or other health care services.

When I had H, I was in my twenties. I didn't really know anyone who had babies then, didn't know anybody who had given birth. I ended up having him in hospital. And I was induced, so I had a fairly terrible time of it. I didn't feel supported. I didn't feel listened to. I felt like a lot of my birth choices were quite pooh-poohed in a way. So, scoffed at, when they looked at my birth plan and they said, "Lavender oil? So, does that work?" And I just remember a defining moment of labour, after being induced with pessaries, and it being pretty full-on, to the point where I was actually on a delivery suite, and I was wanting to labour on all fours, and… then the midwife said, "Oh I have to give you an internal." And I didn't know then that I could say, "No, I don't want one." They told me that they needed to do that, and I said, "'Okay. Well, if you're going to do that, and you're telling me I can't be on all fours, you're telling me I need to be on my back, well, then you need to give me an epidural." And that was the moment for me in that birth where things really just did escalate, and then I ended up with forceps and episiotomy and losing lots of blood and so on and so on, and then post-traumatic stress after that, dealing with that, depression. I think it was all linked to that experience. And it wasn't just me wanting to have a wonderful birth experience. It was knowing the way that I should have been able to give birth, and not being supported in that. **Katy B**

Katy's last sentence above states very clearly how the routine practices of maternity services robbed her of bodily autonomy, rather than supporting her to birth her baby. Many women spoke about how professionals, who they had initially trusted, "managed" their pregnancy and birth in a way which undermined their strength, induced fear and left them "afraid to let go."

I had a caesarean the first time in hospital and afterwards I just felt the aftercare and everything… had been really quite a traumatic experience… I was actually quite afraid and I wanted to be in their care and in the care of professionals who knew what they were doing so I did put a lot of trust… I wasn't frightened, I felt really strong when I started on my journey to go there and excited and strong, but it rapidly became very cold and I was afraid to let go and I didn't want to expose any part of myself, so yes I was just told "no" to home birth and it just wasn't possible in that particular area and afterwards I had a visit from a Health Visitor twice and she was complaining about having to cross over fields to get there, so my aftercare I felt was really bad and I felt like I really needed support at that point, and I felt quite angry about this as well because I felt I had been violated and the more I go back over it all, the more I realise I was – I was really, really vulnerable and I was a lot younger then and the way that I was treated and just the whole setup, it just was not conducive at all to a caring environment, so I did feel very violated and I felt very angry for many, many years later…

So anyway seven years later I became pregnant and my doctor was first of all saying, "Oh you are going to be high risk" and my midwife was saying the same thing, "You're high risk and there is going to be basically a clock ticking to see how long you can get the baby out" and I just was like, "Right, really, I think I'm just going to run a mile here."

[In her second pregnancy] I went and did a lot of research myself from things that they were telling me… My doctor who I really felt I quite trusted and respected, her immediate opinion was quite hard, she had told me the reason I am at risk was because I had had a caesarean which meant there was going to be pressure on my womb, that there would be quite a high possibility of my womb perforating during labour and she had actually seen one and so it was not very nice, so I thought like gosh I need to find out about this because if that is the reason they are telling me that I have got a time limit, it is because they don't want my womb to explode because it's got scar tissue, so I did some research and I found some statistics that were saying that actually quite the contrary to what she was saying and it was that that made me think, all that I am getting from you is information that is going to make me want to run a mile and I didn't feel like I had a voice to say anything… and I really wanted the birth to be intuitive, I really believed that it was supposed to be and it is a very intuitive process and right from the word go when I got pregnant, the dreams that I had and what they were telling me seemed really vital and I really, really tuned into myself and I wanted to be able to do that in my labour. I wanted to be able to tune into myself and to be allowed to do that, and just to be given everything that I wasn't given in the first labour.

I went to see my Consultant as well and she was basically telling me how long my labour would be, and also she seemed quite a down to earth woman, and I was really surprised at what she was coming out with, and she asked me if I had any questions and I had quite a lot of questions but I didn't want to ask her anything and did not want to put myself into… open up to anybody about my possible fears or whatever because I couldn't believe she was telling me how long my labour would be. How can you possibly know that? I just felt really strange and so basically what they were saying is you're going to have a caesarean – another one – that is basically what they were saying to me…I knew that the same thing would happen and unless I really had an army of women with me standing at the door and not letting anybody come in with a clock or nothing, what I just really found was that it wouldn't be a safe place to go. **Polly**

Like Polly, many women used the word "violated" in describing their first birth. Others spoke f trauma and alienation.

I had a horrific first birth, and ended up in hospital, and had three days of just, I was just totally violated, and it was completely out of my control, and that was my first child. So, I had a lot of fear… and I was just invisible, I was just this invisible person with no voice and no-one would listen to me at all. **Katuš**

My first birth was, if I could sum it up in one word; terrified. I spent the whole thing terrified. Still battling the vestiges of an eating disorder, the weight gain was scary for me, the whole not knowing what was going to happen and what to expect made me very anxious. I had a horrific birth, with a student midwife who would NOT be quiet and was far too peppy and loud, and a midwife who was pushy. I was repeatedly told that I was "too quiet" to be in established labour and I'd only be one or two cm. Turns out I was eight. I was happily breathing through my surges laid on my side, and she told me I "had" to sit up. Moving onto all fours, she said that wasn't "good enough" and proceeded to grab my shoulders and pull me forcibly back onto my haunches. In doing so, I felt a sharp pain and my son shift inside me. That shift, I feel, changed his position so he was coming through on the widest part of his head, not the optimal part. As a result, he got "stuck", and I "failed to progress." I was blue lighted from the midwife-led unit to a larger district hospital, where two failed attempts at Ventouse (including the cap popping off and liberally splattering the doctor in blood just as my husband walked through the door), and episiotomy no one asked my permission for and forceps, my son, R, was finally born in my blood and my tears. Big bruises blooming across his cheeks from the forceps.

I honestly believe that that disempowering, ten and a half hour birth was a huge contribution to my PND after my son's birth, which also had knock-on effects on our breastfeeding relationship, which was short, full of guilt, and empty of support.

I vowed that I was never going to allow birth and my health care professionals make me feel like that again. **Emi**

I had no say in what was done TO me. I was lied to, I was disconnected from my baby. We have struggled with our connection ever since. **Silva,** describing her first birth

The hospital is like a weird airport where you go and you take your body in this alien world and travel to different doctors who will look at your body in an alien planet, in an alien place, and it's just like an airport I think. It could be somewhere where you can learn about yourself and about the inside of your bodies, it's not supposed to be an alien world is it? It would be good if it wasn't. I think the fact that I didn't have my baby vaginally has always haunted me, it will always haunt me. **Moggie,** talking about her first birth

And I first fell pregnant with my first wee baby in 2020. And then I really wanted a home birth – And I had mentioned the home birth more or less immediately, because it's like this is something that I would love to do... and they're like, "No, no, definitely not. No." It was just an immediate, "No." And I always, to be quite honest, I always felt very upset whenever I would come out of midwives' appointments, you know. I just, it didn't feel natural to me. I didn't feel really heard. But again, it was my first baby and I just thought, "This is what you have to do. Like this is it, you know." But they told me I can have the pool, I can have no lights, I can have all these things. So I was like, "Well okay, this is the way it's going to be. I'll stay at home as long as I can and then I'll transfer." So that's the way that it went. So I went into labour. It was fine, got on grand. But I had to go to the hospital. So put in the car, transferred into the hospital. And the whole car journey, it was so uncomfortable, it was like eleven o'clock in the morning and the sun was beating down and it was April time. And I remember getting to the hospital and there was like a wheelchair there for me. And they were like… and I was like, "I do not need a wheelchair." So I was able to manage to get up the stairs, but they asked me could they just do like an internal. And I was like, "Yep, okay, that's fine." Okay, got that. As soon as that happened, I was like, "What just happened?" It just felt so uncomfortable. It just… from what I had experienced in the house, to get that bad feeling, it was like, "Whoa, no, this doesn't feel right." She said, "Oh, you're eight centimetres." So in a way, to be honest with you, even though it felt quite uncomfortable for me at that time, with it being my first baby, it did help me. "Right, okay, you're eight centimetres, you haven't far to go. You've done so amazing." You know in a way I was able to take a positive from it. Well the Covid test then again I just felt it didn't help me, you know, it was so uncomfortable. And then it was like put into this room. And this room had these like massive windows, you know, even though the blinds were kind of towelled, you know, there was still a lot of sunlight coming in, do you know what I mean. It just didn't feel right. And then from that, things didn't go really well. You know, like I was very uncomfortable. I couldn't get in a position. I just kept saying, "Oh my God, you know. I just don't think I'm going to be able to do this." And then it was the questions, "Do you want an epidural? We'll give you an epidural. Do you want this? Do you want that?" And I was like, "No, no, no. I want a pool of water. Can you get me in the pool?" "Oh no, we can't get you the pool." And I wasn't able to have the pool. So that went from having this really nice experience at home… And I don't like to say I wasn't progressing, but I wasn't. You know, there wasn't really any oxytocin blowing, you know, I was getting examined quite a lot and they were monitoring. And then the heart rate was dropping and all this sort of chaos. That's how I can explain it – chaos. However, I still knew, I still had that intuition going, "My baby's fine, I'm okay. You know, can you back off, I need to do this." Whereas I feel like I wasn't heard. It was completely taken out of my control, do you know what I mean? I ended up having diamorphine. I ended up nearly getting rushed for a C section. "What is going on with this? This is not what I wanted. This is not how it's supposed to be." But long story short, I was told not to push. You know, "Don't push, don't push. We're going to take you for a section." And the next minute, I just felt that urge, that real urge to push and I did. Even though they were telling me not to, I did, I went with my body. And the baby's head crowned, you know, it crowned. So for me, my experience in the hospital wasn't traumatic as such. Well yes, it was a little traumatic, but it wasn't to the extent of intervention and having a section and stuff like that. But I have seen how quickly things can go out of hand in there, and how you have very little control. And oh Lord, I don't know why I'm getting emotional, but it was, it was just very scary how things could have went completely the other way, do you know what I mean. And I just felt so vulnerable in that situation, that I was so close to that happening to me. **Christina**

… and after a while they just said, "Okay, C section."… I guess because I have a history of mental health issues, they thought that so long without sleep would send me into a psychosis or something, because it does happen… I was fine and I was fine after the birth, well, apart from obviously the trauma of being butchered... Anyway, they took me into the theatre and my doula, my best friend... And we were there just, and I felt the weight of the baby come away from my spine; my spine decompressed... Then I heard her screaming. They took the screen down and scarf off my head. I just saw my womb like open and bloodied and this white shiny child screaming... And my first image of her was literally horror. It was like, "What is this?"... It was horrific, and I've never heard a more distressed scream in my life than the sound that baby... made when she came out. And then they faffed around for a couple of minutes and they did put her on my chest...I was just shaking... my arms were literally convulsing and shaking and the baby was being shaken up, it was almost unsafe. You know, they say, "Don't shake a baby," but there I was shaking her around... it's so traumatic... she was born with an Apgar score of ten. I don't see how in any way she was in distress or how the C section needed to happen... Three years later, I got pregnant with her sister and had a horrific breakup in my first trimester with that baby, because my ex-partner impregnated someone else... And I knew from the get-go that the NHS weren't going to come near me... And then I read Unassisted Birth by Laura Kaplan Shanley... the first pregnancy I read every book under the sun. The second pregnancy... it was the only thing I read... And by the end of it, I was just convinced. I was just, like, "Okay, I'm just going to make this happen."... There's not going to be any weird fuckers here poking me in the, you know, the genitals... And there's not going to be any sharp instruments, not going to be any drugs; I'm just literally going to pop the baby out in the pool. **Rose**

The traumatic experiences that influenced these women's plans for their next birth were not all invasive procedures. Some women were traumatised by what would have been recorded in their clinical notes as straightforward normal births. These stories tell of a profound difference between these women's needs and what the NHS maternity services offered. What they experienced as stressful contacts with midwives at routine checks could induce considerable anxiety.

There came a point towards the end of the pregnancy journey where I was so stressed out and anxious from my interactions with the NHS. And I looked at my husband and I said, "Do you know what, the only thing about this pregnancy that isn't easy, that I'm not enjoying, is stressing me out, is dealing with the NHS." Because at this point, my doula had mentioned freebirth and I had been on a Zoom where one of her clients who had a freebirth had shared her story. And I'd gotten the book that she mentioned. Not intending to have one myself, but I was really inspired by her and I got the book and was, "Wow." And I said to my husband, "What would happen if we just took the NHS out of the picture?" And as soon as I sort of chucked that out there as a possibility, everything in me just relaxed and I was like, "Oh. There goes the stress." So my doula was totally on board; she's supported plenty of freebirths. **ME**

One of the things I really wanted with this birth is for me and my husband to not be really stressed out. **Darelle,** after two previous traumatic experiences during births with NHS midwives

I could have just been doing without some of that stuff, you know. I feel like a lot of it's normal and it's over-medicalised and I could have been doing without that stress and stuff, even though it went to plan and I delivered the wee baby and everything, and I didn't need to transfer and everything went quite smoothly. So fast forward then about a year and three or four months later and I found out I was pregnant with my second wee boy. And I said to my husband, "I'm not going near the midwives. I'm not going near them until I have to." Just didn't want the stress of going to the midwives' appointments. I trusted my body; I had researched enough to know my movements, tuned into my body. I just didn't want to be going to midwife appointments and the scaremongering... And just thought that it was a lot of things that were up just to tick a box, basically. So yes, that definitely set me on the path then. I didn't even care if they say to me, "Oh Holly, we've reinstated home births and we're happy to attend." I wasn't, I didn't want them, I didn't want them anywhere near me. And I know there are some lovely midwives, like I had one, as I say, at Z's birth – she was amazing. But no, oh no, it just created negativity when I thought about them, or I just wanted my own bubble for this birth for my baby. And I knew I could do it, so yes, I just... I had to just keep saying to them, "No, I'm fine. This is a service that you offer and I'm declining it. Thank you for the offer, but I don't need it." **Holly**

This time I was just like from the beginning I knew, "I can do this.".. the midwives felt like a nuisance at my first; I didn't feel like I needed them at all. I didn't find them helpful. I actually found they were intruding. Anything negative I remember from my first birth was to do with what they did. So for me, it was quite clear that removing that factor was the way to go, absolutely. And that's exactly what happened. **Carmen**

The reaction of the midwife who took my details was anxiety-provoking. She was shocked that I hadn't had my 12 week dating scan and she had me on the phone for a full hour pointing out my risk factors. She wanted me to come into the hospital twice in quick succession, starting that day for blood and urine tests, and a belated scan. When I came off the phone, for the first time since being pregnant I felt out of control, afraid, and disconnected from my body. Something about the midwife's tone had also left me with the impression that she thought me naive and irresponsible not to have contacted them sooner. Somehow not a good mother, and therefore a worry, even a nuisance to her. But I would forgive her of course if she was the one who would be assigned to me. "Might you be at the birth?" I asked her. I was to ask this question many more times of the various midwives I met or spoke to by phone over the following months. The answer was always either "No" or "I don't know." **Naomi**

Naomi went on to speak of

... my growing concern that the care I was receiving didn't feel like care at all, but disempowering, and that I was becoming increasingly uncertain as to whether I wanted an NHS midwife present at all. **Naomi**

I just remember having my eyes closed the whole time, because I just wanted to stay in my own space. And every time someone asked me to do something or to move for the heart rate check or to do this or to do that, I just felt they were making me come out of myself... It was outwith anything that I needed, which was just my own space; just me and J [partner] together. And so everything was more of a hassle. Everything, everything added was extra particulars that... that weren't needed. Even the birth pool, I would say, was more of a hassle than it was a benefit. Because getting in the pool relieved tensions that I had in my body, for sure which was nice, but then also sort of slowed down my contractions because I was more comfortable. Whereas the gravity, I guess, was allowing the contractions to sort of continue on. **Jessica**, describing her first birth

The need to feel safe is a recurring theme. For some this safety came with the absence of anxiety inducing professionals. Others, like Naomi above, felt they could feel safe if they could build a relationship with the midwife who would attend their birth.

When my first son was about six months old I remember that I started making plans for how things would be different whenever I gave birth again. Even though from the outside it looked like I had had a straightforward home birth, the fight to achieve that had really taken its toll on me. At first I imagined labouring and giving birth completely alone on the first floor of our house, with my friend M sitting on the landing, keeping any midwives from coming up the stairs. This scenario made me feel safe. Because of my previous experience, I knew I would never have "strangers" in my birth space again. I had been completely trusting in my NHS midwives at my son's birth and that trust had been violated when I was not supported in my decision to refuse induction and to birth at home. I spent a lot of time blaming myself for the poor care I received and believed the midwife's behaviour was caused by my own decision making.

Then, when I was discussing birth plans with a pregnant friend in Scotland who was planning a home birth, I learned that she knew her community midwives who would be on call for her home birth. It was a light bulb moment for me, if I knew and trusted the midwives, I could allow them to come up the stairs of my imagined birth scenario. I had a fleeting thought that if I just wrote to the Head of Midwifery and demanded to know the midwives who would be at my birth, then they would have to accommodate this.

Of course by this time I knew enough about the UK maternity system to know that a letter demanding what I later learned is called 'continuity of carer' would not be enough to make that a reality. I became involved with my local MSLC [Maternity Services Liaison Committee] and local and national birth advocacy groups to help improve maternity care. The more I researched how one actually gets to 'know' their midwife at their birth, the more I realised this was very unlikely unless I hired and paid for an independent midwife. This seemed impossible to me because of the financial costs, as well as the issues with insurance that midwives were facing. This was when I first considered planning a 'freebirth' if we had any more children. **Virginia**

S's [first child] birth was textbook, really straightforward and I don't really class it as a traumatic birth, but I was just deeply disrespected. It was a straightforward, healthy, normal birth and I was just peppered with offering of interventions. And we ended up accepting a few, just out of sheer like, "I'm really tired, I'm in a really vulnerable place, because I'm giving birth and it's the first time I'm giving birth, so, okay". And what was really insidious, towards the end, I realised that they kind of roped my husband in…because as much as he was really ready to be my advocate and all that other thing, it doesn't take much, because I mean he's never witnessed a birth before, before the midwife, there's kind of that vibe of, "This is women's business, so you need to help me get your wife to submit to what I want her to do."

… I got turned over, got man-handled over, all the clippy monitory things, of course lost the trace, and she was descending, she was literally coming out… They lost their trace. And I can remember the midwife saying, "Okay darling, we just, we can't hear baby's heart rate any more, so I'm just going to put a clip on her head to make sure, to make sure she's still got a heartbeat."… And it wasn't even like, "Is that okay?"…as she's doing, and she's screwing a thing into my kid's scalp. And she was born so quickly,… it's like the midwife was probably putting counter-pressure on her head as she was coming out, like such a standard birth, why wasn't I allowed to remain on my knees? It had been at that point ten minutes since my waters had gone, it's not like I was pushing for hours. **Jocelyn**

The midwife's approach in their previous births made a lot of difference to many women's perceptions. Some midwives were not comfortable with home births or births that did not follow the pattern to which they were accustomed. A midwife's fear can be highly contagious and marred many mothers' experiences.

And so they got jumpy about A's heart rate. But she was really close to being born… But they were like, "We need to get this baby out!" And decided to sort of give me a fright. And then, when the contractions were there, I pushed and I kept pushing and pushing. And I had some tearing when she was born. I mean, she was fine; she was born into water as I wanted. And she was born peacefully. But the midwives were jumpy about her being born peacefully as well. So they took her out quite quickly and started rubbing her. Which was all just out of the environment that I wanted. But for my first experience, I didn't know what to expect. And the second time, I had a lot more confidence about what I was capable of and what baby would be capable of. And… I didn't make a choice to have a water birth the next time, but I knew that if, oh dear, it was going to take a little bit longer to breathe, there were these techniques I could use, and not to panic but to stay relaxed, and have faith that she'll find her way to it. Oh, that was a good move. So I guess the first time I just felt as if you need someone there in case something goes wrong. **Jessica**

I decided to freebirth because of the experiences from my first birth… that's ten years ago… I was in the prime birthing years, I was a very healthy shiatsu practitioner; I did lots of body work and had counselling and so, on all levels I felt really well prepared. I did hypno birthing, yoga, and I read a lot. I read Sarah Buckley and Michelle Odent, Ina May Gaskin and I read your [Nadine's] *Birthing Autonomy* book… so I decided to home birth… I knew about the hormonal orchestration... I knew... how the body worked best during birth. I knew what the body needed... I found I knew, I trusted my body and I knew what it needed to go to birth safely... We had a birth pool, and we set up a space... and my midwife was happy for me to home birth... I called up when contractions were close together, every five minutes, and strong. I spoke to the midwives for five minutes and she must have thought that I wasn't contracting because I was so calm. So she didn't come for another, maybe six hours. And when she arrived, I knew even before she did a vaginal examination, that I was eight centimetres, and for some reason I was. And she was very surprised because... I was fine really (laughs) I had no pain at that point. And I went into the pool and she examined me again... I know because I'm a student midwife, I know now that it wasn't indicated. It wasn't an hour gap, and she just wanted to check me before I went into the pool. And even though I was progressing well, she got her amnihook out and just said, "Oh, I'm just going to break your waters. It usually speeds things up a little. Is that okay?" And went ahead. And because I was in this zone, I wasn't quick enough to, or prepared enough to say, "Actually, no thank you, there's no reason. I'm doing really well. I'm eight centimetres, there's no reason for it." But she went ahead and did, and I wasn't strong enough to say, "No." And my husband, first baby, he was not prepared to stand up or speak against the woman... And so my waters broke and I was allowed, and I am saying allowed because that's how it felt, into the pool for a short time.

And she made comments like, "God, you're, you're a quiet labourer, aren't you?" And in this tone, as if it wasn't... I felt I wasn't doing it right. I shouldn't be so quiet. I'm not normal, this is not normal. And she kept offering me painkillers, too - gas and air, which I hadn't needed, I didn't need. And then as I got into the pool, what happens quite often, and this is quite a normal thing, my labour plateaued a bit and that's completely normal. But she picked it up as something bad or not okay. So she got me back out, and I had to walk around the room, when all I wanted to do was rest in the pool, and just be gentle. And I'm sure it would have just picked up again if I had been left alone. But she also, as I walked around the room, she had loud mobile phone conversations on the phone - private things and I wished I had just sent her out... or asked her to go into another room. Or asked my husband to do so. But again, I didn't realise I had to be so strong, when all I wanted was to be left alone or be in this quiet birthing zone. So she had her phone conversations and then I trickled blood and I was still very calm and quiet. I didn't seem much in pain because it wasn't that bad. But as I was walking around, it wasn't as mucousy as a bloody show, because my mucous plug had gone already by then, but it was more trickling blood. And it seemed to panic the midwife. And she called an ambulance and... and my body wanted to push. My body, everything in me wanted to push this baby out. And she told me I couldn't, I had to keep it in until the ambulance was in. And that's when I needed gas and air because going against my body was so hard.

And then I was taken to the… hospital… and that ambulance trip was really traumatic…

it was awful, awful. I was half-naked with all of these strange men, and at the moment, it didn't matter really. But what mattered was that I was in pain and I could have had the baby in the ambulance, but I had to do my best to keep this baby inside. And as we got to the hospital, I saw the midwife who had come to my home to approve the home birth and she was lovely. And as soon as I saw her I relaxed again and within a few minutes, between five and ten minutes, the baby was born. And she was worth it all, obviously, so she was very strong and an amazing girl. Truly, just very generous of heart, so she was worth it. But it didn't go as I wished and the midwife who had been in my home, she did come and apologise because she realised it was just a show. I was ready to push, I was fully, I was fully. That that was just normal bleeding. But she was inexperienced and, I guess, she was scared of being at a home birth. As soon as she had come into my home, I could feel the tension. I could feel she didn't want to be there. She felt more comfortable being in a hospital and I did feel it from the beginning. I wished I had sent her away, and asked for someone else, but again, I didn't know I could.

… and she knew it wasn't, it wasn't enough blood. I guess her first instinct probably was that it was a haemorrhage, an antepartum haemorrhage, but it wasn't, it wasn't that much blood. And I know, I'm a student midwife; I have seen that much blood and it's completely normal. Anyway, and then in the hospital, they jabbed me with syntocinon to get the placenta out, which again, I hadn't wanted. It was in the birth plan, but it was shoddy consent again, and I was holding my baby, I was elated and being told that if I don't have this I might have a haemorrhage or, you know…It wasn't proper consent… although I was really happy with my baby, it wasn't what I had wanted. It wasn't as empowering as it could have been.

So when, three years later I was pregnant again, planned baby, and I read more and I had worked through my first birth. I came across a book... a friend gave it to me, of stories, of other women who had freebirthed and Veronika Robinson. I think it's her name, and it was called Birthkeepers. And that was enough. That was enough to make me think, "Oh, women have birthed on their own for centuries." Native American women just go off and have their baby and come back, you know. Or different tribes do it differently, but it's innate. And I knew, I knew my body and I knew how healthy I was. **ST**

Many women wanted more personalised care, to have more agency and to make decisions about what care they felt they needed and wanted, rather than to completely opt out of maternity services. But they found this was not possible within the set menu of care. Some sought care which would be more supportive for them with independent midwives or doulas.

Even though we had agreed that in theory we would have independent midwives for a future birth, in reality it was very difficult for me to go through with it. The person who I'd imagined as 'my midwife' didn't currently have insurance to attend births and I felt disappointed and reluctant to trust someone else. Also, I could not imagine placing the financial burden on my family for care that I felt should be free. My previous pregnancy and birth had been medically straightforward with no interventions and I felt very confident in my body and had been raised to trust birth. I felt drawn to self-care as an alternative to prenatal care with a midwife and freebirthing with a doula friend present.

What stopped me from pursuing this was the outrage that it wasn't a 'choice'. It is difficult to describe, but on some level I felt that if I simply removed myself from the system and looked after myself, without demanding the maternity care that I knew I (and all women) should have a right to, then I would have lost. I felt there was a difference between a self-monitored pregnancy and freebirth where you also have the option to have personalised high quality maternity care with a midwife you know and trust at any point if you choose, and a self-monitored pregnancy and freebirth because there is no maternity system or midwives available to support you. I felt like I was in the latter category.

Finally, because I felt that if I proceeded with an 'unmonitored' pregnancy I was being forced into through lack of choice, I booked with local independent midwives. After our first appointment I was aware I needed a lot of debriefing from my previous birth experience in order to feel like I could trust any midwives. I found this difficult because even though I knew I could trust the medical judgement of the independent midwives in an emergency, I found the practice of seeing a different midwife on the team at each appointment and not knowing which ones would be at the birth stressful. In addition, physical illness (nausea and pelvic pain) which made eating and sleeping difficult started to impact my mental health.

The independent midwives tried referring me to NHS services to address these issues but unfortunately I was faced with fighting within another broken system for physiotherapy and mental health support that did not exist. I despaired that if I, with my privileged knowledge of the maternity system and independent midwives advocating for me, couldn't access services, how impossible must it be for people who do not have advocates or support to navigate the system?

I didn't have a 'birth plan' since I felt that my 'plan' was to have people around me who I trusted so I didn't need a written birth plan. But of course I did imagine how the birth would be. At one of the home birth group meetings that I hosted early in my pregnancy, a mother shared her story of giving birth with just her two-year-old in the room with her, while her husband was ringing the midwives. Since my first labour had been so quick (something I had not been mentally prepared for) I mentally prepared myself for another quick labour, including if it was just me alone with my son. In a way I kind of took it for granted that the midwives would not be there. I didn't intend to call them unless I felt I needed them, and with my previous labour I never got to a point where I felt like I needed midwives. In hindsight calling them had been the beginning of everything that felt wrong.
Virginia

[During her first pregnancy] – I thought about doing it without midwives and I met some midwives… So I asked them about doing it by myself, or without midwives and they said it was illegal, so I just kind of accepted what they said and went, "oh well (laughs), I'll have to put up with having midwives then"… but then I subsequently found out that it wasn't illegal – but not during my first pregnancy.

[During her second pregnancy]... I tried, I tried to sort of explain my point of view to them and I did, for quite a while, want somebody there, some kind of midwife, but I couldn't afford to get an independent one, I couldn't afford to pay for one so I tried to get the midwives to do what an independent one would do and have that kind of point of view, but it ended up that that's not what they're there for, that wasn't their point of view and there's no way they're going to have that point of view so I just realised it was futile in the end...

I wanted somebody there who would support me emotionally, who'd understand my emotional and spiritual point of view and who would only intervene if I wanted them to... and I didn't want to have the gas and stuff there and they said they couldn't come out if I didn't have the gas and stuff there... they couldn't come out... , I just gave up on it at the end... gas and air and the box of bits and bobs, they just said flatly they couldn't come out if it wasn't there... which I understand, if they're used to their gear and that's where they coming from, so, you know fair enough... they don't want to come out...

I never made a decision [not to call services]... if I needed the emergency services, I would have called them, I decided I would go with how I was feeling during the labour...

I think if there was a variety of... skilled people, like not just skilled people who've been trained in the mainstream sort of way of thinking about health and illness but also people who are skilled in alternative methods, like herbalists or... people who are trained emotionally you know, to deal with emotional situations as well, and stuff like that... then I would definitely make use of that... and they're so sure often that they're right...which I mean, sometimes they might be right, but a lot of them have this attitude where they're always right and you're being really irresponsible to try an alternative and I just couldn't be bothered dealing with that, with my second birth, I just didn't want to have anything to do with anything that would be remotely like that, I couldn't... I didn't have the strength or the desire... but not everybody's like that in the NHS... but some of them are. **Charlie**

And as I said, the reasons for me doing it is because when you look at a physiological birth, it's about being undisturbed. And when I would tell them that in my meeting she was asking me, "Right, okay, well when will you let us monitor? When will you let us do that?" And it was like, "No, I don't want it done at all." "Oh no, but you can't." It's like, "Well actually, I think I can. No, I don't want you touching me." You know, that sort of thing. **Christina**

When NHS services are under-resourced, it is often the home birth service, or Birth Centres that suffer. In some cases, while it was not their original plan, women freebirthed because the maternity services lacked resources to respond to planned home births, even before the Covid-19 pandemic overwhelmed the NHS. Sarah W was booked for an NHS home birth.

Just before my waters broke, I said, "It's really getting serious now." So I said, "Well let's ring the triage team again." And we ended up being on hold for 45 minutes [during which time the baby was born] And this is how we ended up having a freebirth. So at the point at which I jumped into the pool and my waters broke, it was like, "Oh there's a head here."

… So maybe there's a bit of me that thinks the only way that I could get my home birth was to have a freebirth. So maybe this home birth that I was so keen to have, maybe that was the way that it was facilitated. And if I'd have got my gas and air, I would have also got whisked to hospital. So it makes me feel like maybe that was the way to get my wonderful home birth, if you see what I mean.

… The things I would change would be just I would plan for that freebirth. I don't think I would push to have a midwife there before, if I could in hindsight change things, I would have probably just not had an ambulance crew quite as quickly, and had a calmer hour. Fair enough, if I needed to go to hospital to have stitches. But I think I would just not have had two ambulance crews in my house. **Sarah W**

Yvonne, herself a midwife, decided to freebirth her twins because there was no home birth service available.

I started looking around at freebirth, because there was no home birth service running at all. And that's been the case for a few months now and it's still suspended in my area due to the staffing situation. So if there were midwives available, I probably would have arranged to have a home birth, because I had a home birth for my first baby and that was a really positive experience. So that would have been the plan, but it just wasn't an option. So we decided as a partnership, me and my husband, that okay, if we got to 37 weeks then we would seriously consider just having them at home if everything else was good. I think that all the risks that people talk about with birth, so many of them are heightened and increased by the intervention that they put on people. And that first intervention is leaving the house isn't it? And that's huge. And people don't realise that and it's such a shame. The evidence is there that it's safe and it's just not the dominant ideology, is it?

[But for] the fact that home birth services aren't on, I wouldn't be in this situation. But I'm actually thankful that it was the case, because compared to my first birth which was a home birth, but was attended to by midwives, there were still elements of that birth that stuck with me in a really negative way, because of interactions with people that I didn't know during that experience. **Yvonne**

Maternity services responses to the Covid pandemic were to increase hospital births whereas other services discouraged patients from attending hospitals. This together with the restrictions caused by the pandemic (such as allowing only one or no birth partner and having to wear a mask) provided further reasons to freebirth for some women.

And neither of us wanted to go anywhere near a hospital in a pandemic. You know, it seemed laughable that they would be saying, in every other area of life, it's don't go near a hospital. Unless you're having a baby, in which case, that's where we want you. And none of this makes any sense. Either there's an international health crisis or there isn't…

They put home birth back on at 38 weeks, but it came with the condition that I could only have one birth partner. And I knew I couldn't agree to that. I needed both. So I knew that if I did phone them, they might make me get rid of either Mum or T. And let alone my doula, who was in the kitchen… how could I possibly choose between my tried and tested established birth team and someone I'd never met. **Beth**

… and then there was the Covid thing because I didn't want people coming in with masks on who I'd never met before, interfering, trying to be helpful. Because I thought that would be so impersonal, didn't want them coming into my space at that time. And there was a strong chance that they could have asked D (doula) to leave, or my partner, which neither would have been acceptable to me… there wasn't any relationship building, I couldn't see my midwife's face, I don't even know what she looked like, she had a mask on the whole time. And she had a uniform on which somehow detracts from the person because you don't get to know the actual person and she had a plastic apron which made it even more inhuman, because of Covid. **Rosalie**

This time I wanted to try being at home. And then a couple of weeks before our baby was due Covid-19 happened, the country went into lockdown and everything changed. Initially the home birth service was still available. However, two weeks before my due date the home birth midwifery service that I had been offered initially, was no longer available. This meant that there would be no midwife present if I gave birth at home at that point. And it was also very uncertain, from one day to the next, their decision kept changing. I went to see my midwife nearing the end of my pregnancy and she couldn't give me a definite answer. She said it's best to expect that we won't be there. This was very frightening for me and my partner. We hadn't considered freebirth and we felt pressured to make the right decision, what with my due date being so close…I felt like my choice had been taken away. I also felt a lot of pressure from the NHS to then go into hospital for my birth. To me, it felt like the preciousness of the birth was being taken away. I was told, "You can stay at home for as long as you need to. Many women aren't in for long. Just pop into hospital to have the baby and then come back out again." Which is not what I was picturing for my birth. It felt insensitive. And also like they didn't have any faith in me, or any real understanding of what a mother needs at that time. To go in and out of hospital in between birthing a baby could be incredibly stressful. From my experience of my first birth, my body needed to rest and feel safe. Not be traipsing in and out of a busy hospital. And it triggered old memories of a negative experience from my first birth that had stuck with me; I remember being transported down two floors to my labour room in a public lift. I remember being in the lift with other people as I was having very intense contractions. And I remember how distressing that felt. So yes, I was aware that I wanted to be at home; I wanted to feel safe and I wanted to be comfortable. So then, my choice was to either go into hospital or to have the birth at home but with no midwife support. We couldn't afford a private midwife… Thankfully I had already booked a doula, M, and she had been supporting us throughout this process, giving information and helping us with 'what if' scenarios. And with not overthinking and over planning either! I talked a lot with my partner T, who is incredibly supportive and together we made a loose plan that would empower me, give me choice but also help me to feel safe. Our doula had been present at lots of other home births. No freebirths that I remember. But she was confident at home births and confident in the power of a woman's body as well and in the process of labour. So I had decided that part of this plan would be to go ahead with freebirth. **Emma**

S, a doula, reflected on the impact of Covid, the reduction in the home birth services and her response to these changes:

With the coming of lockdown, home birth came under threat, in many Trusts, the reaction was to close home birth and think that was the end of it – but the closure of home birth is a reliance on compliance. Women and families were not planning to comply, not in my groups anyway. Instead, I saw my Home Birth Support Group UK members rally around each other – supporting each others' informed choices and sharing how they were challenging their Trusts, refusing to go to hospital consultant led wards and owning their own births. Many Trusts had also closed their midwife led units. Membership has quadrupled, from 2500 to nearly 10,000 at the time of writing, along with 4000 in The Village, my life and parenting support group. This situation led to an increase in freebirth enquiries and enquiries from those who were worried they would birth before a midwife could get to them. Freebirth as an active choice and also what I consider a new type of freebirther, those for whom hospital is no longer a safe space, these freebirthers are just as valid.

"My plan was to call the midwives but after catching Covid I wanted to be prepared in case I gave birth while we were in isolation. I ended up being out of isolation. However when calling up there was no one available as they had to suspend it due to high volumes of women in the labour ward and dangerously low staff levels (my trust don't close the labour ward for any reason, it's open 24/7 no matter what). All the skills I learned from S's freebirth course helped and I managed to stay calm throughout and to calm my husband who was less prepared than myself. The birth was so empowering there is no words to describe how it was for me and my husband. It has changed us for the greater good and we are closer for it." **Cheryl**, group member.

My phone, inbox, WhatsApp, email and all forms of communication exploded. To meet the demand for good quality freebirth information, I set up my Freebirth and Emergency Childbirth Support Group UK, with the support of other birth workers and open minded midwives. This is a unique course in a group based on Facebook and has proved extremely popular. I felt it was important to have a safe space for those who wanted to freebirth, with good quality information and signposting to service provider support if needed. It is also a space used by birthworkers to enhance their knowledge and engage with those giving birth. It is a very special space, a coming together of those preparing to give birth their way and birth workers and professionals who are prepared to support them unconditionally and without judgement.

Freebirth now, instead of being seeing as the risky, pariah option, is being seen as the only choice by some birthing women and parents, who would never have previously considered it. No longer is hospital birth the safe place it had been considered previously. Infection risks and fear of partner separation became bigger concerns for some than the fear of birthing without a midwife. This is also reflected in more positive reporting around freebirth in the mainstream press and journalist enquiries, I have contributed to a number of positive media pieces about freebirth, including in the Guardian and BBC News. **S**, doula

D, a doula, spoke of Covid as hastening a longer term lessening of women's trust in midwives and the support women feel they receive from midwives.

This year with the Covid rules and restrictions and everything else, the women have left it later and later [to call the midwife]. And I think there's lots of factors in there. One of them is they're just not sure if the midwife's going to be okay with their husband and their doula being there, because the current agreement is that they will only have one birth partner, and maybe I've been there for a few hours already, and they don't like the idea of upsetting that flow that they've got going. And I'm sure one of the other things is that the trust with midwives, and the feeling that they've got good support is lessening over the years, and certainly this past year it feels really complicated…

I think that midwives are barely able to scratch the surface of building a relationship. It's heartbreaking for women and women midwives, for all the women involved in it. Because surely, a midwife wants a relationship with a woman, she wants to know her, and the woman wants to be known. You know, people in the groups, they talk about "My midwife," But less and less now, I'm just hearing, "The midwife," and then, "The other midwife," and then, "The fourth midwife." **D**, doula

S also spoke of financial cuts and changes in maternity services pushing women towards freebirth.

I have seen a rise in freebirth, birth before arrival, ambulance birth, car park birth, women birthing alone, or spending a significant proportion of their birth alone in hospitals, everything that happens when birth is underfunded and under-resourced.

"I am due my third baby in 17 weeks. Due to a previous fast delivery, if a midwife is unavailable then I shall be staying at home and birthing, just my partner and I. S's course has given me the opportunity to gather the confidence I needed! "**K,** group member.

The current crisis in midwifery, with midwives leaving in droves, short staffing, high absence rates and high drop out rates of student midwives, is only going to see freebirth rise. **S**, doula

Chapter 2: The journey towards freebirth

Some of the women who told us about their freebirth were having their first babies and these mothers became increasingly aware during pregnancy that the service offered did not fit with their approach to life and to birth.

So when I became pregnant, I hadn't even really considered how things were going to go or what decisions I was going to make. I generally chose things in my life that are fairly autonomous and self-directed, but I hadn't really thought about what I was going to do. When we first went to the GP, F and I - my husband and I - went together. We were so excited and we wanted this energy echoed back to us. We wanted someone to echo back to us what we were feeling and to be celebratory and supportive and we didn't receive that at all. It felt like a real let-down. And she said some things that were such huge red flags for us right away. We said, "Okay, where does it go from here?"... she said... "you're going to be on a conveyor belt from here on out, with all the other pregnant ladies in London, and you will just get directed to your appointments and you'll end up in the end with a baby." And I wanted to throw up!

I had thought about it, but I guess what I hadn't thought about was all of the specifics and how things would... like I didn't end up having any scans in the end. In the beginning, I thought maybe I would. So as I continued on the path throughout my pregnancy, things became revealed more and more. I didn't have a game plan at the beginning. Things became evident as we navigated the system. So then we met with a midwife and she was quite nice but still I really didn't like feeling that I wasn't being assessed as an individual, that I was being assessed... compared to a group of other people. I just didn't feel any sense of being an individual human with a life story and experiences... none of that was taken into consideration and it felt like it was just a pad of paper and set questions and the questions didn't seem to me like questions that were important, like lifestyle besides smoking and drinking – those kinds of things were accounted for but it wasn't like... what mindfulness practices do you have? What's your life like, in terms of how you approach living, in general? That stuff to me seems so important with pregnancy and birth, more so than some of the other questions. So after some lacklustre appointments and after moving house and then ending up registering with a new borough and a new set of midwives and going to the hospital, we hadn't had any scans, and that was at about 20 weeks. And the woman that we met with was really fraught with concern that we'd made this choice and was really going on about placenta praevia as this danger that was going to probably kill me or our child. Like really adamant that this was of huge concern, and when F started to press for statistics and likelihoods, we realised that it wasn't actually that big a concern, so we felt like things were often pushed to the fore and made to be a big deal, but then once you actually dig around and look for numbers and likelihoods and how healthy you are and what your lifestyle is like, they weren't actually, so I thought there was a lot of fearmongering happening. So we started to kind of extricate ourselves from the NHS. Had we had the money, we might have paid a private midwife and gone that route, but we didn't have the money at the time, so we stayed registered with the NHS, but we didn't abide by the standard protocol. **Lacey,** first baby

I guess I always had quite a strong alternative view of things. And in some ways I think through that, I ended up being just much more trusting of myself, rather than the medical model in lots of different ways. When I think about different times, like I got quite sick at one point when I was young, irritable bowel syndrome. But when I had these really full on pains in my stomach, I went to hospital. And I think, because of that kind of experience I had, because basically they didn't find out what was wrong. They just put me on all these different antibiotics. And they just made me so much more sick. And I think maybe that also, I just had quite a strong mistrust in a way. Because then I went to see my own doctor and I did some research for myself, and I realised that it was much more of a kind of psychosomatic experience that I was having with these pains that I was getting, and related to stress and different things. That was not even mentioned to me in any way when I was in hospital. It was so impersonal, my experience, and I was only eighteen, and I was quite scared by it all in a way. I think that was part of what led me on to my spiritual path in a way, I guess as well. Just thinking outside the box a little bit more. Not being in this state of conformity… I was very much in a state of listening to my own body… [rather than] fussing or giving any responsibility to professionals. It just didn't really make sense to me to do that. And I think that's why when it came to me getting pregnant and having a baby… it was just instinct really, that said to me that I didn't… I definitely did not want to be in hospital. And I didn't want anyone to be intervening or having any kind of medication that was very strong from the very beginning. And then when my partner and I went to NCT just to get some more information and find out more. And it just made even more sense, as I learned more about understanding the hormones and what's really necessary in labour. And I got it, why I was having that strong instinct. And it just got stronger. This kind of feeling of not wanting to be disturbed. And I had these dreams as well, where I was completely on my own, while I was giving birth. So it was just really powerful, to have these kind of dreams and it just ties in with the kind of person I am really…

[At] my pre-natal checks, I didn't really get on with the midwives much. I felt like they were too pushy, too much looking at the negatives. Too much telling me about all the risks and making me have more fear than I had before I went… I know they're just doing what they've been trained to do. And I know that a lot of them obviously have seen a lot of things. So they're kind of conditioned in a way to be like that.

But I was also very much like, "Okay, we don't know what's going to happen. And if we need help, then we're going to get help." Like that's okay. **Gauri**, first baby

So I started going into a very natural way of doing all of my health things a handful of years back. I grew up with a nurse as a mom, and she was always very big on the medical industry. And I just always wanted to see other views. And so I looked into doing things more natural and it was interesting too, because the more I went natural, the more I tuned into myself. I would know things before the doctors would. So I remember a time where I went to a gynaecological appointment, I said, "Hey, I have a yeast infection." And she was like, "I'll let you know that." And I was like, "No, I'm telling you I had a lot of sweets, I had a lot of candy and my body's reacting to it. I need to just get this thing cured" And she was like, "Well that's not the case, because if that was the case then all the kids around Halloween would have yeast infections." I was like, "Well how do you know they don't?" (Laughs). It was just like, "I'm telling you, I know my body." And she did her exam came, back, "Well yes, you have a yeast infection." I was like, "Yes, I know." And that became a pretty common thing for me to experience, was this belittling of us as individuals and human beings and it's like this need to tell you what you are and what needs to be done. I started working with acupuncturists, doing herbs and supplements that came from creation, from earth, you know. And then I, this might be a little bit more than what you've heard from other people, but I'm pretty close to God and angels and I've had a lot of direction with them before in my life. And then we got pregnant... I did a pregnancy test, but I just never felt the need to do anything more. I felt so jaded by the medical industry... I didn't want them touching me. I didn't want them being anywhere near my baby. And you know, I just... I think it was about two days after I took the pregnancy test, I could feel his heart beat. And I just said, "Oh that's my boy" you know. Like I immediately was like "that's my boy." And I just wanted to nurture that instinct within myself, I wanted to be present with the true gift of creation from God, you know. And honour that intention that he has. And so I just continued with that. And I knew that's what I wanted to do all the way through. So we never actually had any doctor involved in our pregnancy. And I wanted to have someone present, you know... we knew we wanted to do a home birth and we wanted to be connected in that way, but we... I did some research on what that meant, and I knew once I understood what the midwife's different role was between doulas and stuff, that I didn't even want a midwife around. Because I saw how they were still connected to the medical industry. No offence to any midwife or anything, I just personally didn't want to have that. It didn't feel right to me. And so I reached out to a doula. **Nicole**, first baby

I just wanted it to be really sort of a quiet thing and I wanted to be in control of where I was and what I was doing and I didn't want anybody else to be making suggestions... I would be really hard pushed to have somebody there telling me something who's got experience but if that conflicted with my instincts at that time, then that would be really stressful because I would be thinking, "Well, this person has experience and knowledge that I don't have but my instincts are telling me this" and I thought it would be a conflict, an inward conflict within myself and I thought that unless I was feeling stressed, it would bring on stress so I thought the moment I felt stressed and the moment I didn't feel that I was coping or if the pain got too bad, then I would phone the midwives. I was very sort of central [geographically]. I thought that the midwives would come quite quickly if we said, we're quite far along, could you come quite quickly – I thought they could be there in 20 minutes and first babies take a long time so I thought that sort of timescale would be okay and I don't know, I just didn't get to that stage. Really before the birth, I wasn't confident enough in myself to really let myself imagine that I would cope with labour fine and it would be fine. I just imagined well we'll see how we go and then we'll phone the midwife. I wanted to give birth naturally without painkillers but I did imagine that it could well be unbearable, especially sort of different things that you hear from different people and especially the way the media portray that you think "well who am I to imagine that it's going to be fine" and I don't need to worry so it wasn't a conscious decision beforehand but it was a conscious decision to leave it and having a friend around that was comfortable with that and even supportive of that and even made that choice themselves made then an easy decision for us to make so my partner was free to call the midwife at any point as was I and as was D [friend] but we all sort of decided together that while we're coping it would be nicer without that presence and we coped until the baby arrived so I think also if it would have been a longer labour, I would have probably got more exhausted and phoned the midwife and also I'd read a lot that quick babies are usually fine and the deliveries are fine and uncomplicated and it was quite quick in the end. So, I gave birth without the midwife but it didn't feel like that, I felt like I had had all the support that I needed. **Sarah-Anne**, first baby

Another reason that I chose freebirth in the first place, was I'd been really quite ill before pregnancy with fibromyalgia, and I'd been on very heavy pain medication, which looking back, was not what I needed. I became quite bed bound in the end. I couldn't walk, and so, pregnancy for me was a real catalyst into kind of good health, and to undoing a lot of the harm that had been going on. And so, that was another thing, I didn't want any, kind of, unnecessary medical meddling, which was what was happening with my illness beforehand...I just totally needed my own space during labour.

We didn't want to go to hospital, we wanted to be at home. And that wasn't really looking like a good option for a home birth, because they [in laws with whom they then lived] didn't want that in their home, basically. And so it's not our home, so, that was a bit tricky, we had to sort of figure that out together. And, and in the end, because they've got quite a big garden, we suggested, "Well, why don't we put a bell tent in your garden and have that as our, as our birthing space?" So, they were really open to that, and that's how we got round being on their land as it were. And freebirth was just developing as an idea in pregnancy, so, towards the end, I think I stopped going to most of the appointments. I had the twenty-week scan, and then was just, sort of things were dropping away; I was not going for blood tests and stuff. So, I was sort of slowly getting my head around that I didn't have to do, I didn't have to do anything; I could choose what I wanted to do. And so, we were talking between ourselves about whether we'd be quite sort of open with our plans or not, you know, how we were going to sort of play that, how we were going to come out, as it were (laughs). **Leonie,** talking about the first of her three freebirths

Yes, first baby and our only baby. So we've only got one, and he was our first baby, my first pregnancy, my only pregnancy, and yes, when we got pregnant, we looked into all of the different options for giving birth. We were in Leeds at the time. We knew definitely that hospital wasn't for us, and we just started doing lots of reading and exploring our options. I read quite a lot of stuff by Sheila Kitzinger and then reading stuff by Michel Odent and sort of happened upon the idea of freebirthing. We looked into it a lot; did lots and lots of research and decided that that was the way forward for us... I've not had a bad experience of hospitals. I've never had any negative experience. I've never been in hospital for anything. I've never had a broken bone or anything negative. It was just a really strong sense that I didn't feel that hospital was a place to give birth in. I suppose I associated hospitals with illness or being poorly, or that's where you went if something was broken and it needed fixing. I had a very strong sense that giving birth wasn't something that fitted into those categories. I felt that I wanted to be somewhere that I felt safe and comfortable, and that I could move at will, and I didn't feel intuitively that hospital would make me feel that comfortable. So it just never seemed to be... it was never in my mind that if I got pregnant, hospital would be the place that I would want to go. It just seemed alien – that concept of going into hospital. It was never really an option. I didn't have an unassisted pregnancy. I still had midwives' appointments and I still went to my GP however many times you needed to go, and did all of... what you would maybe class as normal things... went to my regular midwifery appointments, went for my scans, but I just never wanted to give birth in hospital. **Lindsay**, first baby

Many women saw themselves as "working towards" freebirth as their confidence, knowledge and trust in their bodies grew through several pregnancies.

My youngest daughter, A was born at home on the 26th of August 2017. Long before I even conceived her, I knew that with my next baby I would freebirth. It was a natural progression for me, and how I have learnt, experienced and grown since having my first baby 18 years ago. My first baby was born when I was 17 and clueless. A textbook "normal" birth, but far from how I know birth to be now. With my second baby four years later, I knew that things would be different. I began a life long journey of learning, researching, and many, many revelations about having babies. Knowing better I did better. I began to listen to the instincts that I had previously ignored, squashed and thought wrong because of what we are told having babies is like. I birthed that now almost 14-year-old baby girl in my tiny bathroom at home with a sweet young midwife catching her. I still remember her name and her kind gentle manner. Her unobtrusive presence was exactly what I needed and my elation that "I did it!" was unhindered by drugs and hospital business.

My third, fourth and fifth babies were grown and born with a combination of support from IMs [independent midwives] and NHS care. But my dissatisfaction with impersonal, conveyor belt NHS care and uncertainty over midwife availability grew with each pregnancy, as did my knowledge of my own body and birth. I strongly considered freebirth with number five as I could not cope with the uncertainty of who would attend and whether they would attend at all. For all my births I have craved privacy and solitude (two bathroom births and two pool births attest to this!), but I understood that with my fifth baby I was approaching freebirth from a negative standpoint. I was considering it out of fear and mistrust, and out of frustration and anxiety. In the end I was supported by a wonderful IM for this birth, but I knew soon after that I wouldn't need that support again. I was over an emotional hurdle and ready to truly be better off birthing alone next time. **Claire**, sixth baby, first freebirth

In my previous pregnancy with L, which was seven years ago, I'd seen some videos of people birthing totally on their own in the middle of nowhere. I thought that was completely mad (laughs). So it's interesting to think that in that seven year period I've come to a place where I think that sounds brilliant! I think it's just a matter of feeling more empowered and more confident in my own body and having more knowledge of the process. Just trusting the process and trusting my own body. Which I always have done, I think. I've had four children and they've all been natural births without any pain relief or interventions, and I feel like I was able to do that because I've always had a deep faith in nature, evolution, and my body knows what it's supposed to be doing if we can just get out of its way and let it get on with it. So I think I've always felt that way and I've become more and more confident through having my own children and learning more about birth and witnessing other people giving birth as a doula... that actually the human body does know what to do, and women know what to do, and most of the problems that I've seen have come from people interfering with that process, either through pregnancy, undermining people's confidence or chipping away at their innate knowledge, or actually during the labour and birth process, there being systems in place that interfere with what women want to do.

My first birth was in a hospital which was fine, but my next two at home, with one midwife, because the second midwife never made it on time. I spent most of the labour on my own with my partner and then the midwife just came in at the end to catch the baby. So I'd kind of got to the point where I was like, well, I don't really need the midwife. They only seemed like they were there to clean up the mess and do the paperwork. So I had really felt like I'd done it on my own the last two times. I mean, you always do it on your own, you have to pull out your own courage and you have to do it ultimately don't you? No-one else is going to help you! I felt like I could do that. And also, we've moved to a new area since I had my last baby, and I was meeting the new midwives, I just didn't feel like I really wanted to have them, these particular people, with me. It wasn't that I had any difficulties, although the first midwife that I met was quite brusque and quite dismissive of my hippy ideals (laughs). **Elena**

Discovering I was pregnant with my sixth child was a shock, however my primary concern was not the pregnancy or impending birth but how I would navigate NHS maternity services. Like many women I was under the impression that I was somewhat obliged to seek medical assistance. However previous interactions had left me feeling downtrodden and disempowered. My initial discontent sparked the realisation that I didn't definitively know my rights, instinctively prompting further research. I was delighted to learn about 'unassisted pregnancy, wild pregnancy and freebirth' as it aligned with my family's moral principles and values. As an experienced mother who had successfully delivered naturally many times including two babies 'born before arrival' I was confident in my abilities to deliver unassisted. It was to my understanding there was no legal obligation to inform any medical professionals of my pregnancy and so openly chose not to.

I loved my wild pregnancy, it was the least stressful of all my experiences, time usually spent attending appointments was reassigned to personal learning often shared with the other children. I already had an extensive interest and understanding of naturopathy and thoroughly enjoyed broadening my knowledge into pregnancy and birth. It allowed me to confidently maintain privacy and allowed me to choose who I wished to interact with and how often. For the first time I could focus on the nature of pregnancy rather than a predefined delivery date to which I would be herded through a series of checkpoints and scrutinised according to standardised statistics. **J**

… this was private… it was our business only… We only learned, many years later, that this birth would now be called " freebirthing." To us, back then, we just wanted to have our baby born our way, into our arms, in our home, with no interference and we deeply trusted that this would be so.

Our daughter's birth had been fine and quick too but I birthed on a hard "delivery" bed, in stirrups with an episiotomy as I was a first-time mother. This was under the care of the nuns led by the redoubtable Sister Stan. I had firmly declined drugs in labour and was told that I'd want them, "When the pains are reeely bad." "No I won't," I replied resolutely. After she was born the nuns gave us a bottle of glucose water and said we must feed it to her "for energy." We poured it down the sink and they were flabbergasted when we told them that she'd drunk it all! I self-discharged a few hours later, much to the nun's distress and fears that the baby would die, to which we reassured them that all would be well.

Hence when I was pregnant again and no midwives or doctors would countenance supporting a home birth, our decision was made. My partner had helped cows to calve and we had seen goats and horses give birth and I had no fear that my body could not do it and I also had been present as support at local friends' 'freebirths' too. **Caroline B**

It was just a progression I think, when I had my first, I was quite young and I had a hospital birth with her which was not so straight forward because I had pre-eclampsia and I had to be induced. When I had my second, I was quite scared to go into the hospital and I had told my midwife this and she suggested that I had a home birth so, I did that and thankfully that midwife was on call at the time when M was born and then the same with T – I had a home birth with him, but then, when A was born and it was quite late at night and I think I was maybe in a bit of denial that it was actually happening and it happened so fast that it was sort of less than an hour and we had phoned the midwives, but she (A) had come before they got there and then the experience afterwards when the midwives were there and they weren't really very nice to me and I just felt like, I didn't think I could have anybody again when we were having our fifth, C, and so I kind of purposefully didn't phone in time with her although she was really fast and then when we moved here and we were having N, I didn't actually have any antenatal care or anything which was just because of things that had happened before then with various people being involved and so I planned to have an unassisted birth with her which was fine and then again with S, that's what we had planned, so it's just been a progression, I think that I've been a bit more, maybe afraid of having people involved but also a bit more confident in my ability to manage it, although last time didn't go quite to plan. **C**

My birth journey hasn't always been easy with my first four children all being premature (the fourth due to hospital error). It took a lot of faith in my body's ability when the decision was made to home birth our fifth. My husband and I decided we would happily stay at home from 36 weeks and fought hard to get support from the hospital to do so. Having midwives and doctors in and out the room, interfering the birth process and not allowing me to go on to birth as I want were the deciding factors of a home birth and the freebirth. At 37+6 F made a rapid 50 minute arrival after nearly two weeks of prodromal labour. My partner called the midwives as I hit transition, I listened to my body and our son was birthed beautifully into my husband's hands as our other children were upstairs. Our doula arrived ten minutes after his arrival. Midwives arrived nearly 30 minutes after the birth, they stepped back and left us alone, no rush to birth the placenta or any checks. F did a breast crawl and three hours after he was born everyone was away. Just us alone when he entered the world was just perfect, a stark contrast to the previous birth traumas, so when we found ourselves pregnant again just ten weeks later we knew we would plan a freebirth this time. **Sarah M**

And then I always said, "Right, if I fall pregnant again, I'm having my home birth. I'm doing this, I'm doing that." And that's where the freebirth started coming into play. Even when I fell pregnant then with my second baby, I was looking into like the wild pregnancy and all this. But again, especially here in [Northern Ireland] as well, it's like, "Oh God, you know, oh dear, you're not going to go in." So I still was very fifty fifty, do you know what I mean. I don't mean to sound crude, but I was starting to grow my balls, do you know what I mean... I was starting to grow as a person, as a woman. And I was keeping on looking at what my choices was and what my options was, and then I was starting to question them. I was starting to question everything. I went for my appointment and I said, "I'm definitely birthing this baby at home." What had happened the last time, I will not let that happen to me this time, you know. And it was like, "Oh no, no, no. You'll not get a home birth. We're so short staffed, you wouldn't expect us… would you really expect…?" This is what the midwife said, "Would you really expect us to have to come to your home, and we're already so short staffed?" And I said, you know, "That is not my problem." So I always wanted the home birth and then they had told me then, it was like, "No, no, no, look we'll review it, we'll review it." And then that is when I kind of went, "Do you know what, these appointments aren't for me any more." So I started to decline the appointments then. And then I just started to really grow as a woman and rely on my intuition and connect with my body and the baby. And it was a really beautiful pregnancy. And for me, as a woman, too I feel I have grown so, so much from it. Because I went on how I felt and how my baby was feeling. I went on all that. **Christina**

For some women the journey towards freebirth was part of a longer life journey that sometimes began when they were children.

As long as I can remember, I've wanted a very simple life... which was about birth as well. I would never have imagined myself giving birth any other way than completely naturally in how we were meant to do it in the wild, I guess, that's sort of how I work, I think... ever since I was like 12, 11, even younger maybe, I've just wanted this little - little bit of land to be as self sufficient as possible and that came across in every walk of life – like birth as well and I always knew that I would... I was just going to do it when, when I was ready. **Peggy**

My sister and I were born before the midwife arrived. My father caught me and there was a local woman who was experienced in birth present. My Grandma caught my sister, who was born blue with the cord wrapped around her neck. Mum told me Grandma panicked and Mum told her to unwind the baby…

I have always been aware of my Mum's influence in birth, she was very matter of fact, straight forward and down to earth…

I know that when I chose to freebirth, I was wanting to break away from being a good girl and pleasing others / gaining their approval…I didn't want to be a part of the institution or system, I have no interest whatsoever in sitting in hospital corridors waiting for some stranger to call me into a dismal room and take my blood pressure etc. I've always known that if my baby genuinely needed medical help, I would have been the first through the door for help. I also knew that if my baby was not meant to be earth side with me, that was the way it was meant to be. I had had a late miscarriage and held my tiny son, counting his skinny fingers and toes. I also did not want any tests etc because the worry of waiting for results, for what? I am a firm believer in a woman's right to choose, but during my family making days, termination was not for me, so what was the point of scans etc?

It was such a blessed relief though to labour knowing that no one was going to interrupt by asking to monitor the baby, check their position or ask any questions, to be honest. **Caroline S**

My Mum had a home birth in the 90s when I was in my teens. So there's me and then there's a 16 year gap. She had such a terrible experience with me. As a teenager she was not given the opportunity to be informed. So things just happened to her that she had no say in. And she was determined not to do that again. And when she told her GP that she was planning a home birth, the GP struck her off and refused to have anything to do with her. The midwives were fantastic; the midwives were all for it, but the GP wasn't. So I knew from then, I was 16 when this was happening, that home birth was an option, but that also home birth probably came with some kind of fight or at least needing to be assertive about what you wanted. And then I was there for two of my siblings' births. I missed my middle sister by three hours. But I was there for my little brother when I was 16 and really I was my Mum's doula for my youngest sister, for that birth. And I caught her and you know, it was all wonderful. So then when it came to my first pregnancy, I knew that I was going to have a home birth, I always said that if there was a clinical benefit to being in hospital, then I would discuss it. But I wasn't going to fall for, "We think it's best."

… how did I come to freebirth - it's not one event – it's my whole life, all these experiences I've had since, at least since I was 16. But also the knowledge that I'm the only person in my family who was born in hospital. Everybody else was born at home. **Beth**

Well I had ill health before. I had what they call fibromyalgia and I used to take a lot of pharmaceuticals and then through my journey with that I came to realising that ultimately it's a business which thrives off of illness… And I had a friend, she's a doula and I met her some years ago and when I met her I just started asking her about her birth stories, how she birthed. Because I had this dream of wanting to birth with dolphins and (laughing) and then we went from there. And then as time went on, I became less and less reliant upon the NHS. And so when it came to being pregnant myself it was just really natural to not want to engage in any capacity with those services and to just ultimately to actually get help from my friend. And…because she wasn't living in the same country, she was signposting me to information hubs where I could then just educate myself on pregnancy and birth. **Yony**

I've always questioned what people have said to me, when I was about five or something my Dad said, "Always question whatever anybody tells you, everything, whatever anybody tells you," so I've always been questioning of everything, so that's what's led me to question the health system and look at it and observe that it wasn't sort of in tune with the way I felt about the world, so it was just natural for me to want… some alternative way of giving birth than doing it in hospital… it would never, I don't think it would have ever occurred to me to do it in a hospital… voluntarily. **Charlie**

I was kind of looking because, unconsciously or semi-consciously… I've got a much older sister and she has three children and they were all born at home. I remember thinking, because she's fourteen years older than me, so I was eight when she had her first child. And I do remember thinking how strange it was to have this strange lady that you didn't know there, when you're having your baby. It felt odd to me, even without really being able to formulate the thought, but it was there. And then when I came across the idea of unassisted birth as an actual thing, it brought that thought very much to the fore. Does that make sense? **Alice**

I think probably for me, it goes all the way back to I trained as a hypnotherapist in my twenties. And I ended up preferring to work with women who had a fear of giving birth. And so I just focused on that area. And then through that, I ended up teaching hypnobirthing classes and then through that ended up becoming a doula. So I have been present at many births, by the time I was having my own children. And before that I had actually attended four births of one of my friends. And she had to be induced each time with her child, quite early because of medical problems. And so my first experiences of births were this kind of very, very medicalised, all monitored… And it always felt a little bit like the babies were dragged out. And it wasn't as I had imagined it would be… So my first experiences were like, "Oh that's not how I want things to be for me." And then I trained in hypnotherapy and ended up supporting lots of women that way, and then supporting couples. And then being a doula. So I'd been to eighteen births.

By the time I met L, who's my husband, we decided that we were going to have children. And so by that point, I already had very fixed ideas on what I thought would work for me, and what I experienced worked locally and what the hospital was like… I was only going to have my child at home… But I really wanted my husband to have this great experience as well. So I didn't want to have help from anybody who I already had a professional relationship with. So somebody suggested there's a lovely midwife in [place]… So L and I met D. Oh we just loved her. So she supported me through the first pregnancy and birth. And I didn't feel I needed a doula, because she was our independent midwife… And it was great, she came to my home, as you can imagine, it was lovely… it was not how I expected my labour or birth to be at all. But that was our first experience. And it all happened at home and was great, brilliant.

And then, so what, two years later, eighteen months later, we were pregnant again. And obviously, we just wanted D, because not only had I found her amazing – really, really she'd been there for L… But by the time eighteen months went by, D was involved in a big court case… at that point that we wanted her to support us. And she was really wanting to, but… and she thought she would be able to, but it became quite a witch hunt, and it extended longer… And so then, halfway through the pregnancy she said, "You know, what I could do is I could be your doula. I will be your doula at the birth." And we thought that was great. But I thought about that, and I just thought, "Do you know, if something happened and she needed to step up into a midwifery role, she would then face the consequences." And I couldn't have her there, knowing that she might do something in her natural midwifery role that would then put her career in jeopardy. So I said, "We'd love to have you, but we can't do that to you, you know. Your career is so important to so many women." So we then had H, who had been my friend and my doula mentor. And she put me in touch with D in the first place. So we asked her to be our doula. And I think, I said, "Well we'll just see… We'll see how far we get with H, and then we'll just see about the midwives."

[In labour] And I just felt really, really peaceful, really positive. Felt I had the right team.
Cathy S

Like Cathy in her story above, some women learned from other women's experiences.

Well, I suppose it's easier to make a decision if you know somebody who's made that decision before and if you can appreciate their reasons for making their decisions. I think I am quite easily sort of influenced by what's around me and I do feel if I had not met anybody who had ever had a home birth, I think the actual thing that I would have done would have been just to go into hospital. At the time I just felt really like confident at all the things that I had learnt during my pregnancy and made me feel like birth didn't need to be so traumatic and it could be a really nice, gentle sort of welcoming for a new person and I really wanted it to be a family thing and because I'd had some friends that had had home births and were really positive about it – it just made me think, "Oh, we can do this." **Sarah-Anne,** first baby

I was just talking to all the women whose voices I valued. And I had another doula friend who once said that she had never ever been scared at a freebirth. And she now only does freebirths. I was surrounded by women who believed in birth and believed in me…I was good at seeking the voices that I needed. I knew that what I needed was confidence in myself. **Beth**

So the more of birth I experienced as a doula, the more I could see how, when women were undisturbed, it was just a completely normal situation. Therefore, for them there was nobody clinical who could take any responsibility over their care there. It just worked really well. So I knew that if I was going to have another baby, that I wanted it to be like that, and I just knew that I would know if something didn't feel right and I would happily go into hospital if something didn't feel right and bypass the having somebody there. And by that point I knew all of the independent midwives and they were lovely. But because I knew them so well, it just didn't feel right, them being in my space, because it's when, as a woman, you're completely exposed, isn't it?… you're at your most vulnerable, but also, at your strongest. So it just didn't feel that I wanted to have anybody there.

… by that point I was supporting a woman who was forty-two. And the scare tactics because of her age to go into hospital, and the dead baby card, and I just thought, "I can't, I can't have that kind of care/service as part of my preparation to being a parent."

… the big thing that's gone into my choices, is having seen what it can be like with other people come. I've been at births with independent midwives and I think, for me, I'm very aware of other people. I need to be on my own, and having somebody else there, even with C [doula] I did it. I looked to her to ask a question. Now, if I had a midwife there, they have to be aware of the risks, so they might have reflected back, "Well, we can't tell you what's happening, it might be something, it might not be." And just even hearing that seed of doubt, might have made me go in, and I have no doubt if I had an NHS midwife for A's birth, I would have had a caesarean section. Because I had a very, very long labour. I was geriatric, of course, being forty-two, and it was really unconventional, sporadic contractions, nothing following the curve line. So I need to, in order to fully let go, I need to have nobody else there who is responsible for any decisions. And having a friend who's a doula, she's not responsible for anything, other than being there for me, and that is literally it, just being there and that emotional support and holding that space. Holding my wants and my needs, holding that. "What, you want this, but I will do whatever you want," but without putting those questions and that's what underpinned my decision-making. **Hannah**

… it was a friend who'd had D as a doula and she'd recommended it. And then I was thinking, because I'd had a hard time after F [first baby] was born, and also in terms of our relationship and stuff, I'd wanted some extra support after the birth. So I looked online for people who could offer this post-birth support and, and then I'd met D [doula], and then she'd obviously suggested, "What do you want to do about the birth?"… and I trusted her. And because once I'd spoke, learnt more about birth and realised that it probably wasn't going to go wrong, and if it did I knew that I was only like ten minutes away from the hospital in an ambulance. So, it's really not a big risk and also I knew that if I did arrive at hospital, they would let me in straight away… I knew that the most likely reason for going to hospital would be that I became exhausted, i.e. not an emergency… So that's why I decided I didn't really need the midwives there, because I had D in case anything went wrong and, and to guide us through it. And also the other main reason was because of Covid… And the other reason was that I didn't have that personal relationship with midwives because it would have been someone who I didn't know and of course the midwives would have tended to be nice people, but I just didn't want to take the chance of somebody coming in who might have different ideas about things. Whereas I knew that D knew me personally and she knew what I wanted, **Rosalie**

Doulas also learned from their experiences of being with women during their freebirths.

I know the theory, but I'm starting to see it in practice. Like the true nature of an undisturbed straightforward birth. And it's leading me to question a lot about what maternity services is offering, and how, what a big impact it has on that, and how it interferes with that. But of course, even saying this out loud makes me sound like a dangerous person, who's promoting freebirth, which I'm wary of…

I can see myself being at more and more freebirths, rather than encouraging them to call midwives in when I see what a difference it makes. When midwives arrive and they talk very loudly, and they don't know each other, and they've not met the woman before, and they ask her loads of questions, and it's really unsettling for women. **D, doula**

For some women a really positive birth experience, with good midwifery care, led them to decide to freebirth next time.

My first baby was born in October 2010. Her birth was crucial to my future decision making processes and so writing a little about the experience is an important starting point.

When I was pregnant with my daughter, S, I knew nothing about birth and upon reflection feel that I was relatively fortunate with the care I received from my antenatal midwife and particularly, the midwife at the hospital. I don't remember being given a choice about where to have my baby and I didn't know enough to question the idea of hospital.

During labour, the midwives were hands off and rarely in the room, leaving my husband and me alone. I used the birth ball, rebozo and pool in a dim lit room with music and mood lighting. I began pushing before the midwife returned for a routine check (I'd only had one, maybe two checks prior – again, not presented as a choice). When the midwife came back, my husband, D, informed her I was pushing, she quietly remained with us for the hour and a half it took for S to emerge whilst I was on my hands and knees in water. After the birth, I remained in the pool for 90 minutes before the cord was cut (I cut it myself after the midwife asked if I'd like to), then I got out and birthed the placenta, squatting on the floor. S was born within six hours of arrival, weighing 8lbs 8oz.

This experience was pivotal. As I began meeting other new mothers and hearing their birth stories I was shocked at the level of interference and intervention – mostly assisted deliveries or C sections, quite a few inductions. I had made the assumption that all births were similar to my own. I realised how fortunate I had been as I constantly returned to those positive memories in the first, challenging weeks of parenthood. It left me questioning so much and birth was constantly on my mind and I needed to know more…

It [first birth at home with midwife] was a really positive experience and the only thing I would have changed, I've done that this time – I've just left out, and to be honest when I did find out I was pregnant again… it wasn't like a majorly conscious decision to leave the midwives, I just felt… I feel great, we're really busy doing projects and stuff and it just didn't happen, so it just – that's the way it stayed and I haven't felt any need whatsoever to approach – to have any care. **Peggy,** planning freebirth

… when I think back to that birth and how I felt supported and how my body did what it needed to do, it was a bit of a no-brainer, when I became pregnant with A, to go, "Well, I can, I can birth. This is fine. I don't need the reassurance of anyone else around me." **Katy B,** after second rapid birth which was a booked home birth but they did not call the midwife until after the baby was born

I came across it actually before the birth of my first child, F, which was fourteen years ago, almost fifteen. And I'd read some books about unassisted birth. And I was very, just interested in having that kind of empowered experience. And also I'm a massage therapist, I trained in yoga. I've done a lot of movement work; body-based work, movement, that kind of thing. And I was very much interested in like the body's wisdom. And feeling that if we let our bodies do what they naturally do, then that's the best scenario. But when it came to my first child, I'd read the books, but it's your first child and it's an unknown. And I was still a little bit afraid. I thought, "Well I just don't know whether I can do this or not..".. and also, I was in Brighton with my first child, and there was a really great home birth team, and they were really fantastic. And I had a home birth with a pool and the midwife was fantastic, because she basically left me alone. She just said, "Look, I'll be there in the corner." And she just said one thing at one point that was really useful and kind… it was really, really great. So then it came seven years later to being pregnant again, and so I went to the GP. Expected to be referred to home birth team, but I'd moved at this point, so I was no longer in Brighton – I was in Somerset. And they said, "Oh, we don't have a home birth team any more. It could be any midwife. Anyone can attend a home birth." So it's like, it was a new model basically. And I said, "Well I don't really feel very comfortable with that", I said, "for me birth is a very personal experience, and I really want to connect with the midwife and get to know them." And they said, "That's not how it works here." So then I, I wrote to the head of the NHS in Somerset. And I expressed my concerns, and I said, "Look, you know, for me, giving birth is very much like making love, and it's the same kind of process, at the beginning anyway, with the oxytocin. And for me, my fear…" Most… a lot of women maybe their fear is, "Oh I need the support." And my fear was more, actually if I have someone come in who's not pro home birth; who maybe had only done one home birth or two home births, and doesn't even really feel that comfortable with it, then their fear and their desire… their fear of my process might get in the way. And I might end up being taken to hospital when it wasn't needed. It was my lack of trust really in the service. **Rachel**

The desire to freebirth was entirely positive for some women.

There is often an assumption when a woman considers unassisted birth that she has perhaps encountered a negative experience, therefore feels as though she has little choice. I responded to these comments by explaining that my decision to freebirth related to my first birth as much as its connection to any of my prior experiences. I felt absolute positivity, my choices were not made out of fear. **Melissa**

So I didn't freebirth because I had a bad experience. I didn't freebirth because I didn't like my midwives. I freebirthed because I truly yearned for it. I really felt that it is the right thing for us as a family. And since I decided that, there was a complete peace… it came within me, the feeling that I really yearned for it. I didn't want to have somebody around me… I didn't want to think, "You can save me – tell me what to do!" What I really wanted was to tap into myself. I didn't want anybody to tell me how I should breathe or what I can do and give me options. I wanted to find it out myself. So I wanted to have the full experience of what women really feel at the birth of their baby when there is nobody to help. That was the main thing that I really yearned for. I really wanted to feel what is it like when women are pushing? What is it like when the baby is going through the birth canal? What is it like when the head is crowning? I spoke to the baby a lot during the birth. I put my hand there. I navigated the head out. I asked her to turn… so I really worked with the body and the baby and I really felt it. I felt every inch because I really could tune in. I didn't have any distraction from the outside. **Michaela**

I do not believe that freebirth is a choice for everyone and it is something that I worked towards, rather than made hard, fast decisions about but I think it is crucial to stress that my choices were born out of positivity, a deep understanding of myself and intelligent reasoning. **Melissa**

As these women moved towards freebirth, there was a parallel change in how they saw NHS maternity services. Whereas previously these services were seen as the way women had their babies in this country, they were now seen as a safety net which they could rely on in an emergency but which they hoped not to need.

We never called them; we had no intention of calling them. Unless something major was going to happen. But more likely we would have called an ambulance if we found something was really off. **Carmen**

Chapter 3: "Finding your safe place": safety, trust and fear

Different people feel safe in very different birth situations.

There's women that really feel safe in a hospital and great for them, that they do. And I'm saying that, to me, hospitals make me feel really unsafe. In fact, they make me feel quite sick and I don't like them. **Rachel**

… what I just really found was that it [hospital] wouldn't be a safe place to go and other women I had spoken to had said it really is about where you feel safe and that really struck a chord as well – that has to be right…

If I felt safe being in a hospital which, I think of women [who] probably do, then perhaps I would have felt safe in the hospital but not from what had happened before, there is no way. I would feel safe going to a place that was created specifically for that need and really had a lot of creative thought and love put into it – you know, that's the kind of thing, but nothing that's just really institutionalised, it's not safe, it's not safe at all. You're not a person, you're just a kind of number really. So, just being able to be a person who has feelings and rights, and the support aspect of it is really, really big, because the support I got was what enabled me to do it. The support was from the women who have experienced home births and expect it to be a pleasurable, enjoyable experience. **Polly**

And in some ways, I think I had quite a strong fear. My biggest fear was related to unnecessary intervention, and the medical system taking control and taking over. **Gauri**

… people will say, "oh you're having your babies at home that's really brave of you.".. well it's not really brave at all, I don't see that packing things up and finding some way of getting to the hospital to have a baby with strangers around you, is, I don't really see that that's the way it should be so… I think they're braver for going into hospital, through choice anyway, obviously when situations arise it maybe is the best place to be but, if I had the choice then I would never ever, ever go back into hospital to give birth again… **C**

Privacy was of paramount importance for some women to feel safe and that they could give birth. They were very aware of the impact of other people's presence on their labour.

I simply know my body, trust my body, and know what I need as a birthing woman. And what I need is privacy, solitude, and my own space. THIS is what's safest for me. This is how I can allow my body to get on and do its thing. This is how I make as sure as I possibly can that my hormonal cascade isn't interrupted and therefore that my baby and I aren't in danger of slowed labour, stress, or bleeding. Having birthed six babies now I'm very acutely aware of the effect external influences have on me during labour. My husband going out stepped my labour up several gears and his return slowed it again, briefly, but it was noticeable. And this is my husband for goodness sake! I noticed the same effect with our IM's presence in my previous birth, and looking back I see it in all my other births too. I speak as a mother and as a doula when I say this; birth attendants most certainly have their place, but we also most certainly underestimate the effect and potential consequences of their presence in the birth room. The same as the camera affects the subject matter merely by its presence, so does anyone who enters a birthing woman's space. **Claire**

And I remember at the time D [doula] and my partner T were going about quietly and subtly keeping the water temperature constant of the birth pool and even that I was just thinking, "Oh for god's sake, stop faffing around, I'm trying to give birth here." And I couldn't be bothered with anyone doing anything, or T would occasionally ask me a question and I'd just say, "It's fine, it's fine", like I didn't want to think about anything else. So I think that extra interference of people coming in would have just been too much and I definitely in the moment was just like absolutely not. I don't need it, I don't want it, yes. Would be like if you're trying to run a marathon and somebody was asking you about your beliefs or something, you'd just be like, "Oh for god's sakes, go away, I'm trying to run a marathon here." **Rosalie**

Giving birth is a really private sort of thing and I don't manage as well when there's lots of people around and I think if we hadn't had the sort of problem this last time, then I possibly would have not even had my husband present because it just seemed to be easier to do it yourself really than have people constantly (laughs) telling you what you're supposed to be doing and you don't feel that you're supposed to be doing that. **C**

And the reason I pursued it was a sense that I just would feel interrupted by the presence of anybody in my space. It wasn't really a case of being afraid or not having the right kind of support. My midwives for my first baby were the Albany, and we couldn't have really asked for better, in terms of that. And, but there was definitely a sense that I'd be off my stroke and that I would be concentrating on pleasing my midwife, rather than on focusing on the job at hand. **Alice**

In order to fully let go, I need to have nobody else there who is responsible for any decisions. **Hannah**

SK spoke of her insights as a doula:

I'd always been like, I don't really want anyone there while I give birth, the thought, I'm just one of those people that, if people are watching me, I'm terrible at anything. I can't even wash the dishes with someone watching me, let alone give birth. So… this makes sense now, of course women don't want to be observed when they're giving birth, of course you don't want strangers there. It's something we talk about in birth preparation classes as privacy and just staying in your zone and darkness. And the medical system and the way things are set up just doesn't support physiological birth in any way. **SK**

Safety and trust are interlinked and these women trusted their own bodies. They needed considerable autonomy to exercise this trust. The presence of someone who did not share this trust was seen as a negative intervention in the birth process. These mothers were very aware that fear is contagious and therefore wished to avoid contact with professionals who focused on risks or who feared deviation from their usual practices.

… fear is such a huge factor with dealing with pain and the pain is there to be used in a really positive way… Whereas the way it is perceived by medical staff is that there is so much to fear first and foremost, that's where they're coming from. That should be always a possibility that something can go wrong, but they should be able to deal with it. If there is no fear in the first instance, then it's just able to trust. So I really think that whole thing is about the safeness and a place where women can talk to their midwives in their homes, rather than going to the doctors for their five minute check-up which does not even scratch the surface, so that's really fundamental, kind of core. **Polly**

These final days before the birth were the happiest, calmest and stillest I'd had in pregnancy yet. To protect myself from troubling feelings arising from curious, baffled friends and family members, I withdrew from almost all screens and electronic devices. My days felt simple, uncluttered and my sole purpose was to connect with the baby inside my womb, and stay in an oxytocin rich inner state, away from any outside influences or trains of thought that might induce fear, doubt, or negativity. I prayed, meditated, breathed deeply and consistently, and did yoga which promised optimal fetal positioning. I wrote a long love letter to my baby and whispered to it at night before falling asleep. For the first time, I experienced the fetus as a real little human with whom I had a very important connection. My thoughts quietened. With every kick, knee, elbow or hiccup from inside my womb, with every roll, spin, position, my mind focused inwards. My heart swelled with love and relief, a greeting and full-hearted welcome to my little one. My trust in its strength and vitality grew in that final week. So did my certainty that I could birth this child and that it could be birthed and that together we could rise to the challenge of birth with everything it needed to survive and thrive. I had a visceral and embodied sense of my connection to all the women in my maternal ancestral line - all the many, many mothers who had given birth and brought forth life way before the days when society had come to view birthing as a risky and complicated procedure which required a hospital, a vast array of pain medication and machinery, and a host of medical professionals for any hope of finding successful consummation. **Naomi**

I find it really interesting that there's always been a psychological letting-go moment, where I allow birth to happen, and I can switch and go, "Right, okay, now." And I could imagine if you were not able to get into that switching state, how difficult it is and can be. And he's [baby] been very happy and chilled. And I guess that helps, having the two older siblings. Just hang out and be looked after and play. But yes, I'm really grateful that I was able to give birth in that way and trust in my body. And in some ways, I think it's a shame that I've had to put some of the medical establishment at arm's length, because I know not all people want to practise in that way. But I guess that's where a lot of my reasoning came from for wanting to birth unassisted… And people ask me that, because I run the H [London area] Home Birth Support Group, which is a group that I went to when I was pregnant with A, and then I took it on. And people come and share their birth stories. And so sometimes I share mine, particularly if no one's come back to share their birth story. And people often look a bit horrified when I say I chose not to have the midwives there, and I chose to have a fairly hands-off pregnancy as far as monitoring and so on is concerned. And I always knew that, had someone arrived, I didn't want any internal examinations and all those things. And people just go, "Why? Why?" I think they really like the reassurance of knowing someone's there. For them, that's reassuring. I think that's the thing about birth, isn't it? It's finding your safe space, the way you want to birth, that enables you to both birth reassuringly and safely. And mostly I say, "Well, actually, I feel that birth is best not watched, certainly not by the clock, and certainly not by people watching you really closely." And for me, that meant not having people there who I felt would be watching me unnecessarily or monitoring me for things that I felt would be unhelpful in the birthing process. And certainly my experience of having one accidental unassisted and one planned unassisted birth is that, absolutely, my body knew what to do, and the letting go was really important, and allowing my body and my mind to do what it was designed to do was the most important thing; and that was by having the right people around me or not around me, and creating the right birthing environment as well; and for me, doing a lot of the work psychologically beforehand as well. **Katy B**

... a lot of women maybe their fear is, "Oh I need the support." And my fear was more, actually if I have someone come in who's not pro-home birth. Who maybe had only done one home birth or two home births, and doesn't even really feel that comfortable with it, then their fear and their desire... their fear of my process might get in the way. And I might end up being taken to hospital when it wasn't needed... I trust, because I gave birth once, I really know my body. And I know I'm going to be fine. So, and I'll know if there's a problem. So I kind of just was in that really trusting place.

I just want to be by myself; I don't need anyone else there. I know this whole idea of someone delivers your baby. It's like – no, I'm giving birth to my baby. Someone might be there to catch it... But no-one's doing it – I'm doing it. It's like I always find this really hilarious, where you know someone goes, "Oh you know, they didn't get to hospital and this person delivered the baby." And I was like, "No-one does that. It's the woman that delivers the baby." Like this whole crazy notion that... I really respect midwives and I think there's definitely a place for an expert to be in the room just in case there's a problem. Because I'm not a fool to think there aren't risks. But... I had a very easy first birth. And I knew... I thought, "I'll know if something's not right. And I will, I'm not going to be a fool. I'd go and have a caesarean if that was what my body was telling me, if the baby was stuck." But I was pretty convinced I'd be okay. **Rachel**

What I found difficult was that there is clearly also a very political aspect to these choices. Birth is shrouded in a political climate. Whilst I had an intellectual interest in this arena, I found it difficult to establish these boundaries and felt very misunderstood by my antenatal midwife who constantly engaged in the single focus of the perceived medical risk in birth.

I decided to opt out of NHS care at approximately 30 weeks. Disengaging was a natural process; it was the next step of my turning inwards and preparing for a more spiritual experience of birth. Defining the conditions that were right for me, in my circumstances, as an individual and what I personally hoped to learn and achieve through my investment in the safety of such a holistic birth journey.

I had come to trust myself more than I had previously; not just through experience but through research, stories and information that supported my understanding of the science behind mammalian instinct, physiological birth and the undervalued, overlooked role of the hormonal and emotional processes. **Melissa**

The first midwife I went to see I had spoken about it – having a caesarean the first time – and she kind of just brushed it aside… well basically it was because I think my son was really quite a large baby and I am quite small but the explanation I got was… I cannot remember the actual term but disproportionate head to the pelvis and I really went deeper in that myself to try and feel if that was actually true or not, but I just kept thinking more and more, learning more and more about active births and making as much space as possible and optimum positioning and all these things that I had picked up from reading and doing my own research, and it was like, well that has to be a way. I understand that there are hospitals and that things can go wrong, and I never ever took that out of my mind but it was really hard not to let that prevail and so really I surrounded myself with women who trusted the process of women's bodies being able to do it and just being inspired by that. It really, really inspired me and I think that's where, I think when you're pregnant you can really tune into yourself a lot more than normal times, so I really tuned in to what I believed to be true and what I believed was right for me and I lived really close to the hospital so I knew at any point I needed to go there, I knew that I would trust my own instincts to go there in time if I didn't feel… but as soon as I knew I was in labour, I knew that being at home was the safest place and I was so happy that I had the freedom to choose that, and basically it was the women around me who said that it was my choice and right up to the very end I was still… I had made no arrangements for community midwives for a home birth so I just still felt that I would have to go into hospital but you know I got the birthing pool and I just knew that that was my nest, it was my place and I didn't want anything to take me away from that so I knew when I got in there, that is where I wanted to be and I felt wonderful and I felt like this is really safe and it is going to go fine and I just knew it, I think I had prepared myself for it, to trust my own instincts. **Polly**

And I, so in the back of my head, I thought, oh, that would just be the ideal situation, where you don't have that medical pressure, you know, of conforming to policies and timelines and having examinations and having monitoring every five minutes. Because I do really believe that has a detrimental impact on how birth, progresses… my doula experience part made me more confident in birth as a process, but it also made me more fearful of the institution of the maternity services, because of all the things that I've seen.

That's a really interesting relationship I think, my seeing all of these, all the incidents that I've witnessed, and been a part of in hospitals **Katie H**

While some women did not want "anyone else there", others felt they benefited from support from someone they trusted and who they felt trusted them.

… it was really B [doula, retired midwife] that was saying, "You should absolutely do this if this is what you want, and I trust you." And that was really important, that was really important. It wasn't just, like, "Yes, we'll go along with this if you want to," but just, "Do you know what, you're not actually asking enough questions." I said, at one point I said, "Look, I'm sorry, I'm asking so many questions," and she said, "Yes, you're not asking enough questions, never, never stop asking questions…" **Alice**

So I decided not to call them and it was when I was about eighteen weeks pregnant, I thought, "I feel actually quite lonely," because I was still actively working as a doula. So I decided to get an independent midwife to just do some antenatal and postnatal and then it felt that I was looking after myself, because I was getting some support by somebody who's interested in my pregnancy, but not invested to come. When I was going into labour, we had an agreement that she would come soon after or when I wanted her to. **Hannah**

I was vomiting, and I was shaking, the adrenaline I think, but she [doula] gave me honey, just spoonfuls of honey, to give me some energy… and then she told me to get up and walk to the toilet and back, which I was like, "No, I can't, I can't." But then, of course, I trust, because I trusted with her and had that relationship with her, I knew that she was wise and knew what she was talking about, so I did it. And it really helped I think to move him and turn him into the right position to come down. **Rosalie**

Some could envisage a safe place for birth which included midwives who they could trust not to intervene in their labour, but their experiences of NHS midwifery led them to conclude that this was not achievable (see also chapter 11).

I would have just liked to go to a place where there were sort of midwives around and knowing that it's a safe place but still be left to do what you need to do, but actually you know home was a good place and I like the fact that I didn't have anybody trying to check to see if I was dilated or not because that is quite painful and I think kind of stopped the process. **Polly**

I suppose it depends from county to county on what the system is with the midwives, maybe you have that through care of having the same midwife before, during, after the birth, which would be lovely, wouldn't it. In which case there wouldn't be so much of a need, I think, to have a freebirth. But that's not what they do round here… I'd heard about other ones… where midwives had arrived and been very hostile… and I thought, I just didn't want to take the chance. **Rosalie**

For a few women, just the right degree of contact with midwives was possible (see chapter 11).

Section 2: Preparation for Freebirth

Prior to their freebirths, these women put considerable effort into preparing for their labours and births. They sought to take responsibility for both the preparation and the birth itself. They sought out knowledge and what they learned reinforced their interest in and desire to freebirth. They read widely and many took different courses. Some trained as doulas. Many examined their previous labours and births to better understand why they might not have unfolded straightforwardly. Many studied research findings generally, as well as research relevant to their particular circumstances, or read research mentioned to them by health practitioners. They carefully considered how they would deal with unforeseen circumstances should their births not progress as expected, or if their babies needed help during or after birth, looking at how they could best respond to different scenarios. They gradually learned more and more over the course of a pregnancy or several pregnancies and births so that they could prepare the best circumstances for their forthcoming births and parenting journeys.

The preparation took several forms. They learned about the physiology of pregnancy, labour and birth and the factors that support physiological birth. They considered how best to look after themselves through good nutrition and complementary therapies that might support their health and that of their babies. Many emphasised the need to reduce stress, much of which they felt was caused by maternity services and any unfavourable reactions of others to their decisions.

They also sought to "unlearn" the assumptions that go with medicalised birth: dependency on professionals, and the risk and fear that such an approach generates. Emotional and psychological preparation were equally important to them. In taking responsibility for themselves, they worked at letting go of fear and of the need to control birth, seeking to develop awareness of their bodies and their babies, knowing that letting go is essential for the flow of hormones and the unfolding of birth.

Chapter 4: Preparation: learning and unlearning

These women went to considerable lengths to prepare themselves for the birth, researching and "working towards" their aim. They read, gained skills, joined groups and some gained formal qualifications. This involved "unlearning" some previously taken for granted assumptions and exploring many eventualities.

I'd been reading. I had been doing quite a lot of reading and research before I got pregnant... Probably through one of those [online] groups I came across the concept of unassisted birth... then I read Laura Shanley's book and read her website a lot, so that was where I really got my education. **Alice**

I have three children. In my first pregnancy, I found a home birth group through the poster in the hospital. I think I found a waterbirth group first and went to that, and then somebody told me about a home birth group. I looked into it and we weren't sure because of the risks, but then that got me onto researching, and the more I researched, the less intervention I wanted, until by my third I didn't want any intervention at all. **Laura**

My first daughter was born in 2016 and I had planned to have a home birth, but then we transferred to hospital, for failure to progress, a horrible word, and ended up having a C section. So it was just, because my cervix simply stopped dilating around five or six centimetres. And after that experience I decided to become a doula and learn as much as I could about birth and try and help other women. So I'd try and sort of save them from what happened to me because I felt really upset about my birth with my first daughter for a really long time. And so for my second, as soon as I got pregnant actually with my second baby, I started looking into getting a doula, because I didn't have that before and I got quite interested in freebirth, when I was a doula, and I read, what's the name of that book, it's an American author, Laura something or other, I can't remember. **Katie H**

I did the birth classes – the active birth classes at the PPC [Pregnancy and Parents Centre]. And I kept doing the yoga, the PPC and all the information we got there. And I really was reading on the internet. I got a couple of books, of freebirth books. And I really was feeling that I could do it. **Bea**

I'm a birth nerd and an academic. I can read the academic papers as well as the books. And just seeing the statistics and seeing all the different reasons, it's like they can twist anything to be a reason to be in hospital. And like who's comfort is that really for? Is it because it's what's best for me? Is it because it's what they feel more comfortable with? **Beth**

At first, I began watching *One Born Every Minute*. Second, I read *Birth, A History*. This ran simultaneously to the study and completion of The Association of Breastfeeding Mothers Mother to Mother support course and volunteering as a breastfeeding peer supporter at Derby hospital. I also began researching and considering doula preparation courses. I went on to complete one... by which time I was six weeks pregnant with my second baby.

I knew with my second, I was searching for a greater depth to the experience of pregnancy and birth. Something more intuitive, as I had come to trust myself more than I had previously; not just through experience but through research, stories and information that supported my understanding of the science behind mammalian instinct, physiological birth and the undervalued, overlooked role of the hormonal and emotional processes. The reading I had completed (Sarah Buckley, Michel Odent, amongst others), the knowledge and experiences I had gained aided an internal transformation as I began looking for answers and information within. It felt unnecessary to me personally, and I certainly didn't feel I would benefit from routine monitoring, checks, questions and procedures; if anything I felt it would detract and interfere with my pregnancy.

I felt very early on that I wanted to birth unassisted and tentatively began exploring the idea to grasp an understanding of my feelings. I decided to hire a doula to support me with my thought processes and emotions. I booked in with a midwife, declined scans and requested a home birth. My husband was also extremely understanding. We both read Laura Shanley's *Unassisted Childbirth*, amongst other enlightening perspectives (I also found the *Midwife Thinking* blog highly valuable), which really brought into alignment often hard to find information about birth which completes a larger context of the issues women face. Reading became like a process of unlearning many myths perpetuated by our culture that come to be deemed 'normal', it was liberating and freeing to feel as though I was beginning to understand myself and my body, finding my own inner source of strength and knowledge...

A large proportion of our accepted knowledge stems from the cultural evolution of the importance of science and technology as a tool in our lives, frequently excluding intuition as a valid source of information. Think about estimated due dates and how we have come to value the prediction of an ultrasound scan over women's own dates. I think Ann Oakley's description of the pervasive 'unreliable machine' model of viewing our bodies within obstetrics is still dominant. This underpins midwifery education, educational texts, parental advice literature, medical policies and opinion. We are looking at it in purely mechanical and biassed terms, to the detriment of the effects experience and emotion has on our mind and bodies. I believe freebirth to be a valid birth choice on a spectrum, as opposed to a decision 'outside of the system'. Women should be free to access this information, to make up their own minds for there needs to be more than the limitations of the NHS, and more than the limitations of a medical approach. **Melissa**

We were going to have a home birth, for sure. Then there was this nagging thing in me that just... I couldn't sit well with the thought of having more people here. Even though the team was fantastic and I would have loved them at my birth, if I wanted a usual home birth, I just couldn't place it – what is it that I really yearn for? Then I saw an unassisted birth book and I bought it... and when I read it, I just realised that this is what I want. So I didn't freebirth because I had a bad experience... I really felt that it is the right thing for us as a family. And since I decided that, there was a complete peace. And I just knew that there was nothing, other than a real medical problem, that will make me not do it. So I didn't have any fear. We spoke about death as well with the midwife and we knew that this is a possibility. We spoke about the legal side, that my husband mustn't do anything midwives would do. So everything was covered and I did lots of preparation. I'm not going to say that I didn't, because I did. I did lots of mental preparation, I did lots of *Dreambirth* visualisations, I did lots of hypnobirthing, I went for cranio-sacral therapy, I went for somatic experience thing. I did lots of things. I exercised, I did spinning babies and everything to make sure that the baby is in optimal position. So I didn't leave anything to chance. We prepared boxes with things that we might need for the birth. We burnt the cord afterwards with candles as a little ceremony for our family, which was beautiful…

We are actually the most responsible parents (laughs) and the most informed people you can probably find… And we planned it. **Michaela**

So I read this book,… and my [independent midwife for previous birth] midwife in [town], she translated it… even if your birth is not going as you may expect it to, or it's complicated, or there are reasons why things aren't happening as you expect, your body is actually able to deal with that and cope with that. And can do things, if it's in a natural enough environment, if you can be connected instinctively to things. Which I think you wouldn't be able to, if you were in hospital. **Cathy S**

Our decision was not made lightly and in preparation we read the few books that were available at the time: *Childbirth without Fear* by the wonderful Grantly Dick-Read who was the first person to look into the fear-pain-tension vicious circle which impeded good birthing and *Spiritual Midwifery* by Ina May Gaskin which provided us with plenty of practical information. We also used our farm bible *Herbal Handbook for Farm and Stable* by Juliette de Bairacli Levy and prepared herbs for eventualities such as haemorrhage and retained placenta. **Caroline B**

Towards the end of my pregnancy, a friend loaned me the book *Freebirth - Self-Directed Pregnancy and Birth* by Sarah Schmid. The book really resonated with me. I read stories of women who liked their midwives but confidently planned to birth without them. I identified with the stories of 'half planned' freebirthers who had a quiet secret confidence. I liked the positive 'we'll call them if we need them' attitude. The women weren't choosing freebirth because they lacked a supportive midwife who they knew and trusted and who would follow their 'birth plan', they HAD this, and STILL chose to give birth without a midwife. That was exactly how **I** felt! **Virginia**

A few women spoke of learning from NHS health practitioners but this was not easy.

What I did to prepare included asking a lot of questions with the NHS, because there was an assumption, when I went to appointments and when I was offered a service, that I needed to take that service. And so, having M [doula]'s support and talking to my partner and just remembering that I have a choice was what empowered me to feel confident to go against the recommendation of the NHS and follow through with my decision to freebirth. My questions weren't always welcome. Especially with people who hadn't met me before... I did have to ask a lot of questions. I'm not sure I would have been given all that information had I not done so…[freebirth] wasn't given to me as a choice in the beginning. My choices seemed to be; how long I stayed at home before going into hospital. Not if I would go in, but when. There was an assumption that I couldn't have a home birth anymore because that service wasn't available. Rather than respecting my choice to stay at home to birth my baby and helping to prepare me for that. I felt judged by other NHS staff members, as though they saw me as irresponsible and flippant. And that I was putting myself and my baby at risk. I had to ask outright, "What happens if I don't go into hospital? What happens if I choose to stay at home and there's no midwife there? And no midwife can come to me." And then it was, "Well that's your choice. But here are the dangers." **Emma**

Some women spoke of how their learning and unlearning developed with successive pregnancies.

During A's [first baby] birth I wasn't sure at all what to expect and I was intent on following the guidance of all my hypnobirthing readings. I see this now as largely a hindrance because it kept me from really listening to what my body wanted to do. Despite an overall positive birth, there was so much I didn't know. And so much I did, that I had to unlearn. I had no desire at all to use hypnobirthing techniques with E [second baby]. I enjoyed the Ujjayi breath we did in yoga, and how it centred me and brought me always back to my baby. Having refused monitoring, I was unsure how far along I was, or what stage I was in. This was a complete blessing. This felt like a good kind of uncertainty. I didn't know, but my body did. **Kendal**

I was very nervous about the freebirth but also I felt liberated, as this was a choice I had made. I had read a couple of books on home birth and a book on freebirth and chatted to a friend who'd freebirthed before which all helped to improve my knowledge on what the body is capable of and the power of the female body during childbirth. This enabled me to develop faith in myself and my body and understand the process of what happens in childbirth. For example; what is expected and what may be signs something different needs to happen, or when something might be wrong. I used my first birth to guide me with this, remembering how when I first felt the pain of the contractions I became very frightened because I thought it meant there was something wrong, when actually the pain is a really natural part of the process. It helped me to surrender to that knowledge and trust myself. Also, remembering that during my first birth when I reached a point towards the end of the birth when despair arose and I felt that I couldn't do it anymore, that that's quite normal too which I didn't know until afterwards. Those kinds of things helped prepare me for this time. And so T [partner] and I had actually planned, "Okay, what about that point when I think I need to give up, but I don't actually want to go into hospital but I may be saying get me there, because I'll feel like I want to give up." I did some exercises to help me become more present with my body and understanding what my body's cues were. For example, learning how to know when something was wrong or if it was actually just fear and no reason to panic. **Emma**

Many women hired birth pools and other equipment as part of their preparation.

I'd hired a birth stool... I really liked that. And I had my ball, and I had the TENS machine which I started to use which was very helpful for a period. **Darelle**

Some women made particular preparations. ME is a herbalist.

I prepped a whole herbal protocol, all these different bottles of tinctures on it for my husband to use with my doula in case, you know. "If contractions are weak, give me some drops of this. If we need to get things relaxed a bit more, give me some drops of this. If there's lots of bleeding, give me some drops of this." So that was all prepped. **ME**

So I bought this extremely peculiar instrument, but I do attribute this... the success of the birth partly to that. The E… have you ever heard of it?... Yes, it's a good, it's hilarious, it's a balloon with a pump, a hand pump on it. And you basically insert it, insert it where the baby's meant to come out and pump it up gradually. And the first night I did it, I could only get to about two centimetres. And then over two weeks, the last few weeks and you can only use it in week thirty-eight because then you've got the hormones in your system that will allow you to stretch so far. And it can be damaging if you use it earlier. So, by the end of these few weeks, I was up to ten centimetres, without really struggling with it at all, so I was very confident about the birth. **Rose**

Most of the women also booked with the NHS so there was a backup plan in case of problems. A few booked with an independent midwife.

And I was planning a freebirth, got an independent midwife, decided to opt out of the whole NHS system because I found it so stressful in my last pregnancy and my second... She [IM] is absolutely lovely, she's brilliant. I would have been really happy to have her at my birth so that's the thing that's so frustrating about all this [problems with insurance for IMs] **Darelle**

A few women carried out checks that midwives would usually do.

I monitored my blood pressure, probably not as much as I should have, but every two or three weeks. And then in the last few weeks of pregnancy I ordered those urine strips and would occasionally dip my urine in there, just to check there was no protein. **Jocelyn**

Once they started preparing to freebirth, many women found themselves part of a learning community (see chapter 8), sometimes locally and sometimes online which was especially important during the Covid pandemic.

… and then religiously, religiously every night I just listened to these links she [J, hypnobirthing practitioner] sent me, and I would be doing these exercises, and I just shut off from everything, and I'd do it. And, and then in the last week or two weeks before the birth we started having Facetime chats with J again. **Katuš**

I found an online freebirth community in which I became and remain active. It is a wonderfully complex and diverse population. **Melissa**

"I joined S's freebirth course in a group as her home birth group helped me have a lovely hands off high risk home birth with my first, six weeks before the first lockdown. Knowing that my second would be a Covid baby and with the confidence I gained through my first birth, I was keen to do what I could to prepare for any eventuality, including the withdrawal or lack of staff to support a home birth. I knew from previous experience S's groups provide really grounded, good, knowledge based information and the freebirth group hasn't disappointed. It had given me the space to consider what I really want from this birth and how hands off I want it to be. It has also reassured me that I know what to look out for in terms of complications and that I can trust my body. Freebirth wasn't something I was aware of prior to the pandemic and being a part of S's Home Birth Support Group UK, if I had been aware, I may have been more confident in choosing a full freebirth instead of it being a plan B option. I am now, thanks in a large part to the group, looking forward to my birth. I feel knowledgeable, powerful and informed thanks to this group." **Lexi,** quoted by **S**, doula

As part of their preparation, some trained as doulas and learned from births they attended as doulas, and many learned from their doulas.

So when I went pregnant with O, I found out the doula training. And then I was like, "Oh, that is what I need in my birth – a doula, or someone that really supports me and that I really could meet before birth." And I did the training… and then I got really into birth stuff. And I really got informed. And then I came up with the freebirth as well. And it was like, "Oh, people that really get informed and that really feel secure about themselves and about birth and that really think that they can do it." In my other birth… I nearly did it all by myself. Because I didn't feel support. Nobody make nothing for me – I did nearly everything. And then finally to take me to hospital without being needed. So I worked really… read more about freebirth and that was in my head… And then between U's birth and O's birth, I was supporting women as a doula. So I supported, I think, two or three births. So I was really feeling confident with my own body and my own pregnancy… And I was really happy with it… And I really was feeling that I could do it. **Bea**

By this point, I'd also done doula training myself. So I felt I had a great network of other doulas, of people that I could speak to as well. **Katy B**

I remember a birth I was at [as a doula] in Harrogate. And I was with two midwives and the woman was walking around the pool a lot. She kept bringing this leg like this. And I was like, "I don't know what she's doing." And the midwives are, "Hm." And then when the baby was born, he had massive shoulders. And they said she was doing this, she was just naturally doing this movement to help get the shoulders round the uterine canal. And I was like, "That's amazing. She didn't know to do that; she was just doing that instinctively." And I really got the feeling that, even if my birth was not going to be a standard one, and everything was going to take longer, it didn't matter, because my body would still know what to do. And I thought that was... probably what helped me make the decision to go ahead without midwives and doctors. Because I thought, "If things are going wrong, you need the help of doctors and midwives to get it back on track." And I really felt, "Actually no. You've still got it. You can still do it, even if it's not going the way you think it's going to." **Cathy S**

I just learnt so much from D [doula], there was so much that I didn't know about birth, that I didn't know that I didn't know... and from the PPC.. then the active birth workshop, it was amazing, absolutely amazing. So I'd been on a hypno-birthing course, there was a relaxing breath birthing [course, in previous pregnancy], with F, so I thought, "Oh I know about birth." And a lot of the information had been really useful, but it just wasn't as much information as I got from the active birth workshop. So the different stages, what to expect at different stages and the diagrams of the physiology of what happens and knowing about the placenta delivery, loads of things that it missed, D captured with the active birth workshop. And as my doula. So there was absolutely loads to learn. And about the positions for giving birth and about how it's better to tear than to be cut and also that that's rare, that that doesn't need to happen, and I just thought that was... most women tear, but actually it doesn't need to happen, if you don't, if you do it in the right way. And I didn't tear, I just got a tiny graze, which was amazing. **Rosalie**

A doula who works with women who freebirth, stressed the importance of preparation and the time it takes.

It's all in the preparation and I think actually, that's where the work is to be done here... I just say the more, the sooner that you start unlearning this narrative of medical birth, and the sooner you start to get to know your body, the more likely you are to have the undisturbed birth that you want. And to think that women think they can do this at three months, or six months, is a little bit unrealistic and I think that's really setting people up for failure. And maybe that's why, you know, we [most antenatal education] don't do birth education before this time, because they want you to fail... So, yes, it's really wonderful to see pre-conception women coming. And then I sometimes have birth workers coming who just want to learn more about freebirth and undisturbed birth and, yes, I've had women from all over the world come -Australia, America, South America, all over Europe. It's a really mixed bunch and birth, birth is birth, isn't it, and that's the wonderful thing about this, you can teach, it's global and it's just human. **SK**, doula

Though their preparation for freebirthing differed, all the other women we spoke with had planned and prepared for their freebirth. They were upset if people outside the freebirthing community assumed that this was not the case.

I'm amazed that people believe that women are making these choices not consciously, not without research. I can see why people are getting angry, but it just seems to really not have any trust in the intelligence of women. That we'd be like, Oh I don't need that stuff," just on a whim… And I think it's partially to do with people's own experiences and they have to believe a certain story because of what happened to them, or happened to them when they were born and if you pull that rug from underneath them, then their whole belief system has gone, so they get really angry. **Lacey**

Freebirth is such a unique and little understood choice that is unfortunately frequently vilified. I do not believe that freebirth is a choice for everyone and it is something that I worked towards, rather than made hard, fast decisions about but I think it is crucial to stress that my choices were born out of positivity, a deep understanding of myself and intelligent reasoning. **Melissa**

Their preparation and the degree of responsibility they took for their births contributed to the unwillingness of many to discuss their plans with those they saw as unsympathetic to freebirthing.

Chapter 5: Letting go of fear and control: building confidence and taking responsibility

Facing their fear and working to let go of it was really important for many women. Some women worked on inner fears that had come from their experiences of life and how birth is managed.

Well, when I got pregnant… I'd been doing a lot of work on myself… inner work for quite a while before I got pregnant. And I had already related my birth to certain ways of being in me that I had to spend a lot of time unwinding. I was induced as a baby and they got the dates wrong… And I was aware of this tendency in my life, where everything's going fine and then suddenly I'm in kind of fight or flight panic. "Oh, I've got to be there…" And I thought, "God, that reminds me…" in a way I've been patterned into, "It's all fine, it's all fine. And it's suddenly not fine and this feeling of being suddenly pushed." Like I've got to, this kind of fight, flight energy coming on line. And just from doing inner work… I don't know how I came across books on how your birth affects you. But I was like, "Wow."… I'm not going to be induced… I really want to understand what's going on here, and why do these inductions happen. Are they necessary? What's going on?" Because I want to be fully informed. And what I noticed, not just from speaking to some friends… and a friend of mine, who ended up having a caesarean and various things, there's so much fear… And I thought, "Well I don't want this fear to come at me, without me being fully informed." And so I'd started, by researching and looking and this, and then the Unassisted Births book fell in my lap somehow. I read that, and it really spoke to me. And I was like, "Wow, you know, I can… that feels totally right to me." And… I did a lot of work on my fears. Because I was like, "God, actually you know, it is scary." **Rachel**

I'd had a horrific first birth, and ended up in hospital, and had three days of just, I was just totally violated, and it was completely out of my control, and that was my first child. So, I had a lot of fear. It was only through really working on, on getting rid of that fear, that I was able to have a freebirth… and I went to a hypnobirthing, and, and I knew I would be fine. I knew it would be fine, and I just thought, "I'm not letting that fear in."… I met J, the hypnobirthing website midwife, and all that fear I just had to work to get out of me. And I had a lot of fear from the first birth, I had fear from all kinds of things in my life and history that I hadn't realised was sat there, having an impact on me, me and my decisions… self-hypnosis was so, so powerful… it did seem it was all about preparation. When you're prepared for something, it's so much easier, isn't it, when you're fully prepared. And so, things like Somatics and hypnobirthing, and just being healthy always made sense to me, and exercise, and a really relaxed body. I think sexuality as well. **Katuš**

Many women spoke of fear induced by health professionals.

As soon as they [midwives] were there [at her home birth with her first baby], there was fear about everything. So, "We're concerned about this. And we're concerned about that." You know the list of risks that they throw at you. When they turned up at my first birth, they were quite full on… They never asked me whether I felt something was wrong. At least, I don't remember that. They were just telling me how they felt all the time. "So we feel like this is going on. And we feel like that is going on." **Carmen**

Some women found the fear induced by midwives linked with other fears in their past. Naomi's description includes the insight of her work as a psychotherapist and shows how routine monitoring, with all its implications of risk, can trigger old fears and defence mechanisms which could not help towards the birth they sought and might even jeopardise it.

My heart sank to meet her: she barely made eye contact with me for the first five minutes of the visit, choosing instead to communicate with my notes on her computer. I had gone to the check-up keen to be palpated, and she agreed, so I hopped up on the bed and she had a feel around.

Before I knew it, she'd whipped out her measuring band and measured my bump, something I absolutely would not have consented to had she asked. (What would they do with the information they found? What recommendations would their findings lead them to make? What conversations would it mean I would have to have with them?). She swiftly wrote down her findings in my notes, and, before I knew what was happening, she was applying cold gel to my belly and pressing in the hard, cold probe of a doppler. The room filled with the muffled, static sound of my baby's heartbeat, and I froze. K [partner] knew this wasn't something I wanted to be happening (the last midwife who'd tried it had admitted it "makes the baby jump"). He said "what is that? A doppler? Do you want that, honey?" His firm voice helped me unfreeze. "No, I don't." "Oh, I thought you wanted it" said A [midwife] I was very tense when I got to my feet, adrenaline pumping. It was a noticeable change of state from my norm in later pregnancy - calm, soft, feminine and flowing. This is when I met a new part of me for the first time, a part I now call my "Fawner." As a systemic psychotherapist by profession, I think in terms of parts of a whole system. Through my experiences with the NHS maternity services, I was to meet this part of myself several times and always in moments of fear. She is a powerful protector and always acts quickly. When the pressure of the moment with A had passed and I was alone at home, I asked my Fawner about her role. "To befriend the scary ones, the ones in charge, the ones with the most power in the room. To make them like me and think I'm a good girl. That way they won't hurt me." "When did you learn to do this?" I ask my Fawner part. "Age four, first year primary school," came the instant reply, "With Mrs. Jones, who shocked or scared the children she considered bad and rewarded the ones she liked." "You're very skilled in your role", I tell my Fawner part. I could see and feel that this part had been doing her role for ever such a long time, protecting a shocked, scared young part of me. No wonder she was so skilled at it. I sent my Fawner some admiration and appreciation for all her hard work through the years. That midwife and even K had had no idea how shaken and vulnerable I'd felt. Thanks to the Fawner, I had smiled gracefully as I laced up my boots, and nodded politely, wide eyed and unruffled as she explained the nature of the home assessment she'd arranged to make. It had taken all day for my adrenaline-levels to fall and to regain the soft pregnancy bliss that had become my equilibrium. I was spooked by how automatically and efficiently my Fawner had stepped in to blend with me when danger of being overpowered was sensed. Because of my work, I knew that I had to reclaim my honest outrage and sense of agency. To do this I would need to help my Fawner to relax, so that I could own my "No" despite any socially awkwardness that might result. **Naomi**

Many women saw midwives as disempowered by the system within which they worked (see chapter 10). Some were aware of midwives' fears and expectations of compliance, resulting from the maternity services approach centred on risk and routine. This approach did not suit these women who sought to take responsibility for themselves.

All of her communication was about covering her own back. It was always, "Well if the baby's breech, then you'll have to go in to a consultant and you won't be allowed to have a home birth." And I was very much of this like, "Nobody's going to tell me allowed or not allowed. This is my body." **ME**

Some of my friends, I suppose they think, "Oh you're mad. Oh, you're mad. Do they let you?" And this is a big thing too where people say, "Are they going to let you do that? How long will they let you go over? How did you manage that? Did you get..." And then I'm like, this care is only offered to people. None of this is mandatory. They don't own us, where we have to be dragged into a hospital or like this is, it's our decisions to make. **Holly**

Separating themselves from other people's fears was seen as necessary to create the safe space in which to work on their own fears. Having supportive people with whom to work through fears was important, as Katuš found with her hypnobirthing teacher (see above). Their partner helped some women achieve this.

I think for me, pregnancy was hugely about facing fears, because so many things would arise, especially because we decided, as a partnership – F and I together – to go this route of having a freebirth, that we told very few people. We only told people who would be 100% supportive… I didn't talk to anyone who would put their concerns or their fear on me… And I found that really helpful, in just staying protected and then being able to work through my own fears. I think so much of being able to do it for me was facing the fears that I had about birthing and about my preconceived notions of what birth was, and then unpacking all of those societal ideas that weren't necessarily mine, but I'd absorbed them. So it was really work through those and I think that was such a monumental part of me being able to, in the end, do it on my own and feel empowered to do it on my own. **Lacey**, freebirth of first baby

A relationship of trust made a vital difference. Many women spoke of working to build their trust in themselves and their own bodies. Similarly they needed a supporter whom they could

trust and who trusted them and their ability to give birth.

So, when I became pregnant with A, which was a fair few years later, I knew that I needed to do a lot of work on getting rid of those demons, of removing that fear that I was definitely holding around birth, and the trauma of what I'd been through and holding that inside me – the lack of belief I felt I had in my body to… go into labour and birth a baby myself. And so I got a doula, and she helped me go through birth debriefing around what I'd previously been through. And with my partner, who was a different partner to H's Dad. And so for him, it was the first time as well. And he was great at just sort of going, "Well, you tell me what you need." **Katy B**

The kind of emotional support that I found really valuable at the time was the support that you can only get from somebody who is being really positive and I think a lot of the things I got from the midwives were quite subtle things which would undermine my confidence slightly or give me the impression that all might not be well, which they have to prepare you for. **Sarah-Anne**

Building a support network was seen as important preparation for freebirth by many women: friends who shared their approach to birth enabled them to move from fear to self confidence. Feeling safe enough to let go in labour was seen as vital.

I really feel like I worked really hard psychologically at that point, that pregnancy, to remove those fears, to really start to believe in my body, and that I could, I could do it. And I had a wonderful Mother Blessing, where all of my female friends came together. And I really felt a sense of release and letting go once that Mother Blessing had happened, that I was ready. It was really nice. And I was in a completely different mind state for this pregnancy compared to the previous one. I didn't feel like it was so much of an unknown. I knew many more people who'd both had children and were involved in birth as well. And I went along to a home birth group, and I listened to a number of different birth stories. And that was really helpful, because they were not only stories where people had birthed at home, but ones where they'd transferred to hospital, too. And it was starting to help me realise that, if that did happen, that would be okay, if that needed to happen. And I looked round the hospital where I'd birthed my first child, and there was a lot of improvements that had been made to it, so it felt like a different place. So those fears of knowing, like the what-ifs, that was good to be like, "Okay, I'm not going be completely against hospital, if that ends up being a place that I may end up having to go," then that was an option. **Katy B**

Nobody can ask a Mum during the birth to fight for what she wants. You have to allow her to go into birth, and to allow herself to let go. And if a Mum during birth has to fight – things are not going to happen. Because you're in your mind, not in your body. And that is what happened to me the first time, that I was in my mind. I had to be attending to the midwife and to my partner and I was never allowed to be inside my body. And second time, I was just inside my body without having to attend to anybody. And things just happened in a few hours… because I allowed my body to do what it was doing: being sick, having to go to the toilet all the time, nearly at the same time. But it was, ah, free, and the feeling of dancing if I wanted or, or using my ball or lying on the couch. It was how it should be, I think, yes. Because a Mum at birth cannot be fighting. People here have to protect that. **Bea**

Hearing other women's positive birth experiences helped many women see what was possible and this helped to dissolve fear. Positive birth stories made a real difference and were found online as well as from local friends.

I was really, really, really afraid and scared and so I read loads and loads of birth stories and that just gave me so much inspiration and it was being like nourished by these stories and I read a lot of stories of women having vaginal births after caesareans and I built up quite a good picture and listening to my intuition and I really wanted the birth to be intuitive.

… So I just really fuelled myself up with birth stories and that just really inspired me and speaking to women who had had home births and how amazing they were and really getting a sense of the pleasure and the joy of the experience rather than them bombarding with kind of buts, what ifs, what ifs, what could go wrong and I just really started to trust myself but I still felt very scared and I could not speak to the midwife about my feelings at that point, but I didn't want to go into hospital, I just felt that would be the most scary thing.

I surrounded myself with women who trusted the process of women's bodies being able to do it and just being inspired by that. It really, really inspired me and I think that's where, I think when you're pregnant you can really tune into yourself a lot more than normal times, so I really tuned in to what I believed to be true and what I believed was right for me. **Polly**

Other women were helped by pictures and videos.

Perhaps the most profoundly confidence-inducing and educational input we received were the videos and photos shared with us by B. These were of women she had looked after going through the process of birthing their babies. I'm so grateful for all the women I watched give birth for allowing their experiences of birth to be witnessed by me. Looking back, I feel that these images and videos were far more effective in helping me prepare in body and mind for giving birth confidently than anything that was shown to us during the NCT course, or the one we attended run by a midwife at our local hospital. **Naomi**

Many women experienced a gradual process of putting into place the knowledge, support and confidence they needed for their birth.

I had that big freebirth book and, and I started listening to freebirth podcasts and I signed up to a freebirth antenatal course that you could do online, which I never actually, I paid for it and I never actually did it (laughs). Because I found once I became pregnant, I was much less keen on the idea of freebirthing because I felt suddenly quite vulnerable. And my background is actually fairly medical because I'm also a vet. So I have a very strong respect and an understanding of medicine and emergency situations, and things. So when I became pregnant, I sort of put away the thought of having a freebirth. I didn't want to do that because I thought it was reckless or the fear overtook me. So, but it had always been in the back of my mind and when I met my doula, B [retired midwife], for the first time, I just felt so comfortable with her. What I'd thought to myself was, the ideal situation is to have like... you sort of, read, well, in America more, you hear about these sort of like elder midwives or traditional midwives that have lots and lots of experience, but they're not medical as such. But they know a lot about birth and have seen a lot of births. And I, so in the back of my head, I thought, oh, that would just be the ideal situation... **Katie H**

They were also very aware that trusting the process of birth and their body's ability to birth involved letting go of control as well as fear.

There's a really wonderful American doula, she gives this little free download, a pamphlet, it's your birth intentions. So I basically did this three page work book and that was it. But you write your birth plan and that is your instructions about your physical care in labour and birth and that's great, you'll need that. And then your birth intentions was about the emotional side of birth... and it asks some really tough questions, like, "How do you want to feel in birth?" As you birth how do you actually want to feel? And I just want to feel powerful, I want to feel overwhelmed, it should overwhelm me. Like, I've grown a person and I'm birthing them. It should be completely overwhelming and that's not something to shy away from. And things like, what are three character traits that you have that will serve you well in birth. And so that gives you that confidence of - actually, I can do this, I'm educated, these are my things that are just going to allow me to do this. That was really wonderful, and then you come out with this statement at the end... and it prompted you that I want, I trust, I will, I know, I am. So my birth plan was, I want a birth in love and power surrounded by my family. I trust my body, I trust N [partner], I trust my intuition, Mother Nature, and S [doula]. I will meet birth with love, good humour and I will surrender to the sensations and the process. I know I am capable of bringing my baby into the world safely. I am willing, I am willing to surrender control, I am willing to surrender expectations, I am willing to experience birth undisturbed and I am willing to dance with fear and pain. That was mine, that's it, that's my birth plan. **Jocelyn**

In these last weeks, I felt K and I were educating ourselves, and that the effect was that any previous fears we had had of the unknown or of an unmanageable type of pain or intensity was dissolving. I felt K trusted me and my intuition entirely, and that he stood by me in what I wanted no matter what. We felt to me like fellow adventurers about to embark on something which required trust and courage that was growing inside us both now. I spent my days during those final "overdue" weeks of pregnancy at home with K and Mum, and I felt safe. **Naomi**

"Tuning in" to their body and their baby helped many women.

Once I'd decided that I was freebirthing, I got her, "my birthing woman," to record me my own track, that had my imagery in it and things that felt really important. Like when I was picturing my birth. And that was really helpful... I don't think I managed to do it every day, but every couple of days I'd go and do some relaxation and just really tune in to my baby. And she felt very wise, this baby. She felt very calm and I'd walk the dog and just try and listen to her. And try and become a team with her. I didn't know she was a girl at the time. But just really tune in to this person, who knew how to be born. I knew, I trusted implicitly she knew what she was doing. And that it was my noisy, thinky brain that was going to get in the way of that. **Beth**

Some saw their preparation for letting go and trusting as part of their preparation for being a mother.

Birth as a natural, physiological process, as well as a potential spiritual experience - an initiation rite. The powerful love of motherhood through the power of facing physical intensity and surrendering with courage… and certainly something to be allowed to unfold naturally with as much safety, privacy and dignity, and as little intervention and interference as possible. **Naomi**

What I need to work on is my willingness to experience, to dance with pain, to experience discomfort and be open to it. To just really submit myself to the process and just understand that, birth has to break you, it has to break your ego to remake you as a mother of two children, of three children, of four children, every time. You have to have that ego dissolution and that feeling. When I'd have my moments of being a bit scared about, am I really freebirthing, is this a good idea, am I being stupid? That's just a sign that I love my baby, not that it's a stupid idea. Of course I'm always thinking, "is this the right thing for her, is this the best thing for her?" And it's just a feeling and I just need to sit with it and if it never went away, well maybe I'll go and get some medical checks because it's telling me something. Occasionally… and so often it would come to me in the shower, I'd kind of look at my belly and just ask "should I be taking all the checks?", because there's the idea of like, it's better safe than sorry. And well, women aren't safe and they are coming out of the system very, very sorry (laughs). **Jocelyn**

A number of women continued learning about and opening up to the processes of birth in order to help others.

I feel women are so disparaged, discouraged, unsupported in society as a whole, that no wonder we don't believe that our bodies work. We're told every day when we look at the media, "You're too fat. You're too thin." You know, the gaze that is upon us all the time is a critical one. And so when it comes to something like growing a healthy baby and giving birth in a way that is both positive in mind and body to baby and mother – it's no wonder people doubt themselves even subconsciously. So I feel like a lot of the work that I've done throughout my pregnancies has been trying to clear a lot of that away.

Which is why the idea of having another baby appeals, because it's like, I just want to keep doing this work. I can keep doing it and supporting other people, and that's wonderful. **Katy B**

When I hear some of my friends' stories and go, "Oh no, I had to be induced, they had to take me in. And then they told me I needed this. And then they told me I needed that." But I'm thinking, "Oh my God." Sometimes I'd be thinking, "What you probably really needed was a change in position. Or another few days until your baby was ready." But I wouldn't even mind, I feel like I sometimes am inspired to go down the route of birth rights and maybe doula or something like that as well. Because just the stories. **Holly**

SK, a doula working with women with freebirth, spoke of her journey to freebirth as a doula being similar to that of the women we spoke to who had freebirthed. She stressed the importance of preparation.

It really varies depending on the woman and where she's at, some women just need a couple of sessions about what they're afraid of. And we talk things through and there's the usual: oh what if the cord's wrapped around the neck or what if this happens or what if there's bleeding after the birth. And are any of those actual pathologies, have those been created by the medical model to make you feel like you can't give birth? And when we actually talk more about it then they come to their own conclusions. I will say, "you think about this, and do your recommended reading and come to your own conclusions." And, that's a thing, women aren't trusted to make their own decisions, they're just told that someone else knows what's best for them. And when they're given that it's just really, one, surprising and two, powerful for them to, to just be - oh well I'm taking responsibility here and instead of handing it over to a midwife.

And I think there's a whole thing around responsibility and what's happening is people are just getting mixed up, aren't they. The doctors take on responsibility, the midwives take on responsibility, but is the Mum taking responsibility? And once they realise, oh, I'm taking full responsibility for this, and that's actually a really good thing, then that is enough. And then also we have quite a big conversation around death and what does it mean and what risks are they okay with, because risk is such a personal thing. In the UK the NHS will have their version of risk, but is the Mum actually okay with a different level of risk? Because they'll say "oh, you've got cholestasis so you have to be induced at thirty-eight weeks or thirty-seven weeks" or whatever they decide is best. But the woman might say, "Oh I'm happy with the risk of waiting to forty weeks", or forty-two weeks, or whatever, and it's the same with induction and... And why is it that the risk of the NHS is what is the accepted risk? And what are we trying to avoid is this death scenario, mother or baby dying which is the ultimate fear. But this can happen anywhere, in hospital or at home, or without a medic or with a medic present. And how is it to acknowledge that and how would it be for that to happen; because I think that is something I see in women birthing in hospital, they just think because they're birthing in hospital nothing can ever happen. And sadly, loss still happens, death still happens in the hospital and then they're completely unprepared for that scenario. And just how we can walk out the door every day and die, that can happen.

And when families accept that scenario, that whole fear piece about death can really go away. Or there's some acceptance around what the risks are. So you're birthing in hospital, and these are the risks, the cascade of intervention, caesarean, being separated from your baby, versus a small percentage chance of death by birthing at home. And what feels better to you, and of course some parents will say, "Oh I'd rather choose the cascade of interventions" and that's their decision to make. But let them make that decision for themselves instead of being penned into this scenario…

I offer… one to one sessions and then depending on what they need, ideally I have a programme that's eight sessions long and we go through all the sort of typical things that come up. And the idea is that if you do the eight sessions you'll be fully prepared for your birth power. And then I turn that into an eight week online course, with a group of women and then it's also the fact that then they're with like-minded women. And instead of being with women who are afraid and your standard NCT class where they're just priming you for intervention, they're not teaching you how to have physiological birth, they're teaching you whether you have an epidural or not, or what forceps means… just teaching you about medical birth, really, aren't they? They're not teaching you about natural birth. It's been really effective to see, doing the programme but then having like-minded women to support you. And sometimes they're second and third time, fourth time Mums, some of them have had previous home births, some of them have had previous hospital births, some of them have birth trauma, some of them are brand-new first time Mums. They just have so much to learn from each other, which is really wonderful to hear.

…there's a whole range of women from those birthing in hospital, those freebirthing, those who've given birth before, those who are new to this. Yes, people of different ages, I also have women who aren't pregnant yet, who are wanting to learn it for the future. I just say the more, the sooner that you start unlearning this narrative of medical birth, and the sooner you start to get to know your body, the more likely you are to have the undisturbed birth that you want. I've been preparing for my birth for over five years and it's taken me this long to get here. **SK**

While taking responsibility was implicit in many of the women's stories, others talked about it explicitly. They had all thought a lot about responsibility in the context of birth and wanted to take responsibility themselves rather than hand over responsibility to the maternity services or individual professionals within the services. In talking about reducing fear and increasing knowledge, confidence and trust, the idea about taking responsibility was woven through what they told us. Some were very clear about the importance of this.

When people ask, "But weren't you afraid?", they are projecting their own fears and baggage. Their fears are not my fears. The other issue to address with this and many other questions surrounding freebirth is the matter of responsibility. We are in a world where the people in the white coats hold all the knowledge and we are expected to automatically hand over responsibility for outcomes, our autonomy, dignity, and mental health in return for being told how things will happen, having things done to us, and being treated as incompetent, silly children. All in the name of "A healthy baby is all that matters." It's apparently a rather radical notion that women can know their own bodies and minds, and can even retain autonomy and responsibility when they become pregnant. We have this funny thing in our society where the moment a woman becomes pregnant she is seen as incapable of making a rational choice. Suddenly she is the enemy to her unborn baby and we must be mistrusting of her motives and abilities. This sounds like a massive over-generalisation, but if you think about it for a minute you realise that it is everywhere - every time someone says "Gosh you're brave" about home birth, gives you a funny look or the third degree if you decline a scan or blood test, or pulls the dead baby card, they are questioning your ability to make a rational decision simply because you have a baby inside of you. We're somehow selfish for making choices that may not be the norm, when really, how many women do you think make choices about their pregnancy or birth with anything other than their own and their baby's very best interests foremost? No one loves my baby more than me. I would, as most mothers, die for my children if I had to. No one knows a baby better than its mother, and no one knows a woman or her body better than she knows herself. The problem is the systemic undermining of this knowledge and our ability to apply it to our decision making.

So no, I am not afraid that freebirth will lead to death. I am aware that death can occur, just as in any other thing we may choose to do. The difference is that I have retained full responsibility for myself, just as I do so in any other situation. I do not need someone to save me from my own body and I do not need to hand responsibility over to someone with a uniform. I am comfortable with that. Plus, has anyone asked a woman choosing to birth in a hospital if she is afraid of dying because of her choice of birthplace? **Claire**

One of the things that I'm really interested in is what do we do with the information when we gather it? [from antenatal screening and monitoring] Or what are we interested in finding out? So that's what I asked myself. I was like, okay, what information, what's the likelihood that I'm going to get information that's going to really help? What's the likelihood I'll get information that's going to send me in a circle back to I'm fine in the end? If I did find out, would I change the course of this pregnancy? So I just really asked myself those questions. And then I really tuned into my own body. I think a lot of the time your body will express if there is an issue. And so I trusted that. I really trust that, and I think it requires a level of tuning in and mindfulness. You can't just pass your responsibility off to someone else to tell you that you're fine or a machine to tell you that you're fine. You actually pay attention and tell yourself or listen to your baby… And also with things like ultrasound scans, there's a lot of radiation. There's all sorts of things that aren't monitored, even more so in the last… you think it would be getting better now but

I think it's actually getting less — what's the word? — governed, in a sense. Those are the things that I'm thinking about. There were times when I thought maybe I'll go get a scan. And then I was like, okay, why am I thinking that? Is there a reason? Has my body told me? Am I freaking out? Where is this coming from? And so, whenever I started to feel like I wanted to interact with the system, I would really enquire, like what's the reason? And most of the time, I was just going back into that fear place, or also, I had to say to myself, whatever happens, this is my responsibility. I am choosing this course for my life and for my baby and my family, and you have to be willing to take that kind of responsibility. I think most people aren't in a lot of [situations], let alone in birth, because if anything happens, you are responsible. So yes, those were the kind of questions that I asked myself. And... I don't believe that the technology is inherently wrong; I just believe that it's irresponsibly used. It's being used in such a systematic way instead of being, okay, you're super healthy, you've no signs of... you're great, you don't need this. Maybe you need this — you know? Instead of just this blanket approach,... So, I think it's just making autonomous choices actually based on the reality of our unique situations. **Lacey**

Section 3: Relationships around Freebirth

Birth is about relationships. It takes place within a web of relationships and is greatly influenced by them. As a new baby is born, new relationships are created and there is a wide impact on surrounding relationships. Assumptions embedded in these relationships were revealed as the women planned and experienced their freebirths. This was especially clear where the medicalised basis of maternity services was seen as the right or only approach to birth; this view was a place of safety for many professionals and some family members. This created tensions for mothers who did not feel safe with this approach. They often withdrew from or avoided such relationships and sometimes plans were altered where the woman's partner wanted a professional to attend the birth and take responsibility for it.

Relationships take time to develop to a level where there is mutual trust and some of the women in this book would have appreciated being able to get to know and trust a midwife and might have considered having her attend their births. This is why continuity of midwifery carer makes such a difference, but this is rarely available in the NHS. Many women sought the support of friends they knew and trusted. They also developed relationships with like minded women and together they built a mutually sustaining network of relationships.

Relationships with doulas were developed as pregnancy progressed. Some trained as doulas and were doulas for each other. This was seen by many women as a crucially important relationship from which they drew knowledge, security and strength. For some women, doulas were a source of reassurance and support for their partners more than for them.

Many women relied on their partners, some of whom were particualrly positive and supportibve of their plans to freebirth, and during labour and birth. When this happened, the women felt that they and their partner created a strong team and bond where the woman felt safe and protected. Some partners and family members became increasingly supportive as they witnessed the benefits of planning and having a freebirth. Some women found their mothers or other close relatives to be a great comfort and support to them.

The network of relationships that surrounded the women could be a source of support, sustanance and nurturing before, during and after the birth.

Relationships with midwives, however, proved to be complex and often unsatisfactory as women and midwives attempted to navigate a rigid system based on routines that could not easily respond to women's individual circumstances, decisions and needs. The women removed themselves from these difficult relationships that they often felt introduced stress, fear and negativity. Where midwives were found to be supportive, this was greatly appreciated by the women.

Chapter 6: Partners

Some women had the complete support of their partners in planning their freebirth and during labour.

My husband was on board and he would have never said anything against it, because it's my body and it's so clear to him… It's so obvious; it's my body, of course, I make my decisions about it. So he was fully supportive. **ST**

I felt completely encircled by his belief and care. **Melissa**

We decided, as a partnership – F and I together – to go this route of having a freebirth. **Lacey**

I talked a lot with my partner T, who is incredibly supportive, and together we made a loose plan that would empower me, give me choice but also help me to feel safe. **Emma**

My husband K was a hugely supportive influence. He took in positive and empowering films and books with me, such as *Birth in Focus*, *Birth Story* with Ina May, and *Orgasmic Birth*. I felt we were both educating ourselves. I felt he trusted me and my intuition entirely, and that he stood by me no matter what. I spent my days [in late pregnancy] with K and Mum and I felt safe. **Naomi**

And then we got pregnant. We had already also been on the same mindset of doing things as God intended, being natural, and we would listen to different educational podcast talks and stuff. And there was a lot that we already knew, but there was a lot that we also would learn from those different podcasts. And it just became something… it was great to have each other because we both supported that outlook. **Nicole**

Some women described how the support of their partner enabled them to let go and labour.

Allowing your body to do what it needs is truly moving and I know that I was able to fully give into the natural process because I was in a calm protected environment that my husband created. **Sarah M**

My pregnancy ran its course with no cause for concern and when labour began it progressed as had been typical for all of my previous experiences. Active labour and birth occurred in the early hours whilst my other children were in bed. My surroundings were all as planned, my partner was confident and supportive of my birth plan, he remained close, calm and attentive, patiently tending to any request. I trusted my body to guide me wholeheartedly, I was filled with and surrounded by love and the whole process could not have been more peaceful or joyful. **J**

One of the reasons that I chose freebirth in the first place, was because I just know that I need space, and I need, and I only need somebody that I can absolutely trust to not come into that space and, and birth… I just need to be able to get on with it, because I knew that I could, I could do that. **Leonie**, whose husband was the only other person present for her three freebirths

K was everything I would have wanted a man to be - supportive, trusting, humble, respectful and 100% there for me. I may have set some important boundaries, but he firmly held them for me when I didn't have the strength or courage available to me. His presence meant that I could rest into the process and let it take me over. I couldn't have asked for a better birth partner. I feel the trust and intimacy between us has deepened through the experience of giving birth to our beloved C. I feel that through this process he has become more the man he is, and me more the woman. Thank you, K. **Naomi**

I really believed that having a massive heart-to-heart with G, my partner, the night before helped me go into labour. I really felt a strong sense of letting go. I talked to him about how I was really scared of what was going to happen. That was, mostly my fear was around how was I going to cope with three children on my own? How was I going to cope with having a baby? Just, I didn't know. And I talked to him about all of this, and I cried. And he really listened. And I felt really listened to by him for the first time in a long time. And then that night, my mucous plug went, and it was just like, whoof, it was happening. And... I feel that those things are so interlinked. **Katy B,** separated from her partner

… the other most important thing for me about deciding to freebirth and most especially when the emergency arose, was having a fully supportive partner by my side. He never once questioned my instincts/intuition, my abilities or my knowledge, he had faith in me on every level and fundamentally that allowed me to fully relax and feel held and empowered, I never had to explain or verify or second guess, because he trusted in me and it gave me the strength to make the decisions I did throughout my pregnancy, labour and the emergency situation of the birth itself. **Lunar**

For a few women their partner was able to protect them from midwifery services which they found intrusive and threatening.

As soon as the door closed behind her [community midwife], I turned to K [partner] and admitted my anxiety and despair. I said point blank, jaw clenched, that I had no interest in induction, and that I no longer trusted her and certainly had no trust in her assessment of our baby's weight or her prediction that he or she would struggle with a normal physiological labour. I recalled something Ina May Gaskin is want to say: "Your body is not a lemon." K quickly came to clarity and suggested that he call her and let her know not to come back unless we asked her to. We had already agreed that from now on he would act as my guardian of oxytocin and that this role entailed keeping everything that stressed me out or got my adrenaline going out of my space by quickly fielding it. So, from then on we didn't have any further midwife appointments. They did call me though, three further times, using different numbers, which led me to answer the phone to find out who it was. Each time, I told them it wasn't a good time, so that K would call them back and found out what they wanted. Each time, they were wanting to check to see if I was sure I didn't want to consider the interventions or monitoring they were suggesting. K ended up saying very firmly, "I don't think you're hearing what we're saying. We do not want this and we don't want to have this conversation again." After repeating this message with ranging degrees of firmness, to both the community midwife and her supervisor, they finally got the message and for the final week and a half of my pregnancy I had no communication with the NHS whatsoever. This was a true blessing and allowed me to be in a state of calmness, openness, and trust. **Naomi**

I think with O and with M, both those births, A [partner] was very, completely confused, didn't know what was going on and very stressed... but with the baby, with C he was really, I could hear him advocating for me like he's saying what I wanted and things like that. And he was really good actually, really calm, and (laughs) you know. So that was great,... even once we got to hospital… I was really happy to have had that…A, he could just focus on doing whatever I want him to or just, you know, trying to... It was better, it was definitely better. **Darelle**

You know we talk about the pregnancy partner and the birth partner, but also the postpartum partner, somebody who supports you. You need an advocate during the postpartum especially those really early days, and so he did all of that, and he [partner] discharged us, basically, because I just didn't want to see anybody. We didn't see any need. **Leonie**

A few women saw labour and birth as an intimate experience to be shared with their partner.

I've read a couple of birth stories about the way people are, sort of having sex while they're in labour, and that kind of thing. But it's not something that's generally talked about. I don't know how they deal with it in hospitals or anything like that, you know, because it actually just makes perfect sense, like, whether you're having sex or just being sexual or whatever it is, just like the whole thing of, of foreplay, and it's just all good isn't it, it's all going to work, lubricate the passage, going to get that baby out. I just feel there's a part of that education for women that isn't obvious. It should be obviously there, and it, and you have to dig for it, and you shouldn't have to dig for that, I don't think.

And maybe that's why, like, I would feel prudish about having somebody there at birth, because I wouldn't want to share my sexuality with someone just randomly there. Just, even if they were looking the other way, I'd feel a bit, it would make me inhibited, but that's just me. I'm probably just a little bit prudish with…all that, so, I quite like things just to be very personal. **Katuš**

Some women spoke of their partner's needs and doulas helped with this (see chapter 9).

It helped to have such amazing support from my doula and my partner. It was reassuring for my partner to have M [doula] there too. T had shared that he felt a big sense of responsibility, to protect me or take care of me if something went wrong. And because it wasn't his body, it was mine, he felt quite helpless at times. So having M there was a real support for both of us. **Emma**

Some women stressed the need for their partner to feel safe and this involved some compromises for them.

And I was feeling that I really wanted to be special. But it was all in my head, and I was telling people, and my partner, what they wanted to hear. But I was planning what… I really wanted. And then I spoke with N [doula]. And if she was going to be free. And she told me that she had more births, but she was going to be at mine if I needed and if I wanted. And then for my partner to feel more safe, I told the NHS midwife that I was planning a home birth and that I was going to call them. Just for F [partner] to have the birth box at home and for him to feel safe. But I knew that I was going not to call them. **Bea**

My husband was a bit anxious about being responsible, so we decided to have a doula present. So my friend H, who lives in the next village, she's just ten minutes away, she said she would be there. So that lifted D's [husband] anxieties because… I think he was confident in my ability to do it, but he wasn't familiar enough with the birth process that he would know if something wasn't going well or know when we should call for help if help was needed. So he was happy that H was there so that she could just keep an eye on things if anything started going wrong, that she would know that it wasn't normal. **Elena**

… my partner and I had difficulties, because I was very sure that I trusted just knowing I could do it on my own. And he found that quite difficult because he doesn't necessarily have the same outlook as me… in relation to mistrusting the medical wisdom. And I think for him, it was still quite strong this foundation of safety being through the professionals. That the midwives know what they're doing, and that we needed… like he wanted to have a midwife present during most of the pregnancy.

… friend of mine, S, she was a support for us… I think it was actually related to that, having S there was just that bit more reassurance, so my partner W would feel comfortable with us making that choice of not phoning the midwife. **Gauri**

But just two minutes before [baby] came out, I went away from the room from the others and went to the bath tub and overheard [partner] saying to C, "this is not working out, we should call somebody" and you know I just thought "this is quite scary for them" and I thought "this is okay for me because I know she's coming out now" but I hadn't said a word to them. Compared to the first one, I was in a lot of pain, I was just so unrelaxed – it was just excruciatingly painful the two minutes before she was born. I just fell into [partner's] arms and he lifted me up and C caught J [baby], and that was it. I thought "we haven't called the midwives but it's okay." **M**

I was maybe a little bit offhand with L [partner], because he was keen to have a professional, you know, in a professional capacity there. And I think… H's very professional in terms of her doula status, because she will say, "I am not going be here to tell you what to do. I'm going to support the decisions and I'm going to… help you make informed choices. But I am not going to say to you - she needs to go to hospital or you need to do this or… And I'm going to be taking all of my kind of feedback really from how Cathy's doing." So this was a bit scary for L, and I think we went back and forth quite a lot on when are we going to phone the midwives, are we going to phone the midwives. And I was a bit like, "Do you know what, I don't feel I'll need to phone the midwives. But if at some point during the birth you need to phone the midwives, just going to leave that up to you. If you feel you need them, okay." And then, as we got closer to the birth, L was like, "Do you know what, I'm just going trust you. This is your area of expertise in terms of your career [as a doula], what you've done in the past. I know that you trust H. If you feel that you can trust yourself, then I should trust you too." Great. **Cathy S**, second birth, first freebirth

Talking about her third birth and second freebirth, Cathy went on to say.

L had said he did not want to have that experience again without having a midwife. Because obviously, the first time it had been really enjoyable for him. Because he felt no onus of responsibility. Because D [independent midwife] took all that on. And then the second time, he felt this massive onus of responsibility, because H [doula] made it very clear that she was not responsible for me. And really she was just helping. But you know, so I think when L was looking at D the first time around, he looked... she was like, "It's okay." And I think when he looked at H, she was just like, "I don't know what's happening." And I think it really scared L. So he didn't enjoy C's birth at all. And it was just really scary for him, really stressful. So when we were pregnant with F, he was like, "I do not want H. I just want to have D."... I talked to L and I said, "I know last time was not as you wanted it. But we can't get D. I really don't want an NHS midwife there." I reminded him of what the NHS midwife had said when we had C. And said, "Can you imagine," he said it was stressful, "Can you imagine how much more stressful that would have been if we'd gone down the NHS route? If we hadn't freebirthed, it would have been much worse. And the outcome would have been very different." So he agreed, and said, "Okay, we'll get H on board. But if we do feel we need to phone, we will phone." I was, "Yes, yes, we'll phone if we need to phone." I think we all knew there wasn't going to be any phoning. **Cathy S,** third birth, second freebirth

Katuš was more determined despite her partner's resistance.

… he was so resistant. I really, I just insisted, I was just like, "Well, this is what's happening." You know, this is it, I'm having it, I'm having this baby, and it was no longer, like, I didn't feel like I have to say, "Oh, darling, we're having this baby" anymore, because I wasn't having that any more. It was like, "No, this is what I need to do."… And because he, we had that session together, he understood, he couldn't… he understood what it was about… I didn't give him a choice, he just had to kind of go with it… I was about to have this baby, and so, he did just go with it. And if he hadn't gone with it, we wouldn't have had that birth, because we had to be in a state of total equilibrium, and he had to be totally giving to me, and give in, and I had to just be able to give in and trust. And so, it was with her [hypnobirthing teacher] help that I, we could all do that, you know, there was this whole… although she wasn't there, I think we last spoke to her on the day or two days before the birth. She facilitated, she allowed that to happen basically. And she gave him the sort of confidence and, and a role, I suppose. It was like a really clear role. **Katuš**

The dynamic between couples during labour varied and often changed as labour progressed.

So my partner, husband at the time, was around. But my body waited to go into labour when he went back to work, funnily. I did tell him that morning at five o'clock, because I was up pretty spritely having porridge, which at five o'clock in the morning wasn't really my thing, that it does feel like things are starting, but it's slow. I could feel sort of rumblings every twenty minutes. I said, "You know, nothing's going to happen quick, so just go to work and I'll let you know." **Hannah**

Like in that early part as well, my partner couldn't even really... I mean, he would come in and I... at one point I think I asked him not to, just for him to leave. It just felt like it was a distraction to have a lot of eye connection with him. Felt like I couldn't touch him. And I was just very in my own still... And although at the very beginning I said to him that I wanted to be more on my own... As it got stronger and stronger, he was just listening... just was there. Kind of holding the space for me in a way, rather than doing too much. A little like knowing he was there. **Gauri**

Throughout this transition, I had been sending text messages to D [husband downstairs], checking that he and O [child] were alright. D visited the bedroom a couple of times. He held me, swayed with me, offered me reassurance and encouragement. I could feel his enthusiasm and excitement, knowing the arrival of our baby was under way. **Melissa**

I breathed through each pain, no real rest in-between, looking into my husband's eyes. He kept me so focused, he kept me grounded and he was the quiet strong presence I needed. Once again just us in the room that's the heart of the home, bringing our last child into the world. One hour six minutes of the most intense but calming pain. I gave into each surge, I didn't fight it, I let it be. I looked into my partner's eyes, I breathed, I closed my eyes and visioned my baby coming down the birth canal. I embraced her crowning and I watched my partner as he watched her emerge. Once again he instinctively knew what I needed and brought I [baby] earthside onto my chest. **Sarah M**

At one point my contractions stalled, about an hour or two hours in... And then there was a kind of block in me and it was some fear was coming up. And I asked my husband to come and we just talked. After the first birth I had slight depression because I felt so alone with it. My baby had tongue tie and I did breastfeed her for three years, but it was so, so painful in the beginning and very difficult and I felt so lonely. And it impacted hugely on our relationship: between my husband and me. And I was just scared it might... just lack of sleep and everything and if I had breastfeeding difficulties again, I'd have a hard time again in our relationship. And we just talked through it, and he was just wonderful as he is. Just really listened, and he is a psychotherapist. He was only training then, but still he really listened. And I knew we could get through this again,... we got through it before and we knew we could ask for help. And then as soon as we talked about this, contractions just came back, strong and regular. And that was really good learning that emotional fear can actually have such a big impact on the body. And then it went very smoothly. **ST**

Mothers were very aware of the impact of the birth on their partner

Then her head came. And he... ecstatic... he was like, "I have our baby's head in my hand!" I'll never forget that moment and him saying that. And also just the sheer pride and also that Christmas magic feeling. He was just so in awe. And he caught her head and I just stood up and I just caught her body. She just came right out, like this big slippery fish. She came right out and I sat right back down on the toilet. Her cord was really short so I couldn't really lift her up so I kind of put her between my legs but she kept trying to slide into the toilet! And we were laughing – F was like, "My baby's not going in the toilet!", trying to catch her. **Lacey**

And I remember at one point opening my eyes, and I had A [friend] there. And A was like sobbing, she had all these tears. And I remember looking at her... she cries at everything. But she was holding my hand. And I really thought, "Gosh. If this is what it's like for you watching me here, it must be really hard for L [partner]." It was the first time I really had any appreciation that, if it's affecting you this way, and she looked really, really upset watching me…

He [baby] seemed non-responsive; he was sleepy, and this scared L [partner]. Because even on the video, he's a bit like, "Is he all right? Is he all right?" And I'm like, "No, he's fine." He was fine, but he was just slow coming round, because I think it had just been a bit of a shock towards the end. But there was no big cry – it took a while for there to be, and L was like, "He's not making any noise." And I only know all this because it's on a video which I've watched. So that's why I remember it from the video...

But afterwards, I remember a few days later saying to L, like, "Oh yes, I remember seeing A and her being so upset and thinking wow, this must be difficult for L." And it was like I'd invited like the dam opening – he just went, "Oh my God, when you give birth it's just awful. It's the most stressful time ever. I just wonder are you going to die, is the baby going to die. It's just awful. I never, ever want you to have another baby without having a midwife there. It's just awful." And although for me, it's obviously a completely different experience... well we talked about having a fourth, until we'd had three. And I think probably a fourth is probably not in our future now. But we agreed at the time that, if we were to have a fourth child, we actually wouldn't freebirth the fourth child. We would make sure that an independent midwife would be able to support us with a package of care that would suit us and not a full package of care. Because L said, "I just can't take the stress." He's like late forties, you know. "I can't take the stress of having all that... I can't have the faith and the confidence in the process like you can."… So I've said, "Yes, okay, if we did get pregnant again, we did have a fourth child, we'd definitely make sure that it would be with a midwife, for his sake." Because I don't think he would be able to do it any other way. **Cathy S**

And I think as well from my partner, he was very amazed that he was actually there and he was the one that was able to bring her out and I think that has been an amazing thing for him as well, for his confidence. **Polly**

A's [partner] always delighted that he was the first person to hold A [baby] and pass him to me. **Lindsay**

And I love to hear K's perception of it, because he always said to me, "Christina, you always wanted a home birth, but then you went from a home birth, to having a birth with absolutely no midwives." Like he couldn't really… he was a bit nervous, do you know what I mean. Even though he wouldn't… K is really cool as a cucumber sort of guy – doesn't really get too excited much or anything like that. But for him, when you ask him how it impacted him, he just goes, "Oh my God, amazing." He said, "If that's the way she wants to birth the rest of the babies, that's the way we'll do it." Because he loved it, he really did. And he's seen how different it was from the hospital to the home. And he just, he said it was far, far better as well, you know. **Christina**

For at least one woman, her partner's support during labour when she felt at her most vulnerable enabled her to birth her baby at home following a long labour with her first baby, rather than transferring to hospital.

But yes, it ended up during those times where it was really intensifying, I was starting to get nervous… I felt like my body should have moved along quicker. And I was getting concerned that he was stuck. And I was just like, "Oh my God, should I…?" And I was feeling so much and I was really drained and everything, and I told my partner, I said, "I'm scared. I need some help." I was like, I don't know what to do here. I'm really starting to get concerned. And he was so amazing. This is another thing I think that men… you know, partners… men and women, that men can sometimes freak out too. They get nervous, like, "Okay, she said needs help. We're going to go and do this" right. And they forget that they're actually taking away that power, that innate power of adult women and also their own innate power as being the masculine counterpart, right. And so my partner was so awesome, he was just like, "That's not what we want. You can do this. And you know that if you end up going that route, they're going to do things that you're not going to like. Once they've got you in, they're going to cut you open and that's not what we want to do." And I was like, "You're right, you're right." And so I just kept on remembering that. And he was so solid with me and so, he was my rock at my weakest point. I had never thought that I would experience that kind of weakness and… because I'm a strong woman and I know my body and… and I've gone through so many different things in my life, both athletically and mentally, emotionally, you know, all these things. And I was just like, "I can't believe I'm coming to this idea that I need help. But I'm freaked out." **Nicole**

We did not seek partners' views, but Michaela's partner was present during the interview and contributed his thoughts.

It was a very massive experience for me. An unforgettable one… just like she said, we were on holiday and then she gives me this book to read on unassisted birthing. So I had to read about the history of women giving birth without medical intervention, and then there were sections about medical interventions. And of course, we had the meetings with the midwives and everything. But the thing is, having Michaela as a partner inspires that confidence. What she wanted to do, she was very confident about it, and somehow I got that confidence from her. I remember I told my Mum what she was planning, and she was like, "oh my God, she must be crazy!"… But we were prepared.

… when she went into labour about 5am that morning, basically I was just like a robot. I just walked out of the room, went and got the birthing pool, pumped it up and we'd already bought the 26 metre hose so just tried, got it into the shower head and filled up the bathtub, put in the thermometer, got it to the body temperature, 37.5 or thereabout. And then put down the blinds and put on meditation music from YouTube on the TV and put it very low, just the conditions she wanted. So she came in and went into the pool. At some point I found I had nothing else to do. That's why I went to wash the dishes (laughs) from the night before. Yes. And then eventually she just said to me, "Come behind me." And then I came behind her and then I could hear her speaking to the baby, tell the baby to take it easy, tell the baby to turn around… She was just talking to the baby at that point. And I was just near to them and I saw the baby drop into the water. I was frozen! I couldn't do anything. She actually told me, "Pick her up!" And then I picked her up and saw the cord around her neck, and I'm like, "She's got the cord around her neck!" And she just calmly told me, "Just take it off"… she was a bit flopping at the time, and then Michaela just took her from me and blew into her nose and then she blinked and looked around… Yes, and the thing is, we spoke to K all the while, like in the belly, you know. I played with K lots. Most times when I came back from work I might speak to her. She would actually push out on one part of Michaela's belly. So when Michaela eventually blew into her face, it just clicked, and I just started calling her the same names I used to call her in the belly. You could see she seemed to – oh, I've heard this voice before! And so she didn't cry, and it's been like that all through.

She is the happiest baby I've ever seen (laughs). **Michaela's partner**

Yeah. So we had a really good experience and it was a family experience. **Michaela**

Chapter 7: Family and freebirth

Many women were reluctant to discuss freebirth with family members or any of those close to them who did not share their views on birth.

I didn't really talk to my parents about it. I didn't talk to anyone who would put their concerns or their fear on me… And I found that really helpful, in just staying protected and then being able to work through my own fears. **Lacey**, first baby

I remember having a few heated discussions around midwives and with my family, and with my partner's family a little bit. And not being shy about how I felt about things. But I tend to get really quite emotional and I just hated this feeling of pressure. It was so hard to get my message across to people, when they're so set in these ideas about what's safe and what isn't. Who knows best, you know, like I found it so hard people telling me that midwives knew so much better about my body than I did… it would really trigger me, it really would. I'd get really quite emotional. And in some ways, I think I had quite a strong fear. My biggest fear was related to unnecessary intervention, and the medical system taking control and taking over. **Gauri**

I tried to talk to my mother. I thought she might comfort me and then I realised no, she has never been a comfort to me – that was being delusional… I didn't tell many people at all… my boyfriend's parents were more pushy and they were upset by me not getting in touch with the midwives when they found out that I was pregnant and then insisted and put pressure on to me to go and get a scan, so that's how they [midwives] found out.

[After the birth] It was very hard for K [partner]. His family was very square and really hard on him and his Mum and Dad came and they just walked out. They came in and saw that I wasn't dressed enough, you know and just walked out. They just told him it was all terribly wrong that I wasn't in hospital and I wasn't doing it properly you know. My family are all far away so it was all sort of distant and very superficial. **Moggie**

The second home birth was loads better. It was all planned. I'd got more idea of informed choice. I wanted to freebirth that time but for the concerns of my husband, my Mum and my family. **Laura**

For some women it was important to have their mother with them - it was assumed that they would be present and that this would be a positive experience for the family.

It was just so beautiful, it was absolutely amazing. And that's something that you would never be able to achieve in the hospital, having the family, and everybody who I love was there, my Mammy, and that was something that I really wanted to do and show my Mammy, and for my Mammy to be a part of. It just really meant something for me to have my Mum there. **Christina**

Some families had mixed responses.

… the only other sort of difficulty that we've come into contact with is when we originally told people, like family and friends of our intentions to freebirth in the first place. And that was very mixed, so, some of our family members were right there really onboard and totally got it, from, well, from before we even mentioned it really. But some of the family members were really scared, like, "Why are you going to kill your child, not having a midwife there equals death." And it was a very interesting process to work through that together really, so it helped that I'm working in this world as well now, so, through all of my knowledge I can share it with our family, they've got the picture now, now that we've done it three times. They just say, "All right, that's just what you guys do, that's your thing, I get it now." And we've not proved them wrong, because it's not about that, but we've been able to show more and more our reasons for doing that, but we were met with some mixed things, yes. So, like I say, my in-laws, all of their children were born by caesarean… And they just couldn't see why you'd possibly do something different. But slowly, slowly over the years, I think everybody came round and…people have been sharing stuff. So yes, positive. **Leonie**

My Granny… my Granny was having a heart attack to be fair, that there was no midwives going to be attending. And I kept saying to her, "Granny, people in your days or just before you, or your Mammy would have had all their births at home with nobody." But she was just maybe a wee bit old school and… kept finding out about the things that could go wrong during birth and stuff. And it would get like she was… she didn't want to know when I was in labour or anything, because she would have been worried sick. But like my family all along have been pretty positive and complimentary. **Holly**

Some family members gave their full support from the outset, and this was important for the women.

I knew I needed my husband and my Mum. That's my birth team. They've been there for all of them. And I knew that the three of us together are the whole; I couldn't do it with only one of them there. You know, they each give me different things when I'm in labour… We had as a family decided that we were happy freebirthing. **Beth**

… my Mum's been really supportive, my Dad was frightened, I think, a bit, he didn't say much but… he tried to… he was sort of with me in trying to get midwives who would share my point of view and he was very frustrated by the fact that they wouldn't… he just phoned them up and wrote letters and things… and my partner was supportive of me as well… and most of my friends were supportive as well. So I felt very well supported by other people. So I didn't feel I needed the midwives there really. **Charlie**

And when my sister said she was coming, I felt like this, "Ah, great, she's coming." I'd really wanted her there, and I was able to get on with it. So there was partly a feeling of: "This is great. I've got someone coming who's going to look after me." But also: "Oh, my sister's coming. She probably doesn't have very long. I'd better have this baby quite soon." **Katy B**

For those who already had children, the impact of the pregnancy and birth on the children was important.

I loved my wild pregnancy, it was the least stressful of all my experiences, time usually spent attending appointments was reassigned to personal learning often shared with the other children…

Taking personal responsibility allowed the development of a stronger than usual family bond, the children had been able to play an integral role, they were increasingly knowledgeable and excited to greet their newborn sibling. I felt completely in tune with my body and baby, filled with love, and confidence all eventuality had been planned for. **J**

… our son was here and it was just… good… He was a bit bored (laughs). He wanted to watch a fairy tale on the tablet, so he went into another room and said, "Just call me when the baby's born." **Michaela**

It was lovely for my toddler being here too. Like I think it's nice to normalise this [birth], you know, for them as well. So he was up and down and jumping off the pool and stuff before I got in. And he was a welcome distraction at times. **Holly**

T [son] was wonderful to me, it was just so good that he was there and you know he jumped in the bath as soon as she was born. He was just glowing with pride and he is always so proud of her and it has just been wonderful that he was there and that he was involved and very, very connected. They have trouble not being together which is tricky because they have got two different Dads but they are just so great… that was just the best part of it that T was there for his sister and I think it has given him a broader understanding of getting on with other people too, it's not just his sister, just a better understanding that we are spiritual beings and it's been really good for him. I think being at the birth, I think it's really good to do that. I mean I have often heard him like saying that "birth is like worse than dying" you know to other people and I've thought "Oh dear" but I don't know, maybe it is in some cases, there's some truth to it. **Moggie**

I felt connected with him [baby] throughout the whole pregnancy. I had no scans over that pregnancy. Everything just felt very easy and normal and kind of, "Kids, what did you do in your Easter holidays?" "Well, we were there when my Mummy had a baby." It was lovely and it was lovely for them to be there when he was born and actually, of my children, he's the one that's a little bit of a terror, so I think for bonding-wise, it's probably quite good that they were there when he was born (laughs). **Hannah**

And I wanted my daughters to be there as well at the birth. So that was quite a big part of the decision, I suppose, because it was really important for them, for their own journey as women, when they come to have their own children, to know that birth is normal and not something to be afraid of. I wanted them to see it as peacefully and gently as possible, without it being a medical event. So I decided it would be better if there weren't lots of people with plastic gloves and aprons on and… yes, I didn't want it to be like that. I wanted them to see it in as raw and natural a form as possible. So it was actually quite a party, the birth, because my Mum had come over to stay with us and she was responsible for looking after the girls, and then my husband was going to catch the baby and put up the birth pool – that was his job. H [doula] was there just to keep a watchful eye and do the placenta smoothie afterwards **Elena**

Elena's story contains her two daughters' accounts of the birth as they were present during the recording.

N Could F and L tell me their stories?

Elena Do you want to do that, girls? Would you tell Nadine your story of R's birth?

Nadine Would you? Can we tape it? Is that all right?

Elena Yes. I'm sure they'd love to.

Nadine Why don't you come and sit here so that you're closer to it [recorder]? Tell me about his birth.

F Well it was quite funny, because when Granny came to pick us up, she'd usually pick us up for violin, and she'd just got back from Canada, so maybe she'd mistaken the time. I thought she'd maybe mistaken the time and I was thinking, "Violin this early?" And I was asking Granny what was up, and she was like, "You'll see." And I was like, "Is the baby being born?" and she didn't say anything! So we came home. It was really nice and dark in the room because they'd put blankets over the windows and the door. It was a nice blue, calm light. It felt really nice. Mum had the TENS machine on and we got changed, and we got some colouring and some cushions in the corner and a blanket, expecting it to be a bit longer. Dad was there filling the birth pool. It was a quite nice feeling, being there. I was rubbing Mummy's back and stroking her hair. Then when she got into the birth pool, I was there with a cold cloth, even though I got it in her eyes! (Laughs).

Elena You were a little bit vigorous to start off with! You got the hang of it very quickly.

F Yes. I went out of the room to go to the toilet, even though there was the toilet in Mum and Dad's room, but I went out to go to the toilet, and Granny thought I'd heard the door,... and then Granny came running up behind me, "Did you hear the door?" I'm like, "No, I'm just going to the toilet." And then we heard Mum roar as she was having the contraction.

Nadine She roared?

F Yes, like a lion (laughs).

Elena I'd been quite quiet for the rest of it, hadn't I, until the very end.

F Yes.

Elena I turned into a lioness.

F Yes, and we heard it so we came running back to the room and his head was out. His eyes were shut and you could see his head – he was facing the ceiling and he was like [demonstrates] with his eyes shut, his mouth opening and shutting under the water, like he was trying to… like a fish. It was quite funny. And then Mum roared again and Dad was in and out and he came out. It was quite special, and Dad caught him and then Mum went over the umbilical cord. And he was just on Mum and he was having a good little cry. It was really nice and he had all this mucousy stuff on him that made him look a bit alien-ish! (Laughs).

L Did it?

F Yes. They were in the birth pool for a little while, and Mum came out and we cleaned up R and Mum and we snipped off the umbilical cord… Mum was waiting for the placenta to come out and she was just standing here with this big silver bowl. And just some blood came out and then five minutes later, the placenta came, and it landed on the edge of the bowl, half of it in, half of it out. There was a plastic sheet on the new cream carpet, all around, just to stop everything getting on the carpet, but there was only a little bit of blood that got on the carpet. It missed the bowl completely and it was like that and it slopped… and blood was going everywhere and everyone was like, "Ahhh! We need to clean all this up!"

Elena How did you feel about seeing all the blood and stuff? Did it make you… scare you or anything?

F No! I found it quite funny that it missed the bowl. Then when Mum was getting all cleaned up in the bath, R was all clean, and he was wrapped up and Dad was holding him in the bed, me and L on either side, and we were singing him songs. It felt very peaceful… It was just really special to be there, seeing him being born. And seeing him grow now, like almost five months, is quite alarming. It seems like time has flown.

But he's been a peaceful and smiley baby. He's been really peaceful. And he doesn't cry very much and he's just really smiley all the time. Sometimes when we come in Mum's feeding him on the couch and he comes off the boob and his face lights up, and like, yay!

L The funny people are home!

Some considered their freebirth from the viewpoint of the baby being born.

Listen to your baby… I really wanted to instil in her a sense of trust. I wanted her to feel that I trusted her timing, I trusted her development, I trusted the course of her life from the beginning and I really believe that that blueprint will stay with her for the rest of her life, being trusted and allowed to take her own time and steer her own course, and then I just get out of the way, just continue to get out of the way. **Lacey**

Kate addressed her freebirth story to her baby, handwritten "for E's baby book." She conveys to the baby that his birth was a joyous family occasion: "the loveliest time."

It all began on the morning of Wednesday Dec sixth your Mummy woke up needing a pee, which she did a lot when pregnant. This time when she got to the bathroom she found her pyjamas were soaking wet. She thought to herself "I don't usually wet myself in the night." So Mummy smelt it and thought "I don't think this smells like pee." Mummy wiped herself and it was pink. That's when she knew that this was it – her waters had broken. Mummy crept back into the bedroom not wanting to wake up Daddy but he already suspected but didn't say anything and we both went back to sleep.

Mummy slept a bit but also had cramps and was very excited thinking about you and what was about to happen. Then put the hypnobirthing on and tried again to sleep.

At 7.00 Mummy couldn't wait any longer and woke up Daddy to tell him. Daddy was smiling and laughing and Mummy was too and they both had a lovely kiss and cuddle.

That morning Mummy and Daddy distracted themselves with doing normal things. Mummy made a big stew in between having little surges. Mummy and Daddy told A and B [two friends who would be supporting Kate and her partner] what had happened in the night. A recommended a nap, so Mummy and Daddy went to bed and listened to the hypnobirthing.

The plumber came unexpectedly and Daddy showed him round the house so he could check the radiators but checked with Mummy before that it was okay for the plumber to come in. The plumber thought Daddy was mad.

Mummy and Daddy had always planned to go for a walk but it would be dark soon, so they wrapped up well and set out into the rising storm. They went down to the Loch, Daddy held [dog]'s lead as Mummy was having surges. It was wild, windy and exciting. We walked round the Loch as far as we could go and on the walk back saw a man out on the Loch windsurfing and Mummy and Daddy were happy and excited and felt so lucky.

Mummy and Daddy got cosy at home and sat down to watch a film. Dad wanted to watch "Almost Famous" but Mum, of course, had the final say and we watched the first half of "Save the Last Dance." Then Mum had a big surge, got very angry at the film and switched it off.

Mum spent the next while doing her birth dance round the flat. She tried lots of different positions round the flat trying to get comfortable: on the ball, against the mantelpiece, on the walls, but you wanted Mum to stand up and wiggle her hips.

Daddy stroked Mummy's back and hummed lots to remind Mum to hum too, which she did. Daddy stayed calm and breathed slowly and deeply to encourage Mum to do the same thing too. He also said encouraging supportive things when Mum thought it was getting too much. Daddy was completely in awe of Mummy and the amazing thing she was doing in giving birth.

The surges were short and close together and we thought it would still be a long time. They called A for advice on how Mummy might get some rest. She recommended a shower and Mummy's surges relaxed and so she got into bed with Daddy to get some sleep and we all listened to hypnobirthing. Mum still had to breathe through surges but managed to have little naps.

A couple of hours later a big surge made Mummy leap out of bed and the sleep time was over and the birth dance began again now with more intensity.

Some hours passed. Mum drank water and ate snacks. All Daddy ate the whole night was two pieces of toast and spread.

We called A again for reassurance, but still felt there was a long way to go.

Mum tried to have another shower but this time the surges stayed intense so she knew things were moving on.

More time passed. More surges. More birth dance. And then something changed. Mummy got quieter, still having surges but her energy was turned in on herself and her breathing calmer. She didn't need Dad's support as much and rested her head on a pillow on the mantelpiece. Dad saw Mummy was coping well and lay down to get a quick nap on the futon on the living room floor next to Mum. Mum kept thinking "It feels lovely. So comfortable and lovely to open." All the time she felt you moving about and it helped to remember we were doing this together.

Something big changed inside Mum. She felt you move down inside her pelvis and a big gush of water came. She knew something different was happening and felt like she needed to push. (This was about 40 minutes before you were born.) Mummy said, "The baby's coming" and Dad leapt up from his nap. Mum told Dad to call A, which he did and A came even though they thought your birth was still likely to be a way off.

Mum went to the toilet, thinking she needed to do a poo. When she sat on the toilet she remembered her [midwifery] training and realised it wasn't a poo but your head. Lucky, for she got off the toilet right away.

Dad started up the birth pool thinking there was still lots of time in between rubbing Mum's back and humming. Mum told him to put towels underneath her because she knew that you were coming soon. Mum was now down on all fours!

Meanwhile A had lost her car keys and she had to wake B to drive her. So both A and B arrived together about 20 minutes before you were born.

When the surges came, Mum could feel you move down and put her hand between her legs and could feel your head.

In between surges, Mum was chatting to A and B. Mum hummed and during one surge wolf howled.

Dad hummed also and stroked Mum's back. B held the space calm and relaxed, meditative.

Then it was your time. Your head came out in one surge then Mum went up on one

[knee] and with the next surge you were out. Mum caught you in her arms, at the same time as saying "I won't be able to catch him." Her next words were "It's a boy" and you did a big wee and started to cry. Mum lay back on some pillows and put you to her chest. Dad cuddled in close and cried a little and we were both truly amazed that you were now here with us. A looked after Mum and a few minutes later your placenta was born.

B wrapped us all in blankets. Then her and A helped the three of us into bed. A and B made food and golden milk and fed Mummy lots of dates. It was the loveliest time. **Kate**

Some women found their family responded positively after their freebirth.

Well, just really amazing – well my Mum was a little bit concerned, like I should go and get the baby checked out as soon as possible, but she was absolutely…, I think she was so proud of me, and then she said family friends had said that they felt it was amazing and I was really strong for doing that, so very positive… It was really, really positive and of course all the women who had known I had gone through this caesarean before and the trauma of it, were just so happy for me and it made the whole transition into motherhood so much more enjoyable. **Polly**

Some did not tell anyone that they freebirthed.

I haven't really told anybody else that when the babies have been born unassisted that was… how it was planned. **C**

Chapter 8: Friends and the freebirth community: holding safe space

A few women spoke of reaching a stage where they could be open about their desire to freebirth with certain friends and/or their freebirth community.

With number four... I had also reached the stage where not only was I 100% ready to take full responsibility for myself, I had the confidence to tell my partner and my friends my plans: no midwives till after the birth. **Caroline S**

Most of these women did not want to engage with friends who would not be sympathetic to their reasons for freebirthing.

I didn't really speak to anybody else and actually I haven't really told anybody else that when the babies have been born unassisted that that was... how it was planned... I've got one really good friend from church and she's kind of aware of that and she knew that I was planning the same for S, but apart from that there isn't really anybody, because I think that people are so... I don't know if people are so judgemental about it or whether they're just so scared of thinking about doing that themselves but they don't understand because people will say, "oh you're having your babies at home that's really brave of you"... well it's not really brave at all... **C**

We told very few people. We only told people who would be 100% supportive. **Lacey**

It's hard speaking positively about it to other women because there is just such a trauma coping mechanism that they do just have to convince themselves that what you did was dangerous and bad... if they don't it might cause them to actually truly reflect on their own experience and realise maybe it didn't have to be like that. **Jocelyn**

Most of the women we spoke with wanted additional support, especially during labour which could include support for their partner. This support, which was seen as coming from wide experience and knowledge of birth, had to be respectful of the mother's autonomy and to protect, and in no way encroach upon, her relationship with and responsiveness to her body and her baby. The phrase "holding the space" or "holding safe space" was often used and others spoke of the desirability of "a wise presence." To ensure appropriate support the mother had to know and trust the supporter.

We asked her to be... supporting us for the birth as well. But just really hands off, just holding the space for us really. Just as an extra, extra person around. I think it was actually related to that, having S there was just that bit more reassurance, so my partner W would feel comfortable with us making that choice of not phoning the midwife. **Gauri,** freebirth of first baby

... during the birth I think it would be nice to have someone who's been at births you know, who's helped women, but not essential I wouldn't say, not unless I felt it. If I did feel that maybe I needed a bit of help then it would be good to know that there was somebody there that I could call... who had that kind of experience, definitely that would be good...but somebody who believes similar beliefs to me about the way the world works. **Charlie**

They were very aware of the impact of another's presence on a labouring woman and some never found the right person to be with them.

I suppose it's nice to have your husband there... obviously because it's his baby as well but... sometimes I think you need to have... maybe... another woman there just because they've been there and they've done that and they're able to look after your kids, or you can say to your husband, "If you look after the kids and then I'll have somebody who's just able to hold your hand and so that you know that you're not... there on your own", cos it is a really... a really lonely experience... having another woman present is always something that I've thought about with the last two really,... or maybe I've just never come across the right person...I think it would just be nice,... even if the person wasn't actually with you, just to know that there's somebody around... that... if you needed somebody that they were there and... there's somebody there that could make you a cup of tea or something because I know after N was born, she was born at just after six o'clock in the morning and we waited a couple of hours before we cut the cord and stuff and we just had that time where I was sat, because I couldn't do anything else because the placenta was still attached and everything, but it was half past eight and I was making cheese on toast for the kids for their breakfast because my husband's not very good at doing that sort of stuff and if I'd had somebody else here that could have maybe helped out and stuff like that it then would make... that time better, I think, but yes... having somebody that you feel like you would like to have and having somebody that you were able to ask who would do it are two different things... I think most women would probably like to have somebody like that. **C**

… having an experienced brain in the room would have been helpful… but the impact that would have had on my nervous system… It was the right decision [to freebirth]. But it's quite interesting to be able to look back and see how "Yes, right, some input would have been helpful" and I think now, if I was to have another baby now, I would certainly have a doula with me… I have good friends who could fulfil that role… and that feels very different to having a stranger… But I had two close friends for baby number one, who were volunteering, who were more than qualified, they would have been… really level headed and really good and it, it still felt too much to have them. **Alice**

Supportive friends were very important for many women.

I choose carefully what and who I surround myself with, especially when I am pregnant. My body listens. Maybe my baby does too. I am no good at building walls. I am not impenetrable, words invade. But when I choose carefully, what flows in is necessary and good. How do you start a birth story when the story is everything that leads up to birth, too? The women who are friends and who share their wisdom easily. The Blessingway they threw me and the words they gave which made their way in. The kindnesses of a rare community. **Kendal**

I have got really amazing friends who are really so supportive within the process. And I think just the more you can get positive stories in you, when you're approaching birthing, it's really so beneficial. And during the birth there were a couple of women advised, and what they told me about their experiences that really came to me, and really helped me. **Gauri**

… having somebody that you didn't know wouldn't help that situation so in the end we decided that we'd leave it, we'd leave phoning the midwife… so I phoned my friend, D, at the time when a lot of people would have decided to call the midwife but I just thought it would be such a nice atmosphere, just to feel you've got someone holding your hand and kind of meet me, and I know that she's gone through it and she knows what I'm going through and I just felt a lot of support from that. **Sarah-Anne**

In some areas there was a site such as the Pregnancy and Parents Centre in Edinburgh, or a local home birth group where they could find supportive, like-minded friends.

I moved from the area I was living in the north of Scotland and came to Edinburgh so I was really much more in contact and able to do a lot more networking as I had been quite isolated before and all the women that I seemed to be meeting were all a large circle of friends knowing each other but a large majority of them had home births and I really saw that they were very relaxed. I could really see the connection between the birth that they had with their child and just the whole relaxed nature and I just felt I had suffered and because of that, my bond with my child as well had been, I could really feel it in my heart, I just knew for sure that there was something, there was a huge connection between being able to give birth in a way that was actually really, really quite good and I was meeting a lot of them then who had home births, and I kept thinking at the back of my mind well I could do that or I definitely wanted to do that but I always at the back of mind thought maybe I can't do that, and that certainly what was reinforced to me when I first went to see my doctor and midwife really…

[During labour]… all the time I had two women's faces beaming at me with just absolute beauty and love and I just felt so beautiful because what was coming from them I had not a single fear of what is happening here, and all I had was their bringing me on and bringing me on, and I just became more and more confident with myself because they were really strong in giving me that and didn't interrupt the process so that at one point I just wanted to tell them how much I was loving it because it was so beautiful what their faces were radiating – I think what they later said was how I actually looked and that makes a lot of sense because… and I just think that is fascinating and I just think it's so magical and maybe part of me would have grasped on to that. I didn't even feel her head coming out, and I was like "well hang on a minute you know I think the little head popped out" so it was smooth you know and there were no interruptions… the support I got was what enabled me to do it. The support was from the women who have experienced home births and expect it to be a pleasurable, enjoyable experience. **Polly**

And I asked a friend as well to be there with me, and she's not a doula, but she was in my women's group. And she was also at my Blessingway that friends had arranged and I felt... so a Blessingway is so much deeper than a baby shower, and I felt deeply, deeply supported the second time round. The first time round I was the first one of my friends who had a child. And I felt really alone with it, even the home birth was a big step for me. But this time round, they had arranged a food drop for a month after the birth... Yes, I knew I was well supported on all levels. So she was there, H, and my husband and another friend came to just play with my daughter in the garden. And so I started contracting, around elevenish in the morning. And I just carried on and I made lunch for everyone. My friend came round for the play date, she played with my daughter and her two girls in the garden. It was August and sunny and my husband came home. It was very calm. I went and rested in the bedroom, did my hypnobirthing and my friend came round, gave me a foot massage. It was so, just like a lovely, normal, beautiful day (laughs). My husband came, set up the pool. And it was going very well. I knew I was dilating easily. **ST**

I had a wonderful Mother Blessing, where all of my female friends came together, and I felt really looked after and celebrated. And we feasted. Someone made a cake with a hole in the middle the size, she said, that my cervix needed to dilate to. It was a very nice cake. I think she was training as a midwife at that point. And one of the most magical moments, actually, was where I was laid down – here, in fact – on the floor, and they all put their hands on me; and it was a real moment, where I felt that all those women were connected and they were there to support me. Another thing that they did was everyone brought some material and one of the women made a quilt, which is a lovely quilt that I was able to have for the baby and future babies. And there was a nice bit of ceremony and ritual about it as well. And I really felt a sense of release and letting go once that Mother Blessing had happened, that I was ready. But, yes, it was really nice. And I was in a completely different mind state for this pregnancy compared to the previous one. I didn't feel like it was so much of an unknown. I knew many more people who'd both had children and were involved in birth as well. And I went along to a home birth group, and I listened to a number of different birth stories. And that was really helpful, because they were not only stories where people had birthed at home, but ones where they'd transferred to hospital, too. And it was starting to help me realise that, if that did happen, that would be okay, if that needed to happen. **Katy B**

For some the situation was more complex as they felt they needed to protect their friends.

... and at the time C and E (friends) were there... but at the time C thought that we had to call a midwife legally, that we were doing something illegal and that was on our minds,... Compared to the first one, I was in a lot of pain, I was just like so unrelaxed – it was just excruciatingly painful the two minutes before she was born. I just fell into [partner's] arms and he lifted me up and C caught J [baby], and that was it. I thought "we haven't called the midwives but it's okay" so it was crazy. A week later when they came to visit and they found that I had had the baby, I told them that I didn't have anybody with me but T [older child] because I was wanting to protect my friends in case it might have been illegal. I was mad to tell them that, to tell them such a lie, it was crazy, I cannot believe I did it, still to this day, this lie was just so hard, it was just so hard and they were asking details about giving birth by myself... but they took it in and they believed me, I could tell that they were believing me. They sent in a Social Worker to make sure that T wasn't traumatised as well. **Moggie**

For the women who were doulas, or who trained as doulas in preparation for freebirthing, the doula community was very supportive. Some were doulas for each other's freebirths.

[In a later pregnancy] I didn't know I was going to have C... because having had the miscarriages before, I became really, gosh, I really need that, I need that emotional support more than anything now... C was in Australia. I did ask her when I first got pregnant, but she was in Australia... But it's actually really lovely her being in Australia because when I was waking in the night, because I had loads of false labour starts, it was her daytime hours, so I would message her on Messenger in the night. It was just lovely being able to talk... Anyway, she got back on the Wednesday and I went into labour on the Sunday, so she'd had a few days to get over her jet lag. And then, yes, we called her out and it was so lovely and I needed her there actually. I needed that woman there. **Hannah**

Many found a supportive community on social media

… social media is amazing because it connects us all. I mean it's annoying as well. It connects us all with these communities of people that have the same type of outlook and thinking around the world. So you've got the FreeBirth Society podcast. And suddenly, these stories are getting more of an audience, a wider audience than they would do normally. I feel that's why I run a home birth support group. It's around normalising home birth. **Katy B**

Throughout my preparation, I found an online freebirth community in which I became and remain active...I have found it to be a very open, supportive, nurturing community which holds space for women from all kinds of spheres and who go on to experience many different birth outcomes. It is a place where personal growth is supported and difficult subjects are questioned and discussed without judgement or prejudice. There are wide ranging reasons why a woman may consider or embark upon freebirthing but I find the difference in the freebirth community, as opposed to more mainstream models of care, is that there is a greater tendency to respect the individual's history and life experiences as a process that has informed their decision making as equal to the evidence or research. It reconciles these two often opposing positions, allowing greater clarity in the decision making process. **Melissa**

And I've heard from, oh you probably know who I mean, the lady who's Welsh in

England that runs the freebirth... Facebook group or something, she's got long, white hair, do you know who I mean? I did a podcast, the active birth podcast... and there was a WhatsApp group created before the birth and people had told me lovely things that they thought about parenting F [older child], which were really nice to hear and just lovely things about myself that were really nice. And then I knew that I had the support afterwards, and I posted some photos in the WhatsApp group afterwards, of the birth and it was just really nice to know that they were my core support group, and they'd all pledged a way to support me. And they all did... **Rosalie**

... she [doula] informed me of When Push Comes To Shove [doula services]...and then through following that group chat that they have on Telegram,... [she found] information, and sometimes I'd see something and then I'd go to that chat, and someone would have asked the same thing. So then I was just learning all about it through people sharing their experiences or their questions and that was really it. **Yony**

The night I had him [24 days after the due date she was given] I was also on Facebook, on social media. My auntie is a midwife and she had told me that she was advising a placental scan to check the blood flow, because obviously she was a midwife and wanted me to take her advice. So I was talking on a group saying, "would anyone do this scan?" and I was weighing up the pros and cons of that, and I booked it in, and I was still like, "I don't know whether to go to this or not," and I still don't know now whether I would have gone or not. But luckily I didn't have to. **Laura**

I remember actually taking like a wee kind of wobble, I don't know where this came from, for about a month when I was pregnant here with this wee man. And having a bit of a wobble, and I was like, "Oh Jesus, what if the cord's born round this baby's neck." And I don't know where this came from, but I just started to think about it for a couple of weeks. And I was like, "Oh, I wonder what happens now." And I remember writing in there, you know, "I really want to home birth, I really want to freebirth, but there's just a niggle in the back of my head and I can't seem to get rid of it." And then I was just straight away, within 20 minutes, half an hour... it was gone. Because people had sent me the articles and stuff where, as long as baby's still attached to the placenta and they're getting skin on skin... and you know, it was a common thing they were sharing, like it's common enough for this to be born... you know, just basically unravel it. And I was really thankful for that time, because literally, within the space of an hour, like I was fine. So I do think like-minded women, yes I did learn a lot from them. **Holly**

S, a doula, described the online community she facilitates:

This is a unique course in a group based on Facebook and has proved extremely popular. I felt it was important to have a safe space for those who wanted to freebirth, with good quality information and signposting to service provider support if needed. It is also a space used by birth workers to enhance their knowledge and engage with those giving birth. It is a very special space, a coming together of those preparing to give birth their way and birth workers and professionals who are prepared to support them unconditionally and without judgement.

"I ended up freebirthing in the end and without the knowledge I gained through the group, I wouldn't have been able to keep such control, creating an extremely empowering and very positive birth. Not only the birth but also after the birth of baby and placenta. I personally feel S's group gave my husband and I the foundations to a positive birth." **Hannah, group member**

Some of those who do the course decide freebirth is not for them, some join for those "just in case situations" and then see birth through a new lens and approach their hands off, no midwife birth, with newly found excitement. Others use the course, which is excellent wherever and however you birth, to inform themselves and as a reference point once their baby is here. It has all the usual benefits of a Facebook group, a place for asking questions and accessing doula facilitated, peer to peer support in a safe held environment. We are approaching 650 members, since the group's conception in April 2020, obviously some have left with the birth of their babies.

We celebrate all our births on my course, those who freebirth and those who do not. That is true, non judgemental support of birth. **S** doula

SK, a doula working with women who choose freebirth, was also clear about the value of social media for building a community as well as in preparation for freebirth.

I mainly work online with women, so I'm mainly doing coaching for women who want to birth on their own so I don't attend that many births, but I've supported a lot of freebirthing families through my coaching and through my online education classes.

… I'm on Instagram and that's, quite I guess a growing alternative field there, conversations that aren't being had in other places… sometimes I'll invite them [women who have freebirthed] to one of my online groups to share their story because other women find that really inspiring. I have Instagram Live so I'll invite them so then the whole community can watch and it's recorded. The thing with Instagram is that you're always in touch in some way, aren't you, like they're watching you or you're watching them and things come up. And so I guess we do keep in touch but not one to one, really. And I have an online mothers group so I invite any of my clients to come to that and we have a community space there that meets every couple of weeks. And it's all alternative, like-minded Mums who, again, are struggling, they can't go to your average play group because they're still breastfeeding their kids at three when no one else is. And they're doing unschooling and all of these things that maybe other people think are strange. So this is actually really a safe space for them to come to and we talk about placenta remedies and attachment parenting and all of those alternatives. **SK**

Chapter 9: Doulas

Over half of the women asked either a doula or a friend, who had previously attended home births, to be with them in labour and birth. A few others had a midwife, doula or knowledgeable friend who they spoke to on the phone during their labour. About a third were doulas themselves and some acted as doulas for each other.

I did have a doula at the time. It was a friend of mine, I was her doula before and she'd made the same decisions as me, she'd wanted to give birth without a midwife there. And it was just me and her there and I knew that she understood me very well and I understood her very well. **Hannah**

And then any and all questions that I had, I would always just speak to my friend about them, the doula. And, yes, she would give me the information or just return me back to myself, she just basically encouraged me to turn to my intuition all the time really. **Yony**

Some trained as doulas after difficult previous births in order to understand birth and to help others and their experiences as doulas were part of their journey towards freebirth. Several trained as doulas in preparation for freebirths (see chapter 4).

… I do the doula thing full time… I think I did it actually, for my own healing and journey. It's really, really helped. **Katie H**

Expectations of the doula varied. All the women saw their doula as offering support but in no way eroding the autonomy of the mother. Some mothers sought only emotional support from their doula.

I had a doula and we employed her quite early on in the pregnancy, maybe after my first scan. We discussed with her our decision to freebirth and she was supportive of that. We also discussed quite carefully the role of the doula and that obviously it wasn't a medical role and that she would be there only for emotional support etc. So we knew that, because we'd invited her into the freebirth setting, we needed to be clear that we understood her role and she knew that we weren't expecting her to be anything other than a doula. **Lindsay**

… in order to fully let go, I need to have nobody else there who is responsible for any decisions. And having a friend who's a doula, she's not responsible for anything, other than being there for me, and that is literally it, just being there and that emotional support and holding that space. Holding my wants and my needs… that's what underpinned my decision-making. **Hannah**

The doula's presence was enough for some women.

And when I was feeling the time of the baby coming, I called N, and I said, "N, I think baby is here, is going to be here soon." And she came. And ten minutes after she came,

O was born... And it was really, really nice. And N was there, but she never did nothing. And after that, after half an hour, something like that, we called the midwives... And everything was perfect.

I think you can feel the support just to have someone sitting on a chair and you just knowing that is there, but not being intrusive, no. **Bea**

Some were reassured by the doula's knowledge and experience of birth, seeing her as a source of emotional support for their partner as well as themselves.

Our doulas were almost supporting my husband more than me, because we go through all the physical stuff, but the guys just sit there in emotional turmoil, completely helpless, they can't do anything. They're just like stranded. So they were explaining things to him. **ME**

So having M there was a real support for both of us. Just knowing she was there in our home. There were a couple of occasions where I really needed that female reassurance too. At one point I felt like I wasn't progressing and M noticed something about the way I was moving in the water and suggested I move my hips in a different way. Within minutes of her direction, my waters had broken, I started pushing and then he came into the world. **Emma**

In some births the doula took an active role, as was Cathy's experience.

Towards the end... I was lying back and I was in the pool, and L [partner] was in the pool. And H [doula] ended up having to be "Cathy", you know, "What's going on with you?" And I think I just expected the birth to be like F's [her first baby] birth – it would just happen to me, and I didn't have to engage. I didn't want to have to engage. Because I just wanted it to be like it had been last time. And it really wasn't. I had to really be proactive, that's the word I can think of... I needed to be proactive in this birth. And H was like, "Do you think that's the best position? You're kind of lying back, you know, do you not want to use a bit of gravity?" And I was just a bit scared to be, to know I had to do something. But she was right; she kind of gave me a talking to, "You know, you've been a while now and why don't you think about having another position…" She was absolutely right. So I did, I stood up and I leaned forward. And obviously, it was much more intense, but that's what we needed. We needed it to start happening. And I needed to really concentrate and not do what would make it more comfortable, but just do what needed to happen... So yes, his head came out… his body just came out and I kept him under the water. I remember L went to touch him, and I went, "Don't touch the baby." He was like, "Okay, I won't touch the baby." And I sat back and his little hand came out of the water first, and then his other hand. And I lifted him up. And I just remember feeling so relieved, "Oh, it's okay." And I put him in my arms. And I was just looking round, going, "Oh, I'm so relieved. Thank goodness he's here." ... And I looked at him, he was like, (gagging sound). And he had like a throat full of stuff. And she was like, "Give him a rub." I was like, "Oh, yes. Give him a rub. Tip him over and give him a rub." And I'd suctioned some of the stuff out of his mouth. But I hadn't even thought to do that, because I was just relieved that he was here and I didn't have to do any of that any more. But he was fine obviously, he took a first shout quite quickly.

I certainly wouldn't like to have doula-ed my birth. But having H there... such faith in H. And she has been to so many births that she's seen... I feel she's seen it all. So if she's not worried, I'm not worried. But then, at the same time, I take her seriously when she challenged me and said, "You know, come on now. You're lying around, you're not really working with this." And I was like, "I didn't have to work with it last time." She was like, "Well, maybe this time you need to start thinking about what to do." **Cathy S**

Some doulas took on "tasks" nearer to those a midwife would undertake. This doula's story could have been told by a midwife, apart from the lack of gloves, until the last lines.

However, at 5am on Monday June 20, you texted and said you thought you might be in labour. You called and immediately had to breathe through a contraction, and you said they are very manageable but coming quite close together, and while I listened you had two more contractions. I told you to lie down again and see if they slowed down, and about 30 minutes later you called back again to describe a large blood loss, and sent photos. While we were talking, you began to vocalise with each contraction, and they seemed to be coming faster, but you were confused because they weren't "painful." Once I heard you begin to moan and told me about the blood, I said I was on my way! While I was driving, you texted about needing to poo, so I really started driving like a maniac to get to you. I was so thankful for that early time of day on a Monday - I made it to your house in a little over 30 minutes when it normally takes one hour.

When I arrived at about 6:50, I found you in the tiny back bedroom draped over a birth ball on inco pads, with naked T [older child] tucked in the corner watching the film Frozen on the computer, and V [partner] kneeling in front of you holding your hands, looking a little bewildered as you were very clearly making pushing sounds. I sat with you to observe, and between pushes you opened your eyes to talk to me and tell me the things you wanted: water, your yellow scarf. You told me to look and see what was happening back there, so I did with your next push and was surprised to see a tiny curl of pure white hair appear and then disappear back in as the push ended. I was not expecting that at all, so I began rushing from room to room. I motioned to your mom to begin assembling the birth pool, half-knowing that it wouldn't be ready in time. I came back in to ask you if you wanted to give birth in this room, because it would happen here unless we moved now. I suggested the bathtub. You said yes, this room was fine, and then you asked me, "Is it normal to not feel pain?" I said, "Yes, it is all normal, you are almost done! Do you want me to call someone?" You replied that you didn't, and if we had called, the baby would have been birthed in confusion while we were yelling on the phone trying to get a midwife here anyway. The pushing urges were coming about every two minutes.

I told V that he would have to catch the baby if you stayed in this position over the birth ball. You said, "No, you do it!" and grabbed his hands even harder. Meanwhile T was making small noises and you were reassuring him, and he seemed satisfied and went back to watching the movie. You quietly said that you were feeling stuck, should you change positions? You sat up on your knees and looked troubled, like you were trying to think of a better position to get into, but a pushing urge came suddenly and you draped back over the birth ball to push. I crawled behind you and put down another inco pad and waited, reassuring you that everything was moving fast and yes it is okay to not feel pain! I thought to take some pictures here and there. With the next push, the baby's head began to crown fully. I made observations - yes, the scalp was pink, yes, it's coming the right way, yes, it's coming smoothly. I decided to narrate – "Okay I see eyebrows, and ears!" and you yelled, "Don't tell me!" and the baby's head emerged to the chin in that one last push. It was 7:42. I waited for the baby's head to start turning to one side, but it didn't. I had my hands poised to catch but didn't touch the baby at all, but suddenly you tensed up and shouted "Don't touch me!" I explained that you were feeling the baby's head there, the head was out. Suddenly another pushing urge came and I was sprayed with amniotic fluid, and the baby's chin came out the rest of the way, but didn't turn and came no further. The baby was pink, turning purple, moving facial muscles. I hoped gravity would help the baby slide out the rest of the way, but then the baby took one gasping breath. Because of that I decided I should act.

I stood up and touched your right leg, and asked you to lift it up and stand on it in a half squat. I am sure that didn't make any sense, so you lifted your leg and kicked it around, looking for a place to put your foot. I helped you plant your foot out as far as it could go, and then another pushing urge came. Surely the baby would come now! But it stayed firmly face up. At this time it had been over two minutes since the baby's head had birthed. You were asking me, "Help me, I feel stuck, what should I do?" I stood up behind you and put my arms under yours, and asked you to stand up, which you did effortlessly and weightlessly. As you leaned into me, I said, "Okay now I'm going to lay you back down like this," and as I did so, you dropped slowly back and gently down so now you were lying flat on the floor, with your head under my bum and me hovering over you, causing my Arabic gold necklace to dangle close to your face. There was just enough room in that tiny space between the wall, the bed, and T for you to lie down. Then I said, "And now I'm going to lift your legs up like this," and took your legs behind the knees and pulled them all the way back to your ears. Meanwhile V had moved the birth ball out of the way and he was perfectly positioned to make the catch. I said, "Now push!" or something like that. This whole sequence of events took about ten seconds, and I looked down and willed this child to please come now, because I had long fingernails and no gloves and I didn't want to have to go in and scratch you and the baby. As I looked down at V with his hands out preparing to get the baby, I was aware of T to my left and *Frozen* playing... I recognised the tune to *Let it Go* playing quietly as I hoped you'd let the baby go.

And surely enough, this baby's body made that final rotation and the most beautiful little white shoulder appeared, and V caught the baby as the rest of him popped out when I gently put down your legs. (My greatest regret is that I did not think to photograph this moment from my viewpoint.)

A happy (crying) V held the chunky baby up in both hands as I moved from standing above you to sitting on the bed, so he could give the baby to you. He was probably a bit stunned by events as he continued to hold the baby up while you reached for him, and you had to tell him, "Give him to me!" The baby still hadn't made the first cry, so as V laid the baby on your chest, I grabbed a towel and began to rub to stimulate breathing. There were some gurgles, his eyes were open and looking around, and his lashes were caked with vernix, but no big cry. You looked at me and said, "What should I do, help me!" So I lifted the baby upright to sit him on your belly, and this was when you said, "It's a boy!" I tilted him forward and back to clear his airway, but no gasp or breath. Finally I leaned in and puffed hard a few times in his face, a trick I learned in Germany, which caused him to frown and get upset and finally he made a big loud gurgling wail, and I returned him to your chest. I will never forget the slippery, sticky feeling of the vernix on my hands as I lifted him up. I had never felt that before. He cried strongly about five more times, and then in the safety of your chest he settled right back down, obviously breathing this time. All along he had a lovely colour but now he was properly bright pink. You said, "I love you!" and I replied, "I am so proud of you" and squinted to try not to drip tears into your face as I was standing over you again!

I remembered that the placenta was the next task. Most of the baby's amniotic fluid came out gushing behind him, but we did a very good job keeping the mess on the inco pads! I wanted to change the soaked inco pad so I took it out from under you and replaced it with a fresh one. In that moment, a gush of blood appeared. I had never been so close to that much blood at once and I thought quickly, "How do I solve this?" The reality was that I had no training or medication to help with too much bleeding before the placenta. In actual fact it was a tiny amount of blood, probably 200 ml, but I looked up at V and said, "Ok you can call the midwives now if you want!" I think I did tell V that I wanted him to call someone just because of the blood, but no more blood came after that. **Z's birth**

Some women were glad of their doula's help after the baby was born.

M supported us with this understanding that the blood loss was normal. I'd prepared so much for the birth but not prepared so much for afterwards. And so once my baby was born I was elated, exhausted and ready for rest, and then I got this incredible pain – which was just the placenta, nothing to worry about. But I'd forgotten about it. And so my body had tensed up and wanted to rest so I struggled to deal with it, perhaps I'd got to the peak of giving birth and I just didn't want to do any more, or feel any more pain. It had been going on for a while and I was in a lot of pain round my lower back – I couldn't lie down properly. M explained that if the placenta was in for too long there was a chance of it causing problems and asked if I would like to think about going to hospital and getting some help. This was all I needed to hear. It was at this point, when I'd been reminded of my choice, that my body starting moving through the process and within minutes I'd turned over onto all fours and birthed the placenta. M had said what I needed to be reminded of and that helped me. **Emma**

Some doulas had been midwives but had ceased to be registered as midwives

When I became pregnant, I sort of put away the thought of having a freebirth. I didn't want to do that because I thought it was reckless or the fear overtook me. But it had always been in the back of my mind and when I met my doula, B [retired midwife], for the first time, I just felt so comfortable with her... and I thought, "Well, this is exactly what I wanted" (laughs). Someone who'd had a lot of midwifery experience that isn't actually a midwife right now. And then I toyed with the idea of having an independent midwife. Because I thought that was the only way to really get midwifery care that wasn't going to be like obtrusive and interfering. Which is sad to say that that's how I feel after years of supporting other women through birth, which was really all with the NHS. But my doula experience part made me more confident in birth as a process, but it also made me more fearful of the institution of the maternity services, because of all the things that I've seen...

I mean, having B there did feel like, and I said this to her at the time, and I hope that she took it the right way, I said that having her there felt like I had a guard dog at the door of the bedroom. Because she did help sort of letting people in or not letting them and things like that. **Katie H**

I thought it was a job for life when I went into it, it was an absolute job for life and I absolutely loved it. And I loved midwifery and working with, caring for women and supporting them and things. But I realised over the years, I saw big changes in that time, from the late 90s there were huge, huge changes. Probably in what I thought was the wrong direction. More focus on budgets and things. Like when I started training, we gave great quality care – brilliant quality of care. We had lots of time for women. We, particularly postnatally, we had so much time for women postnatally, to sit and talk to them, in the hospital I mean. And that was completely eroded to nothing over that time. Birth had become even more medicalised within that time, although it had always been medicalised but you know, there had been positive things like birthing pools and stuff over that time, but then induction became a huge issue. So I think over that time I had been looking... thinking this is maybe not for life, but I don't know what else to do, because it's what I love. So I started to teach pregnancy yoga. I trained as a yoga teacher so I could teach pregnancy yoga. Started to do a bit of birth education on the side after I had baby number three. Which I took ownership of a wee bit more than my first two births; I just went through the motions of birthing in the hospital where I had my own babies. I knew the people, it all seemed kind of safe. But then for baby number three, someone suggested home birth and I went down a rabbit hole into different, a different point of view. And then I did a doula course for fun, because I just thought it would be really nice to do. And it would inform my birth education, help me support women at my yoga class better. And I just loved it. And I thought, "I think this is something that I want to do." But I had to give up midwifery to do that, because too much of a grey area, you know, supporting women outwith the system, while working within the system...

just all too complicated.

And probably back then, I would have thought that freebirth was probably far too out there for me. But over the time of supporting women who make choices outwith the system, and trusting, really trusting women's decisions for what they think's best for them, I came to a point where I was comfortable enough, comfortable with twin freebirth. So a bit of a journey. I don't know where I stand legally with freebirth, which is kind of complicated, maybe slightly more complicated for me. But although I trained as a midwife and worked as a midwife, I'm not a midwife; I have midwifery training but I'm not a midwife – I don't work, I'm not on the register. I see myself as a bit of a lay person with extra skills. So as long as I don't work as a midwife, I don't use midwifery: examinations, feeling people's tummies, all that kind of thing, then I don't think that I can be called to account. **Eve**

Other doulas told of their journey towards supporting women who planned to freebirth

So I suppose in the past, I would have shied away from being around women who were thinking of freebirthing, and I would have insisted in the past on calling midwives at a certain point in the woman's labour. Because, well, I like midwives, I value their skills, I want them there. But over the years, I've come to realise that it goes better when the women tell me when they want the midwives called, not the other way round. And this year with the Covid rules and restrictions and everything else, the women have left it later and later. And I think there's lots of factors in there. One of them is they're just not sure if the midwife's going to be okay with their husband and their doula being there. Because the current agreement is that they will only have one birth partner, and maybe I've been there for a few hours already, and they don't like the idea of upsetting that flow that they've got going.

And I'm sure one of the other things is that their trust with midwives, and the feeling that they've got good support is lessening over the years, and certainly this past year it feels really complicated. And no woman has ever said to me, "Can we freebirth, and is it okay if you, you can support that?" until recently. Women are starting to say it to me. "How would you feel about being at my birth if we don't call midwives?" And the answer I give is pretty uniform now, and I say, "Well, that's entirely up to you, but you have to understand, I can't give you any medical advice, but I'll be there in support of you. And if you decide that you want to have a midwife there anytime, just let me know, and I'll give them a ring."

So, yes… I wonder if women are planning it in the background, but just not saying. You know, I wonder if part of them wants that, but they don't know whether they can pull it off or they don't have the confidence to start at that point or they're frightened to tell their partners that they're considering that… I'm sure all of those are possibilities, and so, they've perhaps mentioned it, like, this, you know, "What happens if we don't call until after the baby's born?" And I said, "Well, that's okay." And one woman particularly recently said, "Would you get in trouble?" And I said, "Well, no as long as I didn't do anything midwifery," you know, "I'm not going to touch your baby," but I never would anyway. "I'm not going to give you advice," but again, I wouldn't anyway.

So no, I'm not going to get in trouble. But I think we're all aware that women whose births I've been involved in, and the situations I've been in, we're aware that the midwives are quite unhappy about it in most cases… certainly I've had it voiced to me that they feel like I've encouraged it, and that I've taken the role of a midwife in advising them that I will take care of them, and look after them, and that we don't need midwives, and that's been the thrust from a couple of midwives.

So, I mean, it's not true, but I can see why it's easy to scapegoat somebody, rather than say, "Oh, dear, perhaps that woman didn't feel terribly well supported by maternity services." **D**, doula

For some their experience as doulas influenced plans for their own freebirths

When I became a doula, I worked a lot with women having hospital births to start with. And then a woman came along who'd met a lot of doulas and she chose me as a doula and she was having a home birth and I was absolutely delighted supporting somebody having a home birth because it was the first time. And I think I was just really naive because of the experiences that I'd had with my own birth, that I just thought generally, the women who would be midwives supporting women at home would be really positive. Would be just really present for women, and with women midwives. So this woman that I was supporting, she'd planned a home birth. It was her second baby and her labour was progressing really beautifully. And the plan was to call midwives and… every so often I would say to her, "You know, things are lovely, just let me know when you want to call the midwife." And it became very obvious that she didn't want that and I felt I was in a position where I didn't feel very comfortable. Because it's not anything that we'd discussed. And eventually her waters broke and she was just great. She was just getting on with her thing, she was almost dancing through her labour, it was so beautiful. She was just cracking on with it. And so after her waters broke, she said that she's going to get in the pool, and she got in the pool. And I did say, "You know, I think it would be a really good idea," and by this time, I was sort of making that my suggestion. "I think it would be a really good idea if you call the midwife now." At that point, she was in the pool and she said, "Okay, then." I don't think she actually wanted that at that point, but she said, "Okay." Anyway, when her husband called the midwives, she could hear in the other room the midwife speaking very loudly saying, "Well, she needs to get out of the pool." And I was there, and I said, "You don't need to get out of the pool, if you're in the pool and you're happy, it's fine, you stay in the pool."… "Everything's fine, just let her get on with what she's doing." Anyway, quite quickly two midwives arrived. They arrived with a student midwife and they came in, and they turned the lights on and I explained, "She's been doing really well and she's enjoyed having the lights off and that's really working for her, the quietness is really working for her" and I turned the light off. She turned the light back on, the midwife, and it became this scenario that I just had not prepared myself for, I didn't think would happen. It was the midwife who was very frightened by going into somebody's space, who was so far into her labour, a midwife that felt, to do her job properly she had to have done all the assessments using the tool, the… Partogram, that she needed to have that done, in order for her to be able to fulfil her role as a midwife. She said to the woman, "You need to get out of the pool so I can do the VE," and the woman said, "I don't want to." And I said, "You know, this is her choice and, you know, she needs to be able to stay where she's comfortable." The midwife went on about it over a twenty-minute period, so the woman just went, "Oh, I'll just get out the pool." Anyway, after about two hours, she was pushing still, and they called an ambulance to wait outside. And the ambulance stayed there for about two hours. And overall, she probably pushed for six hours. She did have her baby at home, but she had a very, very nasty tear and her baby was eleven pound five. But afterwards I went home and I wept.

I went home and I wept because I had coerced her to call midwives. She didn't want that and because I didn't feel comfortable because it was something we hadn't discussed, I had changed the course of events I felt for her. And I wept because if the midwives hadn't been there I think that baby would have been born very quickly, maybe… it wouldn't have taken six hours anyway. I went back after and she was really happy with me. She didn't feel I'd coerced her into anything. She didn't, she just said, "I do wish I hadn't called the midwives, and I think all along that was my plan. That I didn't want to have the midwives there." And I just said to her, "I wish that you'd talked about that because then I might not, I would have either had time to think about it and said, well, maybe I'm not the right person to be there."

And she was like, "… I got the birth I wanted, my first birth was a traumatic hospital birth and although the midwives were very difficult in my space, I got my home birth, and for that I'm happy."

We kept in touch for a long time. She wrote me an email and I got the emails of the midwives and I forwarded her discussion of how the birth felt to her, to the midwives. And I was actually at a birth with the midwife, another woman who had a home birth a couple of years later. And she took me aside afterwards and she said, "I really reflected on what the woman had told me, and it was, it was really difficult at first, but it did really make me think about how I come across." And she was still quite pushy at that birth, but still she was better than she was, and she was more aware of her own behaviour and fear, I guess.

But after seeing the effect of what somebody could have in the room, I made it very clear to everybody I met as a doula after, "It is not my responsibility to tell you when to call the midwife. It is your responsibility."…"If you for whatever reason don't want a midwife there, you need to tell me now, we need to talk about it."

But then after that I ended up just being at, quite a lot of BBAs, and then I thought, "Gosh, these births are really easy, women having fetal ejection reflex, and it was just so, they were just so easy." I remember one person was a friend. Her partner called me over and said, "Oh, she's in labour, I think things are progressing quite well." And I got there, and [she] was actually on the toilet and I was like, "Mm, do you want to have your baby down the toilet? It might be a good idea to think about where else you can have your baby." And I pulled the mattress off and got everything ready. And then I called to her husband, "I think you might need to come upstairs just now," because the baby's head was there, and he was like, "Have I got time to wash the banana off my hands?" because he'd been feeding a toddler, and I threw a towel over his hand so that he could catch his baby. But there was just so many births like that, that were just so easy. And then there was also lots of lovely births that I was at with midwives there, but they were longer, they were just longer. So the more of birth I experienced as a doula, the more I could see how, when women were undisturbed, it was just a completely normal situation. Therefore, for them there was nobody clinical who could take any responsibility over their care there. It just worked really well. So I knew that if I was going to have another baby, that I wanted it to be like that, and I just knew that I would know if something didn't feel right and I would happily go into hospital if something didn't feel right and bypass the having somebody there… So it just didn't feel that I wanted to have anybody there…

So when I got pregnant with [baby], by that point, it wasn't just BBAs that I had been supporting, it was women who were intentionally calling me saying, "I want to give birth. I don't want to have a midwife there." And then I would say, "I am not a cheap, independent midwife, because I'm not a midwife. I have no clinical responsibility, I do not know if something is wrong. If there is an emergency, I cannot do anything."

"You know, if you were, if you were giving birth and something didn't feel quite right or there was a bleed or something, it, it would be your responsibility to call emergency services. And I could speak to emergency services with you asking me to do that. But I cannot do anything clinically." And it was very clear in my agreement being birth support with people, that that was the case. But again, not all of them were quick by that point, there were lots of births that were longer. But just simple, straightforward, normal… and sometimes as well, I remember when I was pregnant with O, I remember I was at somebody's birth and she was freebirthing and it did, it just took ages [I was] downstairs thinking, "I hope everything is all right." But I would always say to the woman, "How are you feeling?" "Great." "That's great then." Or she would ask me, sometimes women will say to you, "Is everything okay, is it, is this normal?" I'm like, "Do you feel everything's okay?" But it was all great.

So, yes when I was pregnant with [baby], I just couldn't, especially after, having a reputation as a doula who is often at freebirths, I knew I needed to not check in with the NHS. **H**

One doula spoke of how she had moved from attending births to mainly working in on-line preparation for freebirths.

… it's all in the preparation and I think actually, that's where the work is to be done here… Because I think truly to freebirth, like if I'm there, it's not a freebirth, because I'm sort of then acting as a traditional midwife, like I'm not a medical midwife but I'm with the woman and therefore it's not, it's then an assisted birth. Even though I'm not monitoring or measuring or doing any of those things. And that's what most of the women that come to me want is a… truly unassisted birth. They want to feel that they've done it completely on their own, but they have these fears and they have beliefs or they're, what if this happens, or what if that happens, and we have to talk through a few things for them to feel prepared. And I think if everyone had like a certain level of preparation, like anyone can do this. And actually it's much better for them, they feel more powerful, rather than me being there, and when they've done it themselves, they feel better. And then there's only one of me, I can't attend ten births a month, it's just not feasible, really. So, yes it's a bit of a win-win for both of us…

… preparation is just what stands out to me, now, from doing this work. Because when I first became a doula I thought it was all about the attendance and I thought being there, in the moment. And doulas have this thing where it's just like, oh we do two antenatal sessions together and then I'll attend your birth and then somehow, it'll all be perfect. And now when I do have my one to one clients whose birth I'm attending, I just say, we have as many sessions, as many antenatal sessions as you need. Because the more time we put into the antenatal, the less time and the less interventions there are in the birth. So I can put in my hours in the birth and I think about these, you know, twenty-four, forty-eight hour births that I attended in the system with women who weren't prepared, versus four, eight, twelve hour births with women who we've done, yes we've done twelve hours, twenty-four hours of preparation together, but isn't that a much better thing to spend our time on. Yes, so I think that's just what's paramount, is that women feel truly prepared and they're informed, that work around belief and the body. **SK**

Chapter 10: Midwives and "the system"

Almost all the mothers had contact with NHS maternity services during their pregnancies. Many found that midwives were opposed to their views, and assumed they were entitled to attend and exercise control during births, sometimes even describing freebirth as "illegal."

[Midwife in previous pregnancy] she did say that, "It is illegal for you to birth your own baby Peggy" and I said... (laughing), "That seems the strangest thing for someone to say to someone expecting a baby." **Peggy**

[During her first pregnancy] I asked them about doing it by myself, or without midwives and they said it was illegal, so I just kind of accepted what they said and went, "oh well (laughs) I'll have to put up with having midwives then"... but then I subsequently found out that it wasn't illegal – but not during my first pregnancy... I think if I'd known that it was legal to do it without midwives, I would definitely have done it that way.

[During her second pregnancy] I was much more aware of what I was doing and what my rights were and things, and they told me it was illegal as well, they came and said, "well sorry you can't do that" and I said, "No actually it's legal, I've looked it up, I've researched it and here's the stuff off the internet." I gave them this set of stuff off the internet and there was a student midwife there and she was really interested... and once I said that they kind of backed off a bit, because they started off being that kind of - I'm superior to you attitude towards me. **Charlie**

I think it's really wrong when midwives don't know that it's okay for women to not have midwives there and they feel almost like they're entitled to be there and do what they want to do. **C**

Many mothers felt that their views were not heard by midwives who were focused on their routine practices, which for them were imperative.

When I mentioned firstly when I went to the first appointment that I was going to have a home birth, the community midwife was absolutely aghast at this idea, and said, "what about pain relief?" and I said, "well I've done lots of research and I think I'm going to be OK." And she was like, "well, you don't have a clue what it's like to give birth to a child." She said, "you'll never be able to birth your first child at home." I was like, oh, really? I was quite shocked by her response to that. But rather than that putting me off, it actually made me even more determined to have a home birth. And every time I discussed the idea of home birth, she was really negative about it, to the point where I started thinking, "hang on a minute, maybe she isn't the kind of person who I want to discuss what my actual plans are." When it came towards my due date, we had a home birth visit and she came to see me at home. I had my birth plan written out and I had in my birth plan that I wasn't intending to call any midwifery help unless I felt there was an emergency or I felt something was wrong. And I asked her to read my birth plan and she said no, she wouldn't - there was no need to read it. I asked her again if she would read it because I thought there might be some things in it that she'd quite like to discuss with me. And she said she didn't want to read it. I said to her, "what if we decided that we didn't want to have midwives present?" And she said, "that's ridiculous!" And I went, "OK, we don't need to discuss any further." And she was just so closed to the idea of looking at things. She was just not into the whole home birth idea, never mind anything else. I just said, "right, I don't need that kind of negativity encroaching into my birth space. I'm just going to leave it." So it wasn't until after I'd actually had my freebirth when she came round to do the postnatal visit that she was like, "ah, now I understand why you wanted me to read your birth plan." She was actually quite okay about it, even though the first thing she said was, "you know that it's illegal?" Which is obviously not true. But after the whole... that comment... she was actually quite pleasant. But she was very negative about the whole... even just the idea of giving birth at home for a first baby, never mind anything else. So I didn't feel she would be open to discuss that. **Lindsay**

I went for a scan. I wasn't into it at all but pushed into it and then I moved and they still managed to catch me up. They got in touch with me... and this midwife came to visit me to check me out and I said "can you sign this paper for me?" and she said "well, you're not really going along with what I'm telling you about it, it's not a safe thing for you to have home birth, you know, after having had a caesarean the first time" and she insisted that I have a scan to see if it was breech which she was at the time – she was when she asked me to, I knew she was, but I thought that she would turn and she did, she turned the night before we went for a scan, she turned round and I thought "bless you" you know, she is very compliant, she is like she really wants to help, probably because I was in like a dreadful state emotionally which is very helpful. So I went for the scan – I did my bit and then I said "come on, sign my bit of papers so I can get my grant and we can go and buy this washing machine" and she refused, you know, she refused because I was still saying you know "no" to coming into the hospital. She just lost it, she was trembling and K [partner] was with me and she told him, "she's not responsible, she's not responsible, don't let her do it" and she totally got him on her side and I thought I cannot believe this is happening you know, I can't believe it. I ran out in tears and C was there with the other kids and just completely burst out you know emotionally, and things were very tense with K already and then he drove us back home, having no confidence at all into what I was doing, that I could be letting our child die. It was just like the last thing that I needed really so I never got in touch with them again and gave birth without them. **Moggie**

Their appointments with midwives were felt to be dominated by the midwives' need to tell them of the risks of their situation and their plans. This had a negative impact on these mothers.

... my pre-natal checks, I didn't really get on with the midwives much. I felt like they were too pushy, too much looking at the negatives. Too much telling me about all the risks and making me have more fear than I had before I went, you know. I know they're just doing what they've been trained to do. And I know that a lot of them obviously have seen lots of things. So they're kind of conditioned in a way to be like that, I think. **Gauri**

I found my midwife appointments really, really stressful. And I actually always find seeing anyone in the medical profession really stressful. It makes me feel really anxious. And I'm not actually really an anxious person at all. I generally feel quite capable and confident in expressing what it is that I'm after. But I just feel like I lose all my power as soon as I'm in those kinds of environments. And I had said to my midwife that I wanted to have a home birth. And it was very clear that she wasn't supportive of that… it was really not a good match…

I felt like the language they used in all my appointments was really off-putting… being pregnant and going through what feels like it should be, and is, this massive hugely emotional transformative experience… And I would go to my appointments and expect maybe to have a sense of connecting with another person, about this experience. But all I got was, I just felt like all they ever did was talk to me about risk, and try and quantify things that were happening in my body… and actually, you know, I think my midwife wasn't doing that in an over the top way, she was just… it was just clear that she was following the protocols that they had to follow. **Ally**

… the care I was receiving didn't feel like care at all, but disempowering, and I was becoming increasingly uncertain as to whether I wanted an NHS midwife present at all. **Naomi**

This institutionalised approach can erode a woman's confidence in herself and was therefore seen as best avoided when they were seeking to protect their confidence in themselves and their bodies. So some women felt pushed into freebirth by the rigidity and negativity of their midwives' approach.

J, who was my midwife here, she said, "If you're not going to let us do stuff, don't invite us to come. I'd rather you not… you know, don't make the call if you're not going to let us do our jobs" And I thought, "Really then, I don't want to feel under pressure to let you do your jobs. Because I know what that is for you, because I've attended birth." And I, you know, I'm in the birthy circle [she is a doula]. So I knew what she meant by that. And that had to be the decision for them not to come. Because then they would hijack my birth anyway, because I'm so then focused on what they need to do, and what I'm not going to want them to do and you know. There's a lot of talk about vaginal checks and where you are in labour. I didn't have any of that with D [IM booked for her first birth]. It was all completely hands off. If anything, she was encouraging me to check and… not encouraging but said I could. So I was really keen. So they probably thought I might not call. There was probably talk around that. And so when somebody did come out, [after the birth]… And we relayed how things had happened and how labour had taken quite a while and it hadn't got into that standard, that regular. And she said, well, "I think really, you're very lucky to have gone ahead as you had" she said, "because if you'd have phoned us to come and support you, there's no way we'd have let you go that long, contracting like that. Because we'd have just thought this is getting you nowhere;

you're getting tired. Something's clearly going on positionally. And we'd have probably taken you in.".. And I remember feeling at the time really, "This is why you weren't supposed to be here. Because that's what could have happened." And I would not have gone straight for section, but the stress involved in L being told that and, H trying to protect birth space, and me being aware of what's going on would have been really, really difficult. And could have completely sidelined the natural birth I was trying to have. So I really felt I did the right thing. There was a lot of people though who didn't know I was going to freebirth. And lots of people that did know, and thought it was crazy. But I really felt quite kind of vindicated in my decision to do it. Because having heard that woman say, "If we'd have been here, it would have been a completely different birth." I was like, "Right. That's why you weren't here." **Cathy S**

So I got an email and it was from the lady who asked me previously and I told her that I would meet her after I had the baby, you know, to discuss. So she had reached out, she said, "I'm following up from the conversation [about home birth] that you had yesterday. This is about a risk assessment, de, de, de. I was wondering, would you come over and talk to me." So again, very naive, I was like, "Yes, no problem." I thought this was to do the risk assessment. So I went over to this lady... I walked down and there seemed to be a nice wee aura feeling in the room. And you know, sat down with her, started chatting and she gave off a nice vibe at the start. And then as the conversation progressed, I realised that I wasn't there for no risk assessment. She was asking me more why I wasn't coming to the hospital, what could they do to change, do I know the risks. She would need to send someone out to the house to make sure there was an area, so they could resuscitate the baby. This is what she said to me. And I was like, "Whoa, whoa." And I wasn't going to let her see me cry. I definitely wasn't going to let her see me cry. But when I got outside, I bawled my eyes crying. Everything that I was wanting not to happen just happened. I let her in. She got in my head,, she questioned everything you know, even about doing the delayed cord clamping. Anyway, she said to me like... she was like, "Where are you getting this information?" And then I had in my head like why does this have to happen. And I just felt like I was in an interview. I felt like I was in an interview. I was starting to sweat a wee bit, palms of my hands were sweating. And I just thought, "No, this isn't good." And as soon as I walked out from that door, I just said, "That's it." Pardon my language, but "Fuck this. I'm not letting this happen. And I'm not doing it." I got into the car, I rang S, I was so upset. This is a woman, 38 weeks heavily pregnant being left like this. And I just thought, "No. S [doula], I'm done. This is our plan. This is what we are doing [freebirthing]." **Christina**

[After the birth] they had quite a lot of attitude towards me. And they were like, "How much blood did you lose?" And all these sort of things. And I was like, "Well you weren't there. Why should I even give you that information?" Like, "You're here to check baby. You're here to have the utensils to do the cutting of the cord and stuff. But I don't know why I should have to divulge any information further. It's going to be incorrect because I don't know how much blood I really lost or anything like that." It was just guessing... And they just weren't very happy, to be honest. They just came in with an air of, "Oh well done" sort of thing. And they were standing back at the wall, feeling like they weren't welcome or anything like that. But obviously, I don't have any ill feelings towards anyone. I know that it's just their procedure. **Jessica**

Unfortunately it was the same midwives that attended that I had previously sent away earlier that day. One of them was just lovely, the other we found to be very rude, uncaring and messed up repeatedly that night. Some of her actions are going to take a long time to heal from. **Sarah M**

… the next day, the midwives were really on it. They were calling, can we come, can we come? I wanted them to come because I wanted to present her, like, look what we've done! So they came and they weighed her. It was nice to have their support after the fact. Looking back, there were a couple of things they were… She hadn't peed within the first day, and they were like… you've got about five more hours. But it's just that pressure, putting time limits on things. So that wasn't helpful. **Lacey**

Many women told us how the midwives' approach made it difficult to talk with them.

Well, I didn't even ask for a home birth because I thought I would be told "no" and in a way I felt well that's quite bad that I cannot ask… well I tried to think really level-headedly about it and I thought, well I cannot even approach these services because they are going to say "no" to me, but I know that I want to have a go at being at home, but I don't want them to even give me the go at being at home when I have still "at risk" written all over my notes so I still knew there would be that kind of edge on it. So I just wanted to disengage from all of that. But afterwards the midwife had said to me, you know, "you could have asked for a home birth" because she said, "I have attended quite a lot of vaginal births after caesareans" and it was funny, and I was like well, now you're saying that, and I was surprised that never anybody even said, "How do you feel about what happened before and what you expect this time." I really just surprised at that lack of connection. **Polly**

I wanted to have a proper conversation with her about it [having thought through her freebirth plans]. So that was my motivation. And then I realised speaking to her that she didn't get it. And she felt like… which must just be reflective of wider opinions as well, that maybe their perspective is, "Oh there's these kind of rogue doulas out there or these rogue birth educators who are kind of turning people away from maternity services and we're not the problem; they're the problem." Which I found really sad. And also found it sad that then D [doula] reached out to her to talk to her about it and she didn't take that offer. Because actually they just could have learned from that. And felt really kind of grateful, I suppose, to D for being willing to continue walking down this path, knowing all of those things. Because that really can't be an easy thing to do. **Ally**

I started reading up on it quite a lot and found all the information at the Birth Resource Centre and started learning about how I would like to birth and came round to putting together a birth plan. I was not very confident – I had a lot of ideas about how I wanted to have my baby and what seemed to me to be the easiest way of birthing my baby, but every time I brought up the point and a long list of things I didn't want midwives to do, things that I had heard were sort of quite standard, it was quite often brushed aside and it is a couple of years ago so I can't remember that many examples, but I can remember sort of saying that I wouldn't like internal examinations and was probably told you had to do examinations. That's just what they did and I wanted to give birth in the pool and I would have to come out of the pool. I would like to give birth without any pain relief and it kind of sounded like a severe idea to the midwife because everybody had gas and air and it was no big deal, and I felt like that she wasn't telling me that I had to have it, but what it felt like was she was sort of not filling me with confidence that I was able to do it naturally without any gas and air, so it just felt like she didn't have a lot of faith in me to do it really, although I wanted to, and I suppose she was being quite friendly and nice and tried to make me feel like, "oh it's okay if you have gas and air because a lot of women do", but it came across to me that she didn't have a lot of confidence in women to give birth without that sort of thing really. **ME**

My questions weren't always welcome. Especially with people who hadn't met me before. My community midwife less so. I feel fortunate to have had a supportive community midwife who respected my choice to home birth, initially, and then freebirth, as I know that many women aren't as fortunate and can feel immense pressure. I didn't feel judged by her. I think she just got used to me asking questions and challenging decisions. She was honest with me and told me what my choices were. But I did have to ask a lot of questions. I'm not sure I would have been given all that information had I not done so. **Emma**

[After her antenatal encounter with a midwife whose manner robbed her of all agency (see chapter 5) Naomi was]... considering asking for her not to be in charge of my case, I wobbled: "What if she puts 'awkward, demanding, touchy, unreasonable woman' on my notes for my other midwife who takes me on to see? What if the midwife who shows up at the birth is her friend and wants to punish me for excluding her, and then bullies me during the birth, in order to get back at me?" **Naomi**

Yvonne, herself a midwife, felt unable to discuss her freebirth plan with her midwife.

We had a nice plan B packaged away if we wanted to go into the hospital. And that's the kind of birth plan that I presented to my community midwife. And I didn't feel comfortable disclosing the freebirth plan to her, because, well I work in that service and I just didn't feel comfortable with getting, I suppose fear of being judged by colleagues. And then the second thing is that I didn't want the anxiety of having to fight my corner and fight for my rights to be able to do that as a Mum. You know, you're birthing right, and you can choose to give birth where you like. But I just know that through experience, and sort of talking to other people who have been in that boat that you can come up against a lot of challenges from the maternity services about, "Why are you going to make that decision?" You know, all the risks that are involved with that. And I just didn't want to partake in that conversation. Working in that service, you know the risks. You're knowledgeable enough to read up on it and have experienced multiple birth in the past, in different settings. So I guess I just wanted to make that decision without having to fight for it. So one of the midwives called me sly afterwards. Wasn't really that sly. **Yvonne**

Many women spoke similarly of not wanting professionals to judge them and not wanting to have to fight for their choices when pregnant and particularly not when in labour.

… that's hard when you're pregnant – having to fight when you're pregnant and during the birth. Nobody can ask a Mum during the birth to fight for what she wants. You have to allow her to go into birth, and to allow herself to let go. And if a Mum during birth has to fight – things are not going to happen. Because you're in your mind, not in your body. And that is what happened to me the first time, that I was in my mind. Because…I had to be attending the midwife and to my partner and I was never allowed to be inside my body. And second time, I was just inside my body without having to attend anybody. And things just happened in a few hours. **Bea**

Nor did they want to fight in the precious early hours with their new baby.

While I was nursing him, my husband called the midwives… We had talked about this before, obviously - what was the best way to do, are we going to tell them that we're freebirthing? I had all the antenatal care. And, yes, for the preparation, I also had all the blood tests and, just in case of a haemorrhage, that my iron levels were good. I also had scans… so I knew where the placenta was… I wouldn't have gone into this blindly. And we had also discussed what we will say, but because of other friends who had had bad experiences of being bullied when they decided to have a freebirth and told the midwives, we decided to not say anything. And just pretend it was a BBA, Birth Before Arrival (laughs)… that's what we decided to do. Because I, with a new baby and a toddler, you really don't want to have to fight anything. We just wanted to have our baby moon, so he called them and said, "The baby arrived so quick." Well, I mean, to be fair, that was one o'clock, so that's a three hour labour and it was very quick. It could have been a BBA… And so they arrived after the placenta was born, they checked the placenta and cut the cord with my husband, and we kept the placenta and everything was beautiful. No-one had to inject me with anything. Oh, the after pains were so much less painful the second time round. And I had heard that syntocinon can make the after pains more painful…that was a big difference too… the midwives were all right, were very respectful. I don't know. I guess they had an inkling (laughs). They didn't say anything and they were kind. **ST**, a midwife herself

Some spoke of sympathetic midwives who were required to follow the system in a way that prevented them from giving women individualised care.

I actually think I had a really great midwife, she was still very much part of the system. And every time I spoke to her, I was happy to see her and felt like I could be really honest with her and she was honest… she was honest with me, I think, as well. And we had a good relationship. And she still just had to say the stuff that she had to say… she was really up front about all of that as well. But I just found it so off-putting. And it just feels like such a clash, this kind of… even in really sensory terms, you know, all the kind of, the uniforms and the masks and the equipment and the machines and the noise and the lights… it just clashes so fundamentally with everything about, not just the experience of actually giving birth, but with the whole, the whole part of life, of sort of squishy little babies and soft, I can't, I'm not articulate enough to put that into really beautiful words, but it just doesn't work for me. Those two things, they just don't really go together. And so at some point I decided to tell my midwife that I was choosing. I said, "I don't know if I want to have midwives at the birth." And she took it really well actually… I think it's kind of a testament to how she was a good midwife, as in she sat and chatted to me about it for way longer than she had time for… she said, obviously they would prefer to be there. And, but it also felt like she was quite kind of open to almost like a bit of negotiation… And she said that the team leader would want to speak to me. **Ally**

This time I had someone at the booking appointment and from then I had the same midwife every time and for all the postnatal visits as well. So that was good. And she was, I'm not going to say any names, but she was, let's say, it sounded like she's pro-freebirth. Like whenever I hinted at it, she was just like, "We know what you're going to do right" so yes. And she was kind of okay with it. And I thought that was nice, that I don't have a midwife that is anti-home birth, let alone freebirth. And she still repeated all the risks and all those things to me, but I could literally tell whenever she was switching to her script. And she had to say certain things. But yes, just as I was coming to the end of pregnancy, "And you know when to call us if you want to call us." She was sort of joking about it. She knows D [doula] as well, so yes, that was quite nice… So this time that midwife was almost kind of pro-freebirth, although officially she can't be. I never told her that's what we're going to do, but I think she picked up on it. **Carmen**

I knew when I conceived, because it was an accidental conception. We were using condoms, we'd lost a condom and then the following day I went and had the morning after pill but it didn't work. So R [baby]… he really, really wanted to be! (Laughs). But I was absolutely certain of when it happened. And then we went for a dating scan, and they told me that my date was two and a half weeks out from what the scan showed. And it didn't really matter what I said. They were like, "well, no, the scan says this." Thankfully I spoke to a much more mature midwife later on when I went for a blood test for Downs Syndrome – because we have Downs Syndrome in the family so I always get that done, just because I would like to know ahead of time… so when I went for that blood test I spoke to a more mature midwife, who was happy to negotiate my date with me, so she changed the date in my notes to being half way between what I thought it was and what the scan showed. So that made it slightly less difficult to get them to arrange the home birth later on. And I made it really clear with the midwives that I wasn't going to have an induction, but they are obliged to offer me that. And it seemed they were obliged to offer me that repeatedly! And it's a shame because I think that actually they were both very nice women, and they trusted that I'd had three children previously and I knew what I was doing, but it seemed like they were under an obligation to tell me all these risks and to keep telling me what the protocol was, even if it wasn't really what they agreed with or thought that I needed. So despite the fact that I was quite confident in myself and resisting the system a little bit, I did feel like it was always there. But anyway, we got what we wanted in the end. He was born exactly when I predicted he would be born (laughs). Well I thought, it's probably going to be this weekend, and he was born on the Thursday, so I think I was quite right about my dates in the first place. Although it was interesting, because towards the end of the pregnancy, I did start doubting myself. **Elena**

… so I stayed registered with the NHS, but we didn't abide by the standard protocol. One of the local midwives was quite supportive, quietly supportive. She was probably the only person who, once we'd decided that we were going to have a freebirth and not use them but still have them on hand, most of the midwives seemed a little bit nervous of us, whereas she was the only one that was a little quietly supportive. Not too supportive, because I don't think she was probably allowed to be, but she was kind and helpful and she came around a couple of times, and she was respectful of not having scans and I didn't want to have the Doppler, I didn't want to do any fetal heartbeat monitoring or any of that stuff, and she was fine with that. **Lacey**

And maybe my midwife would have actually liked to have helped me, if she felt she was going to be supported too. But she didn't have that kind of support. Not in the [Scottish] area, where I was. **Jessica**

Several women found that midwives who initially seemed supportive, behaved differently as the birth drew near.

J [partner]'s Mum had said something to me like, "Do you not think it would be a wonderful situation to have a midwife or a group of midwives that could support you, so you didn't feel like you had to make this choice?" And I said, "Yes, I think you're right." And I moved forward with engaging with the NHS on that premise. Because I actually had decided, after having A, that I was going to freebirth my next child… So that was where I started to engage with the NHS. And I was always going to work with them to some extent, to make sure that baby was in the right position and the heart rate and everything was in a good rate, coming up to the birth. So I had informed myself as much as I could that baby was healthy, at the right size and all the numbers were good. So that I felt confident to just allow the process to take place when it was happening. So… when engaging with the NHS initially, I said to them, "Look. I'm not sure about having a birth through the NHS. I'm thinking about just freebirthing." And she was like, "Oh okay. Well we want to support your choices, you know. We want to be able to do what you need any time, you know. We're happy to provide the service that you want." And I said, "Okay. Great. Because last time there were some things that happened that I wasn't so comfortable with, that's made me feel that this is going to be the best option for me." And they said that they'd be happy to support my choices. And went along the whole process of my pregnancy saying that they would be happy to support my choices. And I was talking to her, my midwife, who was very friendly and nice, about how it is, where should the midwife sit, should they be in the room, observing quietly and making it quite clear that I don't want them to intervene in the birthing process. But be able to sit back and just sit in the corner with a book or something very quiet, not to intervene. So we had discussions like this. And we had discussions about whether they should be downstairs or how would it go. And the woman was really supportive of the ideas that I was presenting, and asked me to write a birth plan about it. And I did. And then up to the point where I was in my last midwife appointment, this is where they started to say to me, "Do you want to be inspected during your labour? Are you happy to have your waters broken?" You know, all... just the formalities of doing a home birth, they ask you these questions. Like, "Are you happy to have a vaginal inspection? Are you happy to have a sweep? Are you happy to have these things?" Obviously I said no to all of them. But part of those questions was the heart rate monitor. And I was not happy to have that... I decided that I didn't want to have a heart rate monitor check because of my last experience. And so at that point, they decided to say, "Look. We're going to need you, by law, to reserve your consent at every fifteen to five minute period." So I was like, "Whoa. We've just been speaking the whole pregnancy about someone coming and sitting in the space or downstairs... And now you're saying that you must talk to me and you must intervene to say something at every five, fifteen minutes to me." And I said, "Is it not possible for you to do that with J at this point or someone else, you know?.".. So then this is where we started to get into a bit of like a lock. And I was saying, "I want an autonomous birth. I'd like to have an independent birth. I'd like to feel as if there was someone there for baby." So if baby came out in any difficulties, I could be like, "Hey..." call downstairs and there'd be someone there ready to support her. Because I don't know how she's going to come out." And they didn't, they weren't able to do that. And I didn't feel then safe to have them in the space... So they said that they couldn't do that. They couldn't, by law, give me the birth that I wanted. So that meant to me as if the only option, which was the option that I had originally said was going to be the safest thing for me anyway, was going to be freebirth. So then, at that point, I was fighting the case. Because I'd already, even initially, decided that I was going to freebirth. But it would be nice... the preferred option would be to have someone you trusted, someone who was there for you the whole time. Even the midwife I'd been discussing these things with, her personally, her actually coming to my birth and supporting me because she understood from a one-to-one relationship that we'd built, that these were the birth choices that I would prefer. And that this was the mood I was setting. And that this is the environment that I'd like to maintain whilst birthing baby. But they couldn't do it… and then I just decided to have her myself. **Jessica**

Some women decided to freebirth because of how midwives had behaved at their previous home birth.

And I tried to have a home birth with my second and it was all just completely sabotaged really. Midwives didn't really want us to... looking back and you can see, because we actually requested my notes from my previous births and you can really see that they were very much like, they just didn't want to be there, you could tell. **Darelle**

But the midwife, when she came home, it was an NHS midwife, and when she came, she came from another birth. Or she had a really little rest between the other birth and my birth. She came, she checked me and she stayed, but... because it was the first time we met her, my partner wasn't feeling very good. He didn't know if he should attend me, or attending the midwife. And the midwife wasn't really attending me, and I was really coming out of birth all the time, because I was feeling stress about making my partner feeling good at home. And he didn't know if he should be attending the midwife or attending me. So I was really attending more what it was happening in the house, than letting me go and attending the birth. So the birth was really heavy; painful, stressful. And the midwife just started to look all the time at the baby heartbeat. And she was all the time like, "Oh you know, the baby's suffering. The heartbeat is becoming really high." And she was proposing breaking my waters. And at the beginning, I was saying, "No." And then she was like, "Oh, so we maybe have to go to hospital, because the baby looks stressed." And it was something like after, I don't know, twelve, fourteen hours at home. I was feeling the baby okay, but I wasn't feeling attended. I was feeling me out of birth all the time. I wasn't feeling comfy in my own house. And I didn't feel a good feeling with the midwife. I don't know, it was something that, you know, it wasn't nice. And then finally after I don't know how many times her asking me to break my waters, I allow her just to prove if the baby was suffering or not. She was like, "Okay. If you allow me broken your waters, I'm going to see if it's green waters or the waters are okay so we can stay here or…" And she broke my waters; the waters were clear. But she still wanted me to transfer to hospital. So I was like, "No, no, no." And finally, everything... my partner was really getting worried and she was making him being worried. And then they decided, the two of them, decided to just transfer me to hospital.

… We got to hospital. I couldn't say yes or no. I was just... it was at the end of the birth and... I wanted something to happen. I wasn't feeling support in my own home and in my own birth. And then they transfer me. She went... the midwife went in her own car, my partner, took me in our car. And I was like, "Oh, if something is really happening, why you don't take in your car, or why you don't get an ambulance, if it's something really...?" I think she wasn't wanting to be there, or she was tired or... And then they took me to hospital... But the hospital was really busy... but the midwife was nice and she told me, "Okay... I know that you wanted a home birth and I'm going to make you feel like at home." And it was really nice. F just relaxed; my partner relaxed. They give him tea. And he just sat to watch. And then the midwife at hospital took control. The other midwife left us there.

… And in something like twenty minutes, U was born. And something like in two hours, we were back home. So I feel like I gave birth at home. **Bea,** describing her first birth

All this time me with the face in the pillow concentrating on my breathing as I could feel absolutely everything and the pain was very intense and contractions just kept coming and lasting for ages. I couldn't really talk and I didn't want to. My birth plan was downstairs and no one was reading it. Where I wanted hands off birth and no one in the room with me apart from my partner. She saw that there was meconium in the water as everything just kept coming out as baby was coming down so fast and strong like she was crawling out and I could feel every movement in my body and everything what was happening I was so in sync with my baby it was magical but... the midwife kept telling me I need to go to hospital, I kept saying, "No", she said she will call ambulance, I said, "No." She didn't want to be there, she was really pure evil. She kept talking to me only during contractions and threatening, she called the ambulance, I kept telling everyone to shut up and not to turn the light on because I wanted it off and I was trying to stay in the zone with the baby. I was trying to labour and they were doing everything to disturb me, talking between them and I had to waste my energy to say shhhhh. Labour was still so intense and I still wasn't looking up. She kept trying to listen in and it was bothering me so much. She kept telling me I need to go to hospital because they don't have enough space to resuscitate my baby after she's born. I said there is enough space and she doesn't need to be resuscitated, she's fine. She just kept threatening me every time I had a contraction saying that she will be taken away from me, that as soon as she's born they'll bluelight her to hospital and I won't be allowed with her and if I try to stop or do anything they will call police on me as soon as she's born, it's a safeguarding issue. And she just kept saying these things only while I was having contractions. Then she called another ambulance to convince me with the head of paramedics who said he has no knowledge in childbirth and it scares him and I need to go to hospital. At one point I had seven people in the room with me. While I'm trying to concentrate and give birth to my baby who is rushing to get out and is completely fine. Even when she was listening in there was no concerns. They all kept chatting and turning light on when I kept telling them to be quiet. They had no respect for me in my labour, in my bedroom, in my house. If I had more energy and the labour wasn't as intense I would have told them to get out, especially that evil midwife. I won't even put down all the things she said. She also had a go at me for not letting her to do VE. I said my waters are gone, I don't want infection and she doesn't need to know how far I am but she wasn't happy with it. As I was so calm she thought it will be ages. In the end I just wanted them to fuck off so I agreed to go to hospital so they just shut up. **Silva** describing her second birth

Some found midwifery services accepted their decision to freebirth and honest communication then followed which enabled acceptable services to be put in place.

… when I went for the letter from the doctor's – he did actually ask me, the doctor, would it be okay, would you mind if I let the midwives know that you're pregnant and I said, "If you'd be happy doing that, that's fine with me. I don't want any sort of secrecy"... so I did expect a call... I can't say that I wasn't semi dreading it just because I didn't feel like – I'm not very good with confrontation – I didn't feel like I wanted to justify how I was thinking and... to someone who wouldn't necessarily be on the same wavelength as me… but no, it was fine... and they were great as well with it… I made that clear really, we had amazing care [in previous birth]... I was very low maintenance (laughing) for them

I think… I don't think I ever needed to ask any questions or felt like I needed to… so I think they were completely understanding and they said that if you want to, if you change your mind at all or, but I did tell them that I'm thinking of going independent, getting an independent midwife which is sort of true… so they were quite happy, they say they're going to give me a call in early April, just to make sure I'm supported. **Peggy** [went on the freebirth her first baby]

… at thirty-seven weeks I booked in for a home birth. I was very honest about the fact that I was intending to freebirth but didn't want to have to do the admin of trying to notify child and whatever services. I was like, come and do the paperwork, once I birth the placenta I'll give you a call and you can come and do the paperwork… I felt I had a duty to be more open in declaring, "This is what I'm going to do," so the NHS is more aware of it, and to engage with them in the sense of, "This is what I'm going to do and you need to respect that, and when I ask for help, give me the help I ask for, and not try and bombard me with all these other bits and pieces." So I engaged with them in that sense, I went to the Maternity Voices Partnership and I wrote them quite a long letter… although it seems like an oxymoron, I suggested that they should really have a freebirthing midwife. **Jocelyn**

I didn't feel that I need to hide it because it's my decision. So I wanted them to be on board. I wanted them to know it. I wanted to have support, should I need it. So we told them about – when I was around 20 -24 weeks – we told them that we were going to freebirth. They were very respectful, I have to say. It was a really good experience. One of them was assigned to us. We were supposed to have a meeting with the supervisor of midwives, who was supposed to come to our home. After all we decided not to and we just wanted to talk to the midwife that we know. They were offering that they can stay in another room and they don't have to come into the room, but just in case they would be here, and we decided not to do that. Then we had a meeting with our lead midwife; we went through all the risks together, so we knew what to do when… we prepared everything. The only thing I did was to have my blood taken around 35 weeks to make sure that I had enough iron and not at a risk of postnatal bleed. And we were left alone… I mean, it was very, very pleasant. There wasn't any pressure on us at all. The hospital didn't get back to us any more when we cancelled the supervisor of midwives meeting. Nobody pressured us when we cancelled the scans. So it was a very straightforward, easy pregnancy and meeting. Oh yes, we were supposed to go to… see a consultant, which we cancelled as well. Then I was 41 weeks and the midwife called me and offered me a sweep. So we had a great laugh about it and I gave birth eventually at 41+3 [without the sweep] in the sitting room, very straightforward labour. It took about six hours. **Michaela**

I feel like I've done it before, my body knows what it's doing a bit and I think I was in the middle of my pregnancy when I went to the doctors. I had a scan and also I felt so tired and it was quite nice to have it confirmed… and I just had a visit from the community midwife on Sunday and that was nice. She is a midwife that I have met before. She was the midwife that suggested to try the gas and air and she set that up for me and I was really sort of appreciative that she did that – that was a really good idea and this time she seemed a lot more confident that the second baby would be fine and healthy and we don't need to intervene too much with the birth so I felt better this time… She made a joke –she said are you going to phone us this time?… I replied with a lot of questions, so I really do like the feeling of having the midwives on call and having their support there and waiting and I would like to feel that I can phone a midwife but I think that my experience between now and then…that would sort of affect how I feel at the time. But I am aware that it will be a quick birth, or if it's simple, it's likely to be quicker at least; so if I want to phone her… she said best to do it sooner than later. But she didn't seem put out. She didn't seem offended, she seemed really a bit curious but it was okay. She was one of the midwives that I was happy to sort of meet again. **Sarah-Anne,** second baby, second freebirth

We had a final appointment with midwife and senior midwife, where we were able to present our birth plan to the senior midwife, in conjunction with the midwife who was now kind of assigned to me. And we were going back and forth and back and forth about, "If we call, you need to come. Don't try to send me to go in, because I won't." And then they were saying, "Oh but, you know, if resources are already booked out…" etc. etc. And finally, the senior midwife said something along the lines of, "I'm looking at your birth plan and I'm trying to understand what you actually want us to do. Because reading this, it looks like you don't want us to do anything..".. it was basically she was saying to me, "Are you planning a freebirth? Is a home birth your back up plan, effectively?" And I said, in other words, "Yes. That is our plan. That is why it's important that if we call, it means we need you." So when everybody understood that, we were then able to say, "Okay, when you go into labour, give us a call so that we've got you on our radar, so that we know things are in progress. So that we're aware that we may or may not get a call from you." And I wish, I wish that conversation could just be had openly. And I wish everybody could have that conversation, because it makes the whole situation so much easier. And would massively help with resourcing priorities and everything. Anyway, so we got home and I said, "Oh, I feel so much more relaxed now." **ME**

In the end we decided to be upfront about it, and so, I think it was the Supervisor of Midwives as they were at the time, and there was a world of change, but they came round to the home, to do a sort of home assessment, and just to see who we were and to chat about it. And they were quite receptive, actually, it was a really positive meeting. But at that point we hadn't officially said that we want to freebirth, and I was just asking about if we did call them out, what would happen. What was the, kind of, standard procedure, and, and they were talking about, you know, regular monitoring every fifteen minutes and stuff. And I remember very vividly saying, "Well, but what if I don't want that?" And she said, "Well, that's what we do, we have to do that every time we come out." And that was the pivotal point: we didn't; "I don't I don't want that, so I'm not going to call you, basically." And that was fine, it was all quite respectful, and quite straightforward. **Leonie,** her first of three freebirths

So things were unfolding. I emailed the Head of Midwifery at the time, I think I was about thirty-five or thirty-six weeks pregnant, so, very late on really. And I just said, "This is who I am, I'm pregnant, I intend to freebirth again, I've already done that once, no complications, you know. I'm low risk, this is a fully informed choice." Quite detailed, yes, just stating my intention. And I was met with, again, a positive reception, and she just said, "That's great, you know, we're here if you need us, just let us know if you need anything, we wish you all the best." And that was fine, and I'm really glad that I sent that email, because that came to be useful later down the line. **Leonie,** with her second baby in a different area

It was during Covid as well, so, I had to book an appointment over the phone, and that was easy, but then I did go for in-person midwife appointments. And I just thought, "I'm not really getting anything from these appointments, I don't need them, everything's fine." So… when they went to book me in for another appointment automatically, I just said, "I don't want any more, thank you." I declined all further [antenatal] care. And the woman was a little bit sort of apprehensive, if you like. But I think it really helped that it was my third child and my third freebirth experience, and she just respected that, and just said, "Look, you know what to do if you feel reduced movements." We did her thing, you know, the tick boxing her end, and that was it, in terms of face-to-face appointments. And I know that sometimes it can be quite challenging and problematic when you do decline care, but I think it really helped that I'm a white woman, I am articulate, I'm educated too, so, all of these things contributed, fortunately and that was the situation.

I then had an appointment, she came to our house actually, the consultant midwife, because I still wasn't a hundred percent sure at that point that I wanted to not call a midwife. So, she said, "Look, if you are going to call a midwife, I'd really like to be able to communicate your intentions in a positive way to the Community Midwife Team." So, we had about an hour's appointment, where we began discussing birth plans, essentially. And then further by email, and I drafted it up with a very detailed thing, I was very clear, if I wanted somebody there, not in a controlling way, but just very clear about what involvement I would like and, you know, "Don't keep asking me if I want this, don't keep asking me if I'm okay, possibly don't even come in the house, you know, sit in the car outside." But then as it went on, that was a process of learning really as it went on, I realised that I just didn't want them (laughs), I just didn't feel the need to call anybody at all. But that was quite positive, actually. She was not fazed at all by what I was saying, but she just wanted to make sure that her team, because she recognised that the other midwives would have been, tended to be quite anxious about what I was saying, although she wasn't, and that felt quite reassuring. So, I feel good about the relationship with her, and again, it was a different city, so, it wasn't the same Head of Midwifery or, anybody that I'd spoken to the second time. Yes, everything was feeling really positive again, very well received. And I felt confident that I wouldn't get random midwives turning up during labour or be reported or anything. I was just trying to avoid all of those little potholes that had come up. **Leonie,** third freebirth

An independent midwife supported some women who could afford their service but insurance problems prevented them from attending the actual birth.

I had an independent midwife and she was really supportive. She got my previous notes from my birth so that we went through them, discussed them, and she was like, I can't see any reason medically from your notes why it wouldn't be safe to have a freebirth. Like she was completely on board and obviously she couldn't attend my birth. I think if I'd wanted anybody there, I would have wanted her, we built up a really great rapport which is exactly what it's meant to be like, isn't it? **Darelle**

Confidence grew with successive pregnancies for some women and this made honest communication possible.

And my decision to tell them came from a political place really; from a kind of wanting it to be visible that people make these choices and that my baby wasn't just born before you happen to arrive... I am choosing not to call you. And I did feel quite nervous about that. I suppose originally I wasn't going to say to anyone that I was thinking of not calling them. Because it's very easy to just not call them and then they come later and you're just, "Oh the baby was born really quickly." And no one's going to know any different. But I felt like, "Actually no, this is an important thing to do." And I felt more confident and capable than I did in the first pregnancy when I was kind of, "This isn't the time to fight." I felt a bit more like, "I'm not having a fight, but..." I suppose what you would call standing in your power, just, "Let's just have a conversation about this like adults and make this a bit more visible so people can see that people are doing this by choice. And I'm doing it from a place of being well informed." **Ally**

Some women were able to have just the care they requested.

I think my decision to freebirth was always there really, after my last two pregnancies. It wasn't really a consideration. I didn't have any desire to book in with a midwife. And my blood type is rhesus negative... so the only appointment I made through pregnancy... I made one to have my six week scan when I was six weeks, because I've had the ruptured ectopic pregnancy and a damaged fallopian tube, so I wanted to check, obviously, that the pregnancy was in the right place, which I did. Then I saw a midwife at around eight weeks to book a blood test... to see if there were any antibodies because I hadn't had an anti-D jab after the last baby. I didn't want to just have anti-D as a precaution. I wanted to know whether there were antibodies there or not, with it being a blood product. So I had that and I just asked for the results. I didn't want to have any further contact or to be booked in on the system. Obviously, she was surprised by it but she was fine about it. And they contacted me, had that done, and I got the results... and then while I was on the phone to her, I asked if she'd book me in a 20-week scan, which she did, because I've got a history of heart anomalies in my family and I wanted that checking. And when I went for that, they just did a relatively quick scan for the anomaly. I asked them if they saw the sex I'm happy to know it, but I don't need you to carry on the scan to find it or anything, just to check the heart, there's no anomalies, really and things like that, which they were fine with. The next contact I made with them... I'd got to 42 weeks pregnant and I had an episode of reduced movement. So I went into the maternity assessment unit for that... and they just did a scan that I asked for. They offered me some other things but I chose to have the monitors on for an hour, and everything was fine, so I came home again. Me and my husband thought it must be some time soon, and he was born at 43 weeks five days...

Yes, I told them from the very first appointment [that she intended to freebirth]. I think Leeds has quite a good home birth... the midwives from the hospital, they come to the home birth meetings, even though it's like a peer-to-peer support group, it's not a medical group or run by the hospital. They like to get the women to see a familiar face and it's pretty good. Obviously the supervisor of midwives, when I went for the 20-week scan, she did speak to me about it. She asked my intentions, which we told her, and they were happy that I was informed making the decision. I think if I hadn't had a lot of info with me, they might have tried to talk me round. I had that feeling. **Laura**

This time I refused antenatal care even though I am a high risk case. We refused hospital scans but we did go for a couple of private ones. I had five telephone calls with the community midwife over the course of the pregnancy which was enough to touch base with them but all on my terms. As we would stay at home from 36 weeks I felt better having a home birth kit here in case anything went wrong and the plan was always to call midwives after the birth to attend for checks after birth. The day I [baby] arrived I was up the hospital with bleeding and reduced movements after having a very rude midwife in the house. I was seen by a doctor who was telling me my baby could die, I could die and basically putting the fear of life into me. Yet I tuned into my body and I knew everything was fine. A consultant then agreed with me and she sent me home to rest and that's what I did. **Sarah M**

I didn't see anyone after. But I knew everything was fine down there and he was feeding like a good'un. It didn't even sting after. I would have been the first one to go and see anyone if I had... But no, it didn't come up so... The midwives I had with F texted saying, "Congratulations, we've heard about the birth," and, "If you want me to come up any time for a postnatal visit, just text." And they were lovely about it. **Peggy**

We did end up calling a midwife after about two and a half, three hours after birth. And I hadn't delivered the placenta then. And so we needed a little bit of help with that. But we're so grateful, and the midwife that came out was so respectful and was really okay with the fact we hadn't called them yet. One of them, I mean one of the people that W [partner] phoned... it wasn't our local sort of birthing centre, it was a different one. And they were really funny with him. They were really like not okay with us not phoning them earlier. So then actually the birthing centre that's closer to our, where the midwife came from, they were really nice.

… she ended up giving me the injection that they give you, to help to deliver the placenta. And the placenta came out really quickly... by then I was pretty out of it... And I just really wasn't in the space for it in the same way then. And the midwife was trying to check V and trying to check me. And in the end, I asked her to leave because I just wasn't up for it. But she was great, and it didn't matter. We just had some sleep after that and I have to say that the way that the midwives were afterwards, they came to visit obviously like they do. We'd gone through the proper procedures with the midwives all the way up until the birth. So we had a good relationship with them and our actual midwife, once we told her. Yes, they were amazing, they were very, what's the word, I guess, proud or complimentary about my bravery and how I had courage to do that. And you know, they were quite curious about it some of them were. Some of them were a bit funny, and didn't really say much about it. But some of them were quite curious and open to wanting to hear about why, whether we had decided to do that beforehand or not. Which I thought was so great, because some of them were really up for that, really supportive of that. And really kind of understanding... the way they were afterwards was really wonderful, and they were very supportive in relation to our problems, difficulties with breastfeeding. Which was really amazing. I was really happy in the end, really grateful for the support that we got from the midwives, even though that we had gone through the freebirth route, that you know, we admitted that we had planned to do that to them as well. And they were fine with it, which I was very glad about. **Gauri**

I gave birth 41+3 in a pool in the sitting room, very straightforward labour. It took about six hours. The baby was born and we kept the baby on the placenta for five hours and after six hours we called the midwife and asked her to come and check the baby, and check me, if I have any tears, but I felt I didn't. And they were again fantastic, really amazing. They just came, she said, "What do you want me to do?" So I told her I would like her not to touch the baby too much, I would just like you have a look, see if everything is OK. Check me. She did that and left... So it was a very, very pleasant experience... Oh my God, they are amazing! I've been to births with them and it's very... incredible... I've never seen such a good team in London... Some of them I just saw a few times. So one of them I knew [as a doula], and the others I didn't. The one who came after the birth, I didn't know her. But the midwife told us that she spoke to the whole team. She told us what we are doing. She even said she spoke to the emergency services and told them what we are doing... She said if you called an ambulance, they would prioritise you because I've told them about you. **Michaela**

Lacey found an NHS midwife who provided just the support she needed without actually attending the birth.

We actually called the midwives and it turned out F was on call, and we were so happy, because if it had been any of the other midwives, we wouldn't have had them around. F was on call, and we were like, "Hallelujah!" So she came around and she was just really stoic and relaxed, and checked me out. That was the first examination I'd had. I was like, I want to have one, I want to know what's going on, I just want to make sure everything's cool. She was like, everything's fine, you're doing great, just keep going. And that was so reassuring. She could have said the other. She had a lot of power in that moment, and by her just not saying too much, and just saying a little but it being positive, was really… it gave us all a really big lift…and then I just spent the rest of the day trying to get comfortable… and it was just getting super intense… she came around again, probably at around seven or eight, and the same thing, just checked it, and that was the first we listened to the heartbeat, and everything was fine. She was like, you're doing great, you're fine. I was like great! Because she was like, I'm leaving now! We're like, oh, great, see you! And then I went in the shower and had a really long shower.

And then something started to emerge and F was like… and he was applying some pressure and holding. I was like, "I think I have her head", and he was like, "That's not a head! What is that?" I was like, "I don't know what that is. What is it?!" So he took a picture of it and sent it to F. F was like, "It's fine – the amniotic sac, you're okay, keep going." **Lacey**

A few women knew midwives for whom their loyalty to childbearing women was greater than their duty to their employer (if working for the NHS) or their insurer (if independent). Having phone access to a midwife was very positive for a few women who wished to freebirth.

And I have a friend who is a really awesome midwife, called K, who you might know, and I had the great opportunity to just speak to her about some of this stuff. And she let me know things like how often they would like to do monitoring during birth… luckily I had K on the phone at times, who was giving me advice and telling me… she was telling me to do spinning babies moves… that clearly helped the baby's head to engage. **Ally**, describing her second labour.

Many women spoke supportively of midwives who they saw as disempowered.

I work with midwives and I see so much good. It's just they haven't got the choice that they want to give the women. They haven't got it, we have to [carry out] policies and they're so constrained and they're not supported enough. I can't even give completely, not that that's really possible, but give unbiased opinions and choices, is very hard. **ST** herself a midwife

I did feel sometimes that the midwives were kind of doing a job that they're weren't happy with, but just it is difficult to put into words I suppose, but I think that the kind of emotional support that I found really valuable at the time was the support that you can only get from somebody who is being really positive and I think a lot of the things I got from the midwives were quite subtle things, which would undermine my confidence slightly or give me the impression that all might not be well, which they have to prepare you for, but I don't know – I thought they had such a lot of procedures that they automatically do, I don't know how necessary they are really – kind of point to them having an opinion that birth is not an easy thing. **Sarah-Anne**

And I could tell that she wanted to be helpful, but that she was, I want to say extremely disempowered, but that's maybe not fair to her, I don't know because I'm not in her job; I don't know the degree of disempowerment. But you could just kind of tell, because of what she would say and how she would say it, that it was always sort of like, "Mm, it's a bit above my pay grade. And mm, I don't know that I really have the authority to confirm that such and such is an option, or is possible." All of her communication was about covering her own back. It was always, "Well if the baby's breech, then you'll have to go in to a consultant and you won't be allowed to have a home birth." And I was very much of this like, "Nobody's going to tell me allowed or not allowed. This is my body." **ME**

Some women experienced midwives as lacking autonomy which made them fearful when outside their usual area of practice. Women were quick to detect this fear and sought to separate themselves from it in order to create the safe space in which they could prepare for birth.

I thought there was a lot of fearmongering happening. So we started to kind of extricate ourselves from the NHS. **Lacey**

I guess she was scared of being at a home birth. As soon as she had come into my home, I could feel the tension. I could feel she didn't want to be there. She felt more comfortable being in a hospital and I did feel it from the beginning. I wished I had sent her away, and asked for someone else, but again, I didn't know I could. **ST** talking about the midwife at her first birth who transferred her to hospital unnecessarily and later apologised

… the midwife who was very frightened by going into somebody's space, who was so far into her labour, a midwife that felt, to do her job properly she had to have done all the assessments using the, the tool, the… Partogram, that she needed to have that done, in order for her to be able to fulfil her role as a midwife. **H** describing a birth she attended as a doula

Behind these disempowered midwives, women saw a dominant system.

I don't want to say I didn't trust them, but I didn't trust the system. It's not the people, it's the system. I felt like the individual midwives could be trusted, but I knew that they were working within a system that didn't want to allow them to work holistically with me. And I was always worried that they had invisible-to-me lines and beyond certain points, they would be funnelled by their system into pushing me down a particular path. And I was always very wary of that. Yes, bordering on scared…Because there's no flexibility, there's no room for individual professionals to use their professional judgement and their experience and their knowledge of their clients. It's all ticking boxes and - where are the women in this? **Beth**

I was afraid to ask my midwife questions and actually felt she was quite open, quite friendly, quite approachable but I still was afraid because I knew she had so much sort of put on her by the system that I would not know how to break through that – that is what I felt. **Polly**

I can only speak for myself, but my decision to birth without HCPs present wasn't because I don't trust midwives. I just felt like the space and time to birth as felt right to me was far less likely to happen in hospital, and far less likely to happen with midwives in my home. If I could have guaranteed a midwife whom I knew was going to support me in ALL my choices, without judgement, then they could have been there the whole time. But faced with a midwife who told me at the home birth assessment "Well, if you won't let us examine you or monitor you, WHAT is the point in us even being there?!" and proceeded to tell me that if they knew that I would refuse VE's/monitoring, that they would refuse to come out to me. **Emi**

And I said to my husband, "Look, I know…" I wasn't sure about the legality of not calling the midwife. So I said, "Look, just wait till you know it's too late, and then call them." Because I was like, "I don't want someone here that I don't know." And also I don't want… it's become this issue now that I just… I felt like I don't even feel at all supported by the system any more. I don't feel like they're on my side. I don't know who they're going to send. And also, interestingly, this woman who was an independent midwife, she was on the team. They could have called her, they could have had her. And it was all… I felt like almost there was a bit of an attitude of, "Why should she get what she wants?" And I felt really upset by that. Because I thought, "Actually, I'm just asking for my needs to be met. I know what they are, and it's not a big ask you know." And it makes total sense to me. Like, if I was to set up this system, I would have a home birth team, and you're appointed one person and you got to know them. Or two people. **Rachel**

For one mother the rigidity of the system had tragic consequences.

The reason I birthed entirely alone is partly due to the midwives in my borough or trust policy disabling them from simply sitting quietly in a corner until/if I need them. Plus, when I am in pain the last thing I ever want are spectators or strokes on my skin.

If the midwives could have accommodated what I wanted from them then they would have been invited in. If they'd have been there, they'd have noticed twin two's deterioration and I would still have twins and not just one baby. **Reign**

Other health care professionals were part of this system. Some women reported being bullied by consultants, which, in some cases, may have influenced the similar bullying they and others experienced from midwives.

What hasn't changed is the way consultants deal with you… I was badgered from almost 37 ½ weeks when they started calling me. Like it's not even that I was coming in for anything, they started calling me, "So you're coming up to 38 weeks. We'd like… to book you in for an induction at 38 weeks." So I obviously declined all those, because I know that would be my home birth out the window. And I felt really well; I felt much better in myself than the first pregnancy. "What you feel has no bearing on how we assess your risks." They basically told me, "We don't care how you feel. We tell you how you feel. You're 41 ½ years old, this is an IVF pregnancy, you're full term. Your baby is not making any moves of coming to this world" or whatever they were saying. At 38 weeks. That's just far too early to have that conversation. And with such insistence. And you know, dropping the dead baby card at **every** conversation. Different consultants. I have all their names. Maybe I'm going to complain about them, but maybe not. But from 38 weeks, I was, I would say harassed almost continuously by consultants. Even though I had opted out of the consultant route. They said to me that legally they have to. I'm still not sure whether that's even true. **Carmen**

Women were glad that NHS maternity services were there but they saw the service as lacking sensitivity to their needs and so they saw it as a safety-net for an emergency rather than a service they would turn to if things were going well.

In this country we're just unbelievably lucky to have that at our fingertips, it's just amazing and R [partner] and I were blown away by the amount of care, you know but also I did feel that most, that 99% of it was just wasted on me – was just unnecessary, you know, I didn't need all the visits and I didn't feel it was necessary for them to drive all the way – it was amazing, I feel, I'm not being ungrateful…and I've actually explained that to my midwives this time… and I haven't felt any need whatsoever to approach – to have any care… and I did talk to L [former midwife working as a doula]… I suppose for R as well, for my partner, maybe just some support and just to know that she's there, that she'd be on the end of a line, even if I needed to just discuss something. **Peggy**

We are SO incredibly lucky to have a free healthcare system, made up of many midwives who adore their jobs. We are unlucky in that our maternity system, rather like our education system, works on one-fits-all policy, when both education and birth need to be individualised care. The midwives I have had the pleasure of working with as a doula (both community and hospital) have been incredible… Working in tandem with a healthy respect for the different roles we are both there to provide. **Emi**

Along the same lines, some women would have liked a trusted midwife present or nearby but experience told them that midwives could not be trusted not to intervene.

It would be nice… the preferred option would be to have someone you trusted, someone who was there for you the whole time. Even the miwife I'd been discussing these things with, her personally, her actually coming to my birth and supporting me because she understood from a one-to-one relationship that we'd built, that these were the birth choices that I would prefer. And that this was the mood I was setting. And that this is the environment that I'd like to maintain whilst birthing baby. But they couldn't do it. **Peggy**

You know, it would have been nice. Because I don't know what condition baby's going to come out in, to have someone in the space or downstairs that could be a silent observer. But they really couldn't do that without having to intervene in some manner. **Jessica**

Some expressed empathy with the harassed midwives.

The rise in women choosing to birth at home, and choosing to birth without midwives must feel awful to those in the midwifery profession. I can imagine it feels incredibly personal when a woman's previous experience with a midwife leads her to be mistrusting of midwives as a whole. One bad apple spoiling the bunch. And I think often, doulas are contributing to that. I've had so many women ask me "Why do doulas dislike midwives?." THAT'S the vibe we are giving off as a community and that's wrong. It's one of the reasons that I think the presence of a doula can really get a midwife's back up at times. The fact we're providing the one-on-one, continued care throughout pregnancy, birth, and postpartum that they would LOVE to do but can't because of time, resource constraints, red tape also affects that, and the fact that many doulas are openly derisive of the midwifery community. Not ok.

I would love it to be seen more as "Look at these women, making informed, powerful choices about their births!" rather than "Look at these stupid women who don't trust midwives!" **Emi**

For some women, continuity of care from a supportive midwife would have met their needs, but this was rarely possible. For most the lack of continuity, the rigidity of maternity services and the power of midwives to influence their experience of birth loomed as a threat which they sought to avoid. The power of midwives to refer women to Social Services also cast a shadow (see chapter 19).

Section 4: Labours and births

This section contains a collection of birth stories, including two stories about the same birth related firstly by the women and secondly by her doula. The stories cover a wide range of birthing experiences, including the birth of twins. Some of the stories are told by women having their first babies, others are about second and subsequent babies. Within the stories, women describe what they needed to be able to birth their babies themselves, how they coped with labour and birth and what they needed from those around them – if anything. Some of the women describe straightforward births that they found intense but not necessarily painful or difficult, some describe births that were less straight forward and more challenging.

Without midwives and medical management, there were large variations in the lengths of their labours and the frequency and strength of their surges/contractions. While some women talked about long labours and births, others spoke about their babies arriving rapidly.

Whatever careful plans they had made and however labour progressed, the women were well aware of the uncertainties of birth. They knew that there are no guarantees wherever and however a baby is born. Some babies tragically do not survive whether or not the women have midwifery and/or medical care. Rarely, however, when services cannot or will not accommodate a woman's decisions and plans, she may feel forced to avoid maternity and other services and freebirth her baby with sad consequences.

There are no data on how many freebirths take place and no data at all on the safety or otherwise of freebirth. We searched for several years to find the two stories of loss in this section. We continued to search because we felt that the book would not have been complete without including the stories of women who had experienced the devastating loss of a baby.

There will, of course, be experiences of freebirth labours and births which are not included here.

Chapter 11: Labours and births

Different women had different experiences of labour. Some spoke of intensity rather than pain, others described intense "waves of pain" and many experienced contradictions of sensations and emotions. Some had powerful and overwhelming feelings that they could not do it anymore, but as they accepted these feelings, they passed and were absorbed into the process of the birth as no-one suggested pain relief, going to hospital, or other interventions. They described the importance of having a quiet, calm environment in which they could let go, listen to their bodies and babies, move and make sounds as they needed to and be alone or with trusted others as they wanted. These accounts show deep awareness of their bodies and their babies' bodies as labour progressed. They saw their births as embedded in their normal lives: both "amazing" and "normal."

I remembered everything I read in The Birthkeeper, I found faith in myself, my body and baby. Later that night I sat up to go to bed and my waters broke, we laughed, we hugged and we knew she was on her way. I went to the toilet, checked the kids were all okay with one of them still awake beside her brothers. I put on the t-shirt that I wanted to birth in, told my partner he didn't need to worry about the pool as I knew she was coming quick. I moved for as long as I could before the waves of pain became so intense that I ended up lying on the sofa, the exact same position I was in 11 months before birthing my son. I breathed through each pain, no real rest in-between, looking into my husband's eyes. He kept me so focused, he kept me grounded and he was the quiet strong presence I needed. Once again just us in the room that's the heart of the home, bringing our last child into the world. Once again he instinctively knew what I needed and brought I [baby] earthside onto my chest. We quickly kept her warm, skin to skin, towels, blankets but as she was 36+1 I was glad to have midwives on the way. For the second time I experienced the fetal ejection reflex. Allowing your body to do what it needs is truly moving and I know that I was able to fully give in to the natural process because I was in a calm protected environment that my husband created. **Sarah M**, sixth baby

And then it went very smoothly; I went into the pool. And friends of ours, we dance a lot, and they had made, not just for me, but they had made a CD with live music and it's a dancer takes you through a journey. So it starts very soft and flowing and then it goes into stronger beats and more staccato and more linear and…with purpose, and then it goes into chaos, where you just let go of it all and then it goes into very light, lyrical, joyful music and then, ends with something meditative and I danced to that. We put it on and it took me through the birth. So that's about an hour long and it seemed like my birth was following that pattern, and during the chaos the second stage, the roar, you know, he crowned. And I didn't have an orgasm, which was a shame (laughs). I thought this time for sure, but I didn't, but it was so blissful. And the sun was streaming in. There was a light breeze. Actually, just before he crowned, I was pushing maybe three times and without me being able to feel his head. So I did say to my friend and my husband,

"If he, if my baby doesn't crown in two pushes, then I'd like them to call the midwife just to be on standby. Just in case the cord is wrapped around his neck or, something is not right." But I think that was that fear of dying before the crowning. But also just putting things in place just in case. But then, after I said that, after one push, he crowned. And I could feel his head. His lots of hair and he was just looking around really calmly with his head out. And there were a few minutes, just utter peace and silence with quiet music playing by then and I rested and we all breathed. I had to reassure again, that he can breathe through his cord. There wasn't a hurry and after a few minutes, after another push, his body was born. And very different from the first birth... when my daughter was born she came out and I was on all fours on the bed, but as she had slipped out, she had her eyes tightly shut, she didn't want to see anything. It was bright in the room and there were people and she didn't want to see, she had her eyes tightly shut and cried... whereas this time round, it was so calm, he slipped out. I lifted him out of the water and he looked into my eyes and it was utterly beautiful. I will never forget and I'm so sad if women can't have this, I mean this is a normal birth. It can be like this. He was so... he seemed like he'd recognised me and he looked me deeply in the eyes just to check me out. He had a little look around. He was so content and I just held him. I was helped out of the pool, so I could birth the placenta as it was coming. But because I didn't have any more contractions in that time, I just sat on the sofa and I nursed him... he nursed, he came to the breast and yes, as he was simulating my breasts, oxytocin was flowing again and I birthed the placenta within fifteen minutes or something like that. Very easily, I went on my knees. **ST**

… so it was very clear that I didn't want to be in water. And actually, I couldn't really receive any touch or anything. I felt, my body felt so like anything was a distraction... when you actually go into describing it, it's just so intense. There's not really any words to describe the sensations of it. And it's everywhere in your body... my favourite position was probably just sitting and just pushing down with my arms and my hands into the earth. It felt like there was a real kind of grounding going on, and connecting to the ground beneath me. And I did kind of go into this meditation with some of it, I tried to do a bit of my birthing stuff a little bit. Because you need that to relax. And I couldn't really connect to it that well when I was actually in the labour. I was definitely very aware of my breathing. That did help... when you don't have a midwife, you don't have someone seeing where you're at, you don't really know how far along you are... it didn't even enter my head actually to think about the midwives, about whether we should call them or anything. I just knew I didn't want her there anyway. And it wasn't talked about at all... we just knew that we weren't going to call her unless there was really a problem. And it certainly didn't feel like there was any problem. It felt like I was handling it…

I mean, the actual birth itself is so hard to put into words exactly how it was, how it felt. And I think it's just so animalistic, that you just go into this, it's so beyond anything. It's not coming from your mind at all. It's just your body totally taking over. It feels like it is spirit. It is you that's doing... or the combination of you and your baby that's like, that's just happening. There's nothing... It's definitely a massive journey of surrender and... just going with it. Just totally going with what's happening and being present with what's happening in your body. **Gauri**

I had a sort of… slightly nauseous for no reason whatsoever, and I just thought, this is the start of things, I think. I went to sleep, woke up Monday morning… they were more than Braxton Hicks [contractions]… I just knew something was happening. R [partner] went to work that day. I didn't tell him that baby was on the way (laughs). I wanted him to be safe up a tree (laughs). So it was a beautiful day. Me and F [child] were outside all day and they were just getting slightly stronger, every time they were just, just very steady, slowly and… Then R got back about three – it was a short day – they were slowly getting stronger and stronger. Then F had a really early night, about half six or something, and I knew obviously that I would be labouring through the night, and I knew L was working. So I said to R, "Would you feel better if I just phoned L [doula, former midwife] and said to her, if you wanted to phone her any time in the night…?" And he goes, "Yes, go on then, let's just let her know." So I phoned L and she said, "Yes of course, I'll keep my phone on all night if you need…" I definitely felt more active in this birth than F's birth. I was just walking around a lot. But I made R have an early night because I knew, obviously, that… he doesn't have gazillions of hormones to keep him awake, and adrenaline going! I have no trouble keeping awake when I'm in labour, funnily enough! (Laughs). He woke up about half twelve. We have no hot running water or power up at ours, so we had both wood burners going and we'd got some big pans heating up water, big pans. I've got this big tree planting tub that we have baths in in the front room. It's a big tub about that big, which we can just squat down in and have a bath. F loves it as well. So he filled that up in the front room and I was in it for a couple of hours, I think, just topping up with hot water. Gradually getting more and more intense and I was definitely fully dilated at this point, I think, when F woke up about four in the morning. R was on the sofa and I was just squatting at the edge of the bed, and I could tell by R's face that F had woken up, because he was behind me. He just sort of clambered over the bed and came and sat next to me, and said, "I want a Mummy cuddle," and just put my hand round him and he knew I couldn't give any more than that at that point. I just said, "The baby's coming." And he just completely chilled out and just instinctively, he latched onto R. He just went and clambered on R. All the candles were lit and stuff at that point. It was sweltering, so R and F were just in nothing and sweating (laughs) and I was fine! F got in the tub and was splashing around for a bit. Then he got out and they went and made porridge and got on with breakfast. Because we live in one room at home. We've got a little kitchen area with the other wood burner off it, but they're all open together. So everything's in that room, our beds and everything, and the burners. So they were in the little kitchen bit getting on with breakfast and I got in the tub again. R tells me it was about half five, when O was born. I have no idea! R told me all these timings. I have no idea what timings were (laughs). You lose track, don't you? I just remember saying when I was in the tub, I remember saying to R "bring F over to look at the head!" And he brought F over and F saw O's head out. I remember feeling the little ear. Then you started moving your head. I was like, ooh! Kicking inside me, obviously to turn himself.

It was a very strange feeling. Then within a few minutes, he was out. The next push, you were out, weren't you? I remember thinking, straight away, you're definitely smaller than F was! It was all just… ever since I can remember, the birth I wanted, ever since I was a teenager probably, thinking I'm definitely going to give birth like that. Do you know what? I can honestly say there was not one point throughout the whole labour, that I wanted anyone else there, that I felt I needed anyone else there, that even entered my head that - should someone else be here? And R was so chilled out, because I was so chilled out. He was so chilled out, and he said after, "It was so nice, not to have anyone else there, just to know that it was just us and not have to worry about another fire going, making a cup of tea, or having anyone else in the house." He said it was just amazing. And it was just the dream, even down to F seeing everything. It was amazing. Obviously, I probably would have chosen less pain (laughs). Everything else was just perfect. We can all dream of one of these pain-free births (laughs) but it definitely wasn't pain-free. Maybe the next one, if it happens! So I got out of the tub with O then, after a few minutes, and went and sat on the sofa. We just draped this bit of canvas that we've got over it. And then F came over for a proper look at you, didn't he? And he was feeding within minutes, latched on and eyes wide open. And you were as content as Larry, weren't you? I don't know how long after I birthed the placenta… I birthed the placenta and then it was sat on the thing next to me in this tub thing, on the sofa next to me. And then you were feeding away. A while later I noticed how cold the cord had got, so obviously that had done all it's meant to do. It had gone stone cold, and as it touched me I thought, gosh, that's amazing. It had gone stone cold. Then I just reached over and R cut the cord and put one of these food clips on it, and it worked brilliantly. It was all really clean and lovely and that was it. **Peggy**

I didn't feel any pain, I just let it go. And then, it was like, all of a sudden, we'd already put sheets and plastic stuff down everywhere with blankets and everything on top. So, I was free to deliver wherever I wanted. And there was a little toilet, bathroom in the room as well that adjoined it. So everything was there, and I had some candles lit, and, and I just suddenly realised about three or half three in the morning maybe, that really, he was working his way out. And I was going to the toilet quite a lot. It didn't matter, it's fine, it's just pooh, and it's just coming out. And, and I remember being able to visualise really strongly everything that was actually happening, because the midwife had explained it to me in such a clear way. And my partner said, "Well, I'll put some of that music on that you found." So, he put some music on, and lit the candles, and he said, "Shall I call the midwife?" I said, "No, no, it's fine, I don't want anyone here." And I said, "Maybe you should warn your Dad," because his Dad was upstairs. I said, "Maybe you should call him in case there's any kind of noise or something." But actually, it turned out I didn't ever make any noise. And I think it seemed like all of a sudden I was on my knees on the floor, and his head just came out, and then once his head's out, the rest of him was coming. So, it was just me, the baby, and his Dad, and we were there… She [midwife] arrived after the whole birth, and, and the placenta was still… I just remember saying, "You've got to keep me warm now, keep me warm so I can get the placenta out. And kiss me, just kiss me, so that we can get this placenta out." And the whole thing was an incredibly sensual experience for the two weeks even before the birth I was really conscious that I had to feel sexual, at this time, it was all a sexual process as well... there was no rush, and there was no time. There was no thought about time. **Katuš**

It's a soft, misty spring morning in... Ireland. I had planned to plant out the spring cabbage seedlings today in the garden on our wild green land at the southernmost tip of the peninsula. Today is April fifth and I, a young pregnant woman of twenty-five years, awoke knowing that my baby was on the way. I had had a "show" and knew that my labour would start before too long just as it had for the birth of our daughter some three years previously.

I kept this delicious secret to myself and my partner as we lived in a community at the time but this was private, our baby was coming and it was our business only.

The cabbages were planted that day, with me crawling on all fours up the rows, carefully planting what would be welcome greens in the "hungry gap" before the main crop of vegetables became ready in the summer.

By evening time I felt very tired and although I had no contractions that I was aware of, I decided that I really didn't actually want to have my baby right now and would much rather sleep so after a bath in the tin bath in front of the open fire, I slept deeply and peacefully.

It wasn't until the early hours of the next day as dawn came, that I was woken by immense and powerful contractions that I had to focus deeply on as I breathed through them as they surged through my body.

I quickly woke up my partner and asked him to hurry as the baby was on the way. He leaped up, lighting candles and paraffin lamps and got a fire going. He carefully put the prepared cord ties into a little tin with methylated spirits in, as this was our way of cleaning them.

Our daughter, who had a little bed at the end of ours woke, startled. "What you playing?" she asked in surprised innocence. "It's okay" we said, "we're just having the baby."

Soon came a massive urge to push. "Stop" "yelled my partner - "I'm not ready!" But there was no way I could stop as incredible primal urges overtook my body and I roared our baby out. Such a wild feeling as his hot, wet body slithered down the inside of my leg, propelled further down the bed in a torrent of amniotic fluid. "It's a BOY!" said my partner with excitement. "Is he okay?" were my first words as boy or girl didn't matter to me at this stage, I just needed to know that he was okay and I scooped him onto my chest while our daughter snuggled into my arms. **Caroline B**

And I woke up at four or five in the morning with a sensation of my waters breaking. Water, you know, wet all over the bed. It woke me up straight away. I woke up and I realised it had started and I'd planned for, you know, darkness, candles and soft music and water. And you always plan it like this and then it ends up being the opposite, not in terms of the C section, but just in terms of the sun's coming up. People are going, the windows are open because it's hot. There are people talking on the street outside, cars, ambulances, whizzing past. And it's happening too quick to get the water in the pool. I tried, woke up, had about twenty minutes of just kind of prayer and realising it was going to happen now. Even though I didn't particularly, I didn't want to be pregnant for a second time and I didn't want a baby at that time, but I did a baby. And I did want a sister for E, so… It just wasn't the best timing for me… "Oh, my God, I need to call my friend who's my doula." And she was just, like, "You know, it's going to be slow, so I'm just going to go back to sleep for another half hour." I was like, "I don't think you are, you need to come round now."

So, whilst she was getting herself ready, I tried to make breakfast, it didn't work. I tried to have a shower, it didn't work. I tried to get the water in the pool, didn't work because I kept having these intense contractions. So I realised, I didn't realise how quick it would be, but anyway. So I ended up on the yoga mat, where I'd been doing my stretches just before I'd gone to bed… It's a great birth aid. Because it's a really thick one, it was all spongy and good for my knees. I was just on this birth yoga mat, and I don't think I really moved from there, to be honest. I think I moved to the toilet to, kind of, empty your back passage that you get, push down and then that happens. And I was even embarrassed to do that in front of my friend, can you believe, we're so bloody English, aren't we like, but pooing in front of someone is worse… than having sex in front of someone… to me that's like the worst anyway, but we did that. And she was just, like, "Oh, it's all right, darling."

And then, and then I was gripped by what looked like a surge of adrenaline and I was gripped by the idea that I was turning inside out, because I could actually feel the baby's head, but that's on all fours… daylight sort of pouring in through the window. Sirens sailing past the Velux windows and we're on the oak floor… On a yoga mat and there's like blood dripping down my legs. And the sensation's intense and I just keep remembering to breathe. And it's overwhelming, but not kind of, oh, totally within, I mean, like on the edge of my comfort zone, put it that way. Like on the very edge. Like much more of it and I'm, I'm not going to handle it. But then you've got no choice but to handle it. And the head was out, and I was feeling the head, and realising that there was no sensation when I touched the head. Thinking that that part of me was dead or something and it, and it had prolapsed, it was falling out, that something had gone terribly wrong… and C said, "No, darling, that's her head." And one more contraction and the body came out. And literally, I looked down and saw the body come out, and then C literally just passed her… through my legs, up to my arms. I came up, came up on my knees. I held this shimmering, shiny, little baby, and she didn't even cry. Kind of spluttered a bit (choking sound). And she opened, her eyes were wide open. I've got pictures of all of this. Bits, like covered in blood and white stuff and C wrapped her in a towel and it was then, I couldn't believe how uncomfortable it was, because I had the cord… hanging through my legs, so I couldn't really sit on it. It was really uncomfortable.

I was naked and started getting cold, so she wrapped me in a blanket. And, but I was still on my knees, holding, and holding this like tiny little creature. And it wasn't that, sadly it wasn't that immediate like overwhelming love I felt for my first. It was much more of a slow burner, because I hadn't wanted another baby. But I breastfed her and everything was perfect and she was quite big. And it's just, it was actually the perfect birth. Apart from the fact that I didn't really want to give birth at that time. I mean there was nothing about it that could have been more amazing, apart from being in the pool. And then we climbed into, it's so amazing to clamber into my own bed after the birth. Unbelievably comforting. I couldn't imagine there's anything better. **Rose**

The flexibility of freebirth was particularly valued where there were other children, whether or not the mother wished them to be present for the birth. It also enabled partners to continue with their normal activities around the needs of the labouring woman and the woman to choose who she wanted present at any point in her labour.

And then I was like, "Yes, okay, out-of-office on. Now, now's time." And then I just really went into myself, and I didn't want anyone around me. I didn't want G [partner] near me. I was listening to classical music, which I hadn't expected to want to listen to. You know, we spend all these times talking about playlists and making playlists. And I didn't want any of the music that had been put on my playlist. There was something that I didn't want any words or, or associations, I think, with things. Whereas just some classical music that I didn't really know, piano music, was just there, gently flowing in the background. And as I was going into myself, I was kneeling on the floor, holding onto a birth ball, just being loose and with it, and allowing all the sensations to run through me. And it was like I was a vehicle, like I was a receptacle for all of these strong waves and feelings that were just sort of taking over me, and my job was to let go as much as possible, to allow it to do that. And I was just thinking about being open, holding my jaw open, making loose noises with my jaw being open. I think I started to listen to *BD*, whose tracks are I guess a bit like hypno-birthing, but it's more like... I would say, like, positive coaching, where she says things like, "Having a baby is the most natural thing in the world." And it's about having a little cheerleader there to tell you, "It's all good. You're doing fine. This is all natural. All these feelings are right." And I think maybe G started to set up the birth pool. I remember him asking me to move at some point, and I just said, "Just work around me. Like, I cannot move." He was sort of being all practical, birth pool, duh-da-duh-da-duh. And I think he got it all set up, and then there was a moment where he went, "I'm just going to go upstairs and fill it up." And I said, "No. No, you can't. You've got to come here." And I needed him to come to me right then, because I could feel like something was changing and happening, and it was, there was something very intense going on. And so he came behind me, and he was holding me on my hips. And I think at that moment, I knelt down, clenched up, and sort of went, "I can't do this." And he was like, "Yes, you can." And then I knelt back up. And then... I can only really describe as a feeling of like I was sort of like vomiting or, she was expulsively shot out of me within a couple of contractions. And I just sort of felt myself

emptying out, and there was nothing I could do. I don't even feel like I was bearing down. It was just like whoof. And then she dropped down onto the floor, which had been padded with some cushions. And... I think we grabbed some of the inco pads and set them under me. And then G said, "Pick her up, pick her up." And I was just kneeling and looking between my legs, looking at her. And he said, "Pick her up, pick her up." He knew that I didn't want anyone else to pick up the baby. But that wasn't my first instinct. I was definitely just looking. And, and then I did pick her up, and I brought her to me, and she cried. And then I was just shaking. I was just shaking, shaking, shaking, and trying to sit down. And he's putting towels over us. And then we called the midwives.
Katy B, second baby, first freebirth

I really started feeling like I wanted to be in the pool. I'd not got into the pool with any of my other children. And they filled it up enough that I could get in there. I was listening to BD again. She was telling me it was the most natural thing in the world. It was all good. And the eye mask was on. Yes, I was in another state. I got into the pool, and I stretched out sort of froggy-style: legs on my tummy, arms over the edge. And it felt amazing. It felt like I was being held and I was floating. And I really don't remember being in the pool very long before it seemed like there was a big shift in the contractions, and there was a massive pause. And I felt the pause, and I thought, "Ah, something's happening. Something different's happening." And again I felt that fear. And it wasn't a fear of giving birth; it was a fear of everything that's coming ahead of us.

And I needed to be... I was holding tightly onto their hands. And they were telling me... I think they weren't saying much, but... if I needed that reassurance, they were saying, "You're doing great." And, and then I started to feel a real sense of bearing down, and like I had to support that bearing down. It was, but it wasn't quite that expulsiveness of A's birth. It was definitely like a baby's moving. He felt bigger. I could really feel his head moving through me. I remember, there was a moment, and we've actually recorded the last minute of the birth. I wanted to be filmed. And actually, when my sister tried to set up the camera, I didn't want it in my face. But she managed to just sort of turn it on right at the end. It was interesting. I definitely felt the lens on me, when she tried to put it on... So even though she knew I wanted it, it was really hard to have it there. But with this, it was like I could just... again, it was just like mouth open. I felt like I was like, "Aaaagghh," with every... drawing down, drawing down. I can almost feel it again. And him coming down. I remember I said, like, "It feels really funny." And I put my hand back and his head was out. And that's what felt really funny. And it took a few contractions for him to come out. It was the head and then it was the body. And I remember my doula saying, "Reach down for your baby. He's there," And I was going, "I don't think he's out yet." He wasn't fully out. He was half out. And it was that... yes, the feeling funny, and then the body... And it was the strangest sensation, birthing a baby in water. Because I felt like his body was trying to bob up back to the surface, and it was floating. But he was half out of me. So I could sort of feel this baby moving around, half out of me. But it was definitely... he wasn't going to just shoot out like A did. It was definitely like a one, and then another one, and then another one, and he was in the water. And then what felt like an eternity, but it really was maybe a second. I was just sort of there going, "Oh." And they said, "Reach for your baby." And I had to manoeuvre from being on my knees to... I felt like I needed to move onto my back. And then I wasn't really sure where to put my legs. But this was seconds. And then pulling baby out. And then I was just looking at him again, and I said, "The cord, the cord." And he had the cord around his neck. And I knew that wasn't scary, but I wanted, I needed someone else to do it. I couldn't think myself to unloop it. I got someone else to do that. And then I just brought him to me. And he was very quiet and still, and just eyes open and looking at me. And I think I probably sucked on his nose, because I felt like I needed to unblock any mucous there. But he wasn't really, he wasn't crying, but I wasn't, it wasn't like he was meant to be crying or anything. And he was just there, like he is now, but looking up at me. And, and then we were just there in the pool. And it was so peaceful. And I think maybe he went on the boob quite quickly. And G had been downstairs for all of this. I said, "Happy for you to be there." I didn't necessarily want him in the birthing space at that moment, because I didn't feel like it was the right support for me. But I said, "Oh, go and tell G the baby's here." And he came up. And then, I think he went and got A, who was over the road. So she always says, "Oh, I was there when A [baby] was born." because she came in when he was in the pool and I was in the pool. And we stayed in there, had the towels over us. And then I could feel the cord was still inside me. The placenta hadn't dropped out like it had last time. I felt like I'd torn, so I asked my doula to call the midwives, because I felt like I wanted them to check us over – not right now, but in a bit. Because I felt like I'd torn, and I thought, "I just, I want that reassurance, actually." And then we stayed in the pool, and I actually, I sent everyone away out of the room again, so we could just be me and him in the pool, with towels over us, so it was keeping him warm. And just feeding and... again, making the same sounds I'd been making in labour, through those contractions, that were allowing that placenta out. And it took over an hour for the placenta to come away, which surprised me, actually. **Katy B**, third birth, second freebirth

I call N (doula) and I tell her, "You know, I'm in labour. I'm fine. You know, I want to be by myself." And she came from another birth, so she was like, "Okay. So I'm going to go and rest till you call me, if you want." And I never call the midwives. And then I was labouring all night by myself. I remember that night is really beautiful. It was in summer, the fourth August, and it was one of those nights that nearly don't get dark. And then when it is starting to getting dark, it is starting to get light again. And I remember looking through the window, and I was being sick all night and pooing. And dancing and with my music and it was really, really beautiful and magic. And when I was feeling the time of the baby coming, I call N, and I say, "N, I think baby is here, is going to be here soon." And she came. And ten minutes after she came, O was born. We just get up F, the Dad, and he cut the cord in my living room.

And it was really, really nice. And N was there, but she never did nothing. And after that, after half an hour, something like that, we called the midwives. **Bea**

Two days before he was born, I decided a good exercise would be to write down G's birth story as if it had already happened. Reading over it now, I am surprised (and not) by how much of it happened exactly as it is written.

When I woke up on the ninth, sometime before 8am, I thought to myself, "Wouldn't it be funny if I felt my first contraction now?" I went into labour around 7am with both A and E. Like clockwork, I felt a surge. I remembered that during the night I got up to go to the toilet and felt certain I would give birth the following day. The surge felt different, but not strong. Another followed a little later, but they were very spaced apart and no stronger than any Braxton Hicks, so I wasn't sure they meant much. But I had a feeling.

H (doula) messaged me to see how I was and I mentioned maybe, maybe something was going to happen. H had a knack, throughout my pregnancy of knowing exactly what I needed to hear and when and I recalled how she was one of the first people I had told I was pregnant. I didn't even have to ask her to be my doula – we both knew she would be.

But I wasn't sure that labour was close to starting. At 10am, feeling restless, I decided we should go for a walk. We walked for an hour, stopping off at the shop to get snacks. I had a strong desire not to engage in small talk with the over-zealous checkout lady, so I waited outside with A. Occasionally, I'd feel another surge, but they were very irregular and still not so strong at all. So we walked. Close to home, I felt one which was stronger and stopped me walking for a moment.

At home, I went upstairs to lie down, wondering if I should try to get some rest in case labour was imminent, but I felt restless and uncomfortable. I wanted to keep moving.

I took off all my clothes, which in retrospect should probably have been a good indicator of what was happening, but I still felt like, if things were indeed beginning, it might be days yet till I birthed.

H (partner) was updating H (doula). When either of my kids tried to talk to me I felt irritated – another sign, in retrospect. My only thoughts were that I really wanted to move my body and that I absolutely did not want to eat anything.

About ten days before G was born, for the first time since early pregnancy, I felt inexplicably tired. I had so much energy during this pregnancy, and for so long, that I was surprised by the sudden sheer force of exhaustion that overcame me. I slept on and off for two days.

And then, I felt inexplicably sad. So many emotions seemed to rise up at once, and every time I tried to find where they were coming from, or what they were about, I was lost. I had no idea.

I still don't. I drew, and I wrote. I meditated. I walked and did my best to ground myself, thinking often of the strange and beautiful reiki experiences, the symbols and visions which had arisen from them, that seemed connected to these big feelings.

Fears rose up too, and I was instinctively aware of the need to let these feelings be felt, to give them air. I wrote the fears down and sat with them, and then I tore up the paper.

I cried, sometimes wept, and felt a solid sense of grief. Then it seemed to pass quite suddenly. I don't fully understand what happened, but I know that this was an essential and important part of preparing to birth. Maybe it was the first part of letting go.

It wasn't until noon that I started to think I was most likely in labour. The surges were still quite spaced apart but they were stronger. I danced through almost every one. I stood in the doorway and swung my hips back and forward and did a kind of squatting belly dance. A big, swirling naked lady humming and dancing.

The dancing felt so good. I almost felt like I could have gone for a run. When I felt a surge, I focused on it and imagined my body opening up. I could feel the bones in my pelvis loosening.

H started to inflate the pool, although I really had no idea if I was being premature. I threw up into a metal bowl and felt mildly annoyed that despite having not eaten (I never want to eat in labour), I still ended up being sick. Being sick, even once, is absolutely the worst part of labour for me.

Just before 1pm, I had a surge that was pretty intense, and I thought "I hope this isn't just the beginning and I keep having these kinds of surges for days – what if my labour lasts a whole week and I can't cope?"

I breathed. I felt pretty happy that the surges were so focused at the front because I knew that meant G was not back to back. Then, at 1pm, I got into the pool and H called H to let her know I might want her soon, despite me voicing concerns to him that I didn't want to call her until things were really on their way.

I felt a pressure and a pop and realised my waters had broken as I saw a gush of slightly darker water in the pool. There was a lovely sense of relief after this, which I thought was pretty cool since A's waters had been broken by the midwife, and E's had gone just as he was being born.

H arrived at 1.30pm. I was moving a bit around the pool, still enjoying the feeling of being active. I think I said to H that I hoped I hadn't called her too soon. I remember that A did not want to leave the room, so she sat next to H on the couch. I remember that H took her hand. I remember feeling completely calm and present and wanting, needing to feel every single sensation.

I remember the light in the living room, the fullness of the birthing pool and the distinct sharp feeling of my pelvic bones opening up.

I remember A saying to H that G was going to be born in two minutes and H replying that it might take a bit longer, yet. Then two minutes later, G was born.

The amazing thing about birth is not how extraordinary it is, but how completely and utterly ordinary and normal it can be. At ten am I was in our local shop buying Oreos.

At two pm, I birthed a baby, and at 6pm, I was eating lasagne that a friend had dropped round.

G was born about two feet to the left of where his brother was born after a couple of hours of labour. From the photos, I can see that after his head came out I raised my left leg, as if I am preparing to propose. I don't remember doing this, but I do recall knowing I needed to move in the moment after the head was born but before the rest of him popped out.

H and E heard me say, "Oh, hello G!" and came through from the dining room.

After a few moments the water began to feel cool and I wanted to get out as I was still shaking a little.

I moved to the sofa which was covered in towels. I always forget how clumsy this part of birth is – not wanting to let go of G but trying to get out of the pool with the umbilical cord dangling between my legs, still fastening us together.

The afterpains were incredibly intense. I knew I'd have no bother with the placenta and it came out with a slight push. Since we intended on having a lotus birth, the placenta had been placed in a glass bowl, inside a towel, with the cord still attached to G. After a while, G nursed and then I felt like I wanted to go upstairs to bed.

H had made me some peppermint tea since I hadn't eaten and that helped me to warm up. She helped me clean up whilst H held G and then her and H covered the placenta in salt to help it to dry out. H brought me toast in bed whilst G was wrapped up against my skin.

Later, after H had left, I told a few people. The kids came upstairs and showered G in excited kisses and a little curious prodding. I ate lasagne. The cord had gone stone cold and every time we moved it annoyed me, and G would flinch when it touched his skin. We cut it and tied some sterile floss around it.

Then we hunkered down and stared at G and his dark hair and dark eyes and familiar smell, and it was almost just like any other day. A sense of home welled up around me, and I was thankful to be in my bed, surrounded by my people – now five bodies, instead of four. **Kendal**, third child, first freebirth

Chapter 12: Three first labours and births

On the morning of April 14th, 2021, I woke up feeling different in a subtle way. I ate poached eggs on crumpets with marmite in the bath, and then decluttered my laptop desktop and added more songs to my Labour+Birth playlist. At 3pm I drove out to attend an acupuncture appointment, and this time she applied small electrical charges through each needle via probes on crocodile clips attached to a handheld battery pack. I drove home and started tidying the house; the tightenings in my belly were beginning, and I wanted my nest to be tidy. I was filled with a soft, pleased excitement. I knew this was it, and it wouldn't stop this time until the completion.

K [partner] came home... I sat beside him... every nine minutes I took a break to get onto my hands and knees and breathe steadily through the ever-increasing intensity of the womb-tightenings. My Mum made dinner and we sat down around 8pm. My Mum and K began chatting about things unrelated to birthing, and the lights in the kitchen were brighter than upstairs. It felt like altogether the wrong atmosphere, and besides, I wasn't the least bit hungry. I left them to their food, while I went upstairs and put on music to help me shake the tension out of my hips and pelvis with a pelvic rotation to the rhythm of the beat. I was very restless and full of an electric energy and the pain of the contractions was now increasing steadily each time along with an accompanying feeling of being giddy and drugged, floating away from my normal state now.

I called M [retired midwife] between contractions and sounded perfectly normal to myself. She asked whether I would like her to come over, and I told her, "yes" politely, letting her know that there was no hurry other than that I would value her reassurance in light of the increasing intensity of how things felt in my body now. It was by now around 9pm. She told me that she'd take a shower to wake herself up, and head on over shortly afterwards. I hung up, and then called my doula, K too. She said unless I was very urgent to have her there, she'd head over after finishing a late supper. I said that was perfectly fine. I texted B [retired midwife and friend of the family]: "Glad it's begun at last. A bit nervous. Uncomfortable. Restless. Farty. Nauseous. Spacey. Shaky." She texted right back: "A perfect description. Well done Nao. Your body was made for this. Let it happen. Eat and drink while you feel like it. Use leaning forward positions. Remember all is normal. Xxxxxxx"

The contractions now felt like a unique mixture of nausea and burning - an aching wave - and, when they came, there was nothing to do to find any relief but to be on my hands and knees taking long breaths in and out. They were like the worst period pain I'd ever had to the power one hundred. K had finished his supper and came upstairs to join me now. We found together that it helped greatly to have him support my belly using the woven fabric sling my sister had given us for the new baby. When the full force of each contraction hit, K would lift the weight of my bump upwards using the sling, greatly easing the intensity of the pain, making it feel manageable to handle.

This is how my doula K found me, and she entered into the scene silently, respectfully, sitting on the carpet at my level, some metres away. I looked up into her eyes mid-contraction and saw calmness, respect, and love. An atmosphere of stillness and sanctity was gathering now, and I could feel it amongst all of my supporters as they quietly and lovingly went about their activities of holding space for me. At my husband's request, K readied the birth pool and whispered that I could enter whenever I wanted. I realised that I was afraid to leave the combination of K and the wrap-sling, in case the pain that felt only-just-containable escalated to a level that felt scary to me without the safety of this coping strategy that I'd found. I did want to try the pool, though, and was sure that I couldn't handle even the short time it would take to walk from one room to the other. I therefore instructed K to keep the sling in position while I crawled along the corridor and into the living-room. I was helped into the pool, immediately missing being on all-fours with my bump-sling-support. I tried to embrace the warm water as my new safe haven and pain-reliever.

As I wholeheartedly dove into the unknown and intense experience of giving birth, my body was producing the exact chemicals I needed to cope. I was being shown moment by moment - through my intuition and my embodied awareness - the tools I needed to reach for and hold onto with all my might. Somewhere in the transition between all-fours-on-the-carpet and the birthing pool, making sounds became a vital part of my pain-relief arsenal. Every time a contraction's new burning wave of sensation began to crash upon me, I found a deep, dark, low sound somewhere at the back of my throat that exactly matched the frequency of the pain's impact. I uttered each continuous breathy moan with complete focus, experiencing it as a lifeline. The sound gave substance to my breath, and kept me exactly in the present, and firmly, even sternly, away from any future fear.

M entered shortly after I found my way into the pool and found my voice. She entered with the utmost respect, wordlessly taking her place on the sofa beside K. The labour began to take on an element of performance, and a part of me enjoyed that, receiving energy and encouragement from being the centre of attention. Someone had lit the row of beeswax candles I'd set up all along the shelves and bookcases and the room was aglow with a warm, soft light.

Although the warm water provided a lovely way to relax and let go completely between contractions, I was starting to find that, when the contractions hit, I kept wanting to clamber up to standing. This seemed to give me a sense of control and power: I was standing over the pain and intensity - somehow looking down upon it from an elevated position and therefore somehow better able to be with the pain when it hit. I felt I needed to make my body as tall and wide as I could so that I could embrace and contain the pain. As the contractions continued and dilation increased, I found I wanted to encourage my pelvis to expand in width and breadth, even if only in my mind's eye, as I prepared to open my mind to what lay ahead. I therefore found myself seeking support from K to raise one bent leg all the way up to rest on the taut, hard inflated wall of the pool. K stayed standing from then on, meeting me every time I stood to meet a contraction, holding me in his arms as I half held, half pushed against his strong body. I recall him looking into my eyes and moaning and mooing along with me. He rode each wave of burning, churning, nauseous pain along with me through mirroring me at it.

We got into a groove by saying "Yes… Yes…" together. The invitation in the word was to open to this experience and keep opening to it - keep relaxing into it despite any temptation to resist it, shy away from it, tense up against it. The word Yes said again and again with K's support became a new lifeline, a mantra… Something about saying each extended "essss" provided for me an opportunity for controlling my breath and my mind, and gave me a focus into which the wild intensity of each moment could be channelled.

At one intermission between contractions, I remember being filled with rage towards K. How come I had to go through with this massive feat and he got to become a Dad as a pain-free onlooker? It didn't seem at all fair to me at that moment. I got an intuitive download that my years of ambivalence about becoming a mother had been tied up with an unaddressed subconscious awareness of the fury and intensity of childbirth, as well as perhaps fears and doubts as to my capacity to handle it. I believe I spoke some of these thoughts and feelings out to K, M, K, my Mum… whoever was listening. I'm not sure how coherent I was at what I was trying to express, though, and the strong emotions seemed to pass as quickly as they'd arrived as I dove with abandon into the next contraction. I was unsure on some level whether my abandon to meet each contraction as wholeheartedly as I could came from courage or foolhardiness. Either way, I kept finding myself facing and going into the experience of each one with the same open "Yes" to feel it all.

Through listening to women's experiences of birth through podcasts and my NCT teachings, I had learned of a moment of clarity that can come at the transition point between ending cervical dilation and the beginning of the head entering the birth canal. I've heard that it can be a moment of panic for women, when they lose the knowledge that they are equal to the task at hand. I felt myself falter here too. Inside my body, I could feel a corner that wanted and had to be turned to proceed. I could also feel some strongly fearful parts of me holding back from the turning that wanted to turn. I wanted to go back, it felt too hard all of a sudden. I felt suddenly crushingly aware that the burden of responsibility to carry this all off on behalf of myself and my family all lay on me. I had no idea how to do this. I'd always relied on my mind to figure out obstacles that lay in my path, and it terrified me that my mind was no use at all. I sensed that the answer was to soften and allow, but the fearfulness held me back from doing so: what if I wasn't able to handle the intensity and became flooded and overwhelmed? What if the process were to injure me and the pain was overwhelming?

I asked someone to call B and put her on speakerphone so we could talk. I wanted to borrow some of what I'd always experienced as her total and unfaltering belief in women's capacity to give birth on their own strength… At this stage, I was faltering… I was even beginning to touch on the painful depths of a familiar underlying insecurity that's often haunted me and which I've often carried with me through much of my life: a sense that I'm inherently incapable of being successful and where others emerge victorious. The intensity of the 'transition' phase was bringing up some beliefs about myself that had been formed during unhappy, even traumatic, events in earlier life... I knew that I couldn't be alone with these self-doubting thoughts and that energy was beginning to rise out of my body and into circling thinking. I tried to express some of this to B, between bouts of deep, mooing moans. Okay, I was coping so far and had got to this point okay, but what made her think I could follow through to the very important completion of this task?

For whatever reason, I was daunted by what lay ahead. I knew I had to take a leap of faith, and I was afraid. The fear was activating a self-critical part of me. My birth experience so far had been one outside time. I couldn't tell you what time it was, or how long I had been in labour, whether minutes or hours. However, this judgmental part of me was beginning to have me focus on time now. It was trying to dissect my experience of giving birth so far into slices of time, past and future. It wanted to compare them against one another in impressiveness level and level of challenge: what I'd achieved so far was *nothing* compared to what I would need to handle going forward. I was in danger of a negative mental cycle: It seemed that this part of me was both fueled by and causing fear and self-doubt in me. It was trying to rather harshly and unfavourably weigh up my capacity to handle what was to come, fear and self-doubt coming out through whispered labels of me as a person: "You're weak. You're cowardly. Others before you may have been up to the task, but you're not."

I remember B's words gently challenging what that self-critical part of me was trying to do. She said "You're doing it." And... "you'll have your baby soon".

When I hung up the phone with B, M said: "You've already done a lot." Simple words, but powerful in their effect. My inner-critic quietened, and I knew I had to sing. God has often put songs into my mind at pivotal moments in my life, with a message or a metaphor or just for encouragement. The one that sprung to mind this time was *I have confidence* from the Sound of Music. I knew I wanted to not just sing the song inside, but to perform it to my audience K and M, seated on the sofa beside my birth pool 'stage'. K tried to join in, but I quietened him: I knew this was a solo performance and the words were just for me. "I have always longed for adventure, to do the things I never dared. Well, now I'm facing adventure... so why am I so scared? Oh I must stop these doubts, all these worries: if I don't I just know I'll turn back. I must dream of the things I am seeking: I am seeking the courage I lack."

I didn't remember all the lyrics of the song, but the line that felt like a lifeline to me formed a rope to hang onto and take me back to courage: 'I have confidence in sunshine... I have confidence in rain... I have confidence that spring will come again. Besides which you see, I have confidence in me.' Something about the reminder of the strength of the elements: fire, water, the inevitable cycles of nature. I couldn't believe in my own strength at that moment, but I could place my faith in these. Looking back, it makes me think of the moment of Buddha's enlightenment. On the brink of realisation, all his demons come up to taunt him: "What makes you think you're so special that you can do this?" Realising himself powerless in the face of this harsh self-doubt within, the Buddha recounted reaching down to touch the earth beneath him. This gesture represented a call for help and the help that came. All the support he needed was available to him at that moment as he acknowledged his contact with something far greater than him: his connection to all of life.

M suggested someone fetch a bag of frozen peas and hold it against my forehead and across the back of my neck. This felt extremely good. It somehow balanced me, and helped me feel comfortable all over. Extra heat that had built up was released, and I felt cooler, calmer and more collected. From here on, it seemed that everything happened very quickly. My focus quietly, calmly and completely rested with pinpoint precision onto something I hadn't been aware of so acutely before: the shape of my baby's head. The process was like a shutter closing: the focus narrowed until it centred on just the fully-open cervix, the baby's head moving down and the finite tracking of every sensation as the dense parting tissues of my vaginal canal met the steadily moving shape of the head along its passage. I felt like a witness to the interplay between vagina and head, rather than in any way instrumental to what they were doing. The words that best describes my part in the process now is 'allowing', and 'focused witness'. I would not stand in the way of this perfect union and the progress they inherently and intuitively knew. I felt I trusted it completely and my mind was steady and calm.

Within what felt like moments, I could feel the head resting at the entrance of my vagina, and a little fear returned. I had heard that most women tear during vaginal deliveries. B had ended our conversation cautioning me to go gently at the end. I realised I didn't know *how* to go gently. The head had taken on a momentum and the only way my vagina seemed to know how to hold it back at this stage was to stay tightly closed and prevent it from coming out at all, which I knew wasn't a sustainable course of action. Suddenly it all felt rather 'all or nothing': keep the baby in and stay unharmed, or open up and plop it out, and tear yourself in the process. A burning feeling was starting to spread out from my perineum bowed and stretched tight over the head that was insistent in its downwards/outwards trajectory. I remember someone saying I should take small panting breaths at this stage, so I tried that out, but it didn't seem to do anything helpful so I stopped. M said that, if I wanted a water birth, I should crouch down in the water now, but I didn't really understand what she meant and for some reason that didn't feel like what my body wanted to do: I wanted to stay standing...

I asked whether M would... hold my perineum against the pressure of the head so that the burning would ease and it could stretch and hopefully no tearing would occur. I'd seen a photo of this in 'Birth In Focus' so I knew it was possible and I pictured it in my mind's eye now. I wanted it for myself and for my vagina: like a strong, pink balloon with a slit of baby-hair filling the air-hole.

A flannel soaked in warm water was fetched and M knelt by the birth pool and stretched her arms across the inflated walls to between my legs where I stood with my back to her. Her support holding the tight perineum was just right, though even with just a little too much pressure on her part the burning returned and I yelped out for her hands to hover in place.

I think it was at this moment that K chose to leave. Unbeknownst to me, he had gone to fetch my Mum from the kitchen, sensing rightly that the birth was imminent and that she would miss the moment unless she came right away. I felt naked and alone without him, and had no explanation of his sudden disappearance. K [doula] took his place holding me up, and she was strong and solid despite being much smaller and shorter; I could tell her whole heart was in this task. But I missed K. My mind threw in a fleeting fear: had he decided he didn't want to be a Dad after all? Had he lost courage and wanted to abandon the mission? I knew his mother had given birth to him and then had immediately left the hospital to prepare the rest of her seven children for an important annual event in the town. I couldn't help wondering at this moment whether the trauma of being abandoned himself as a baby meant he couldn't be available for this mother and this baby now, when it mattered so much? A very determined part of me took over and decided that I was going to go through with this with or without him. I turned my focus back to inside my body and leant my full weight against K [doula], but my heart felt as though it had sprung a hole and there was a feeling of sadness, loneliness, emptiness.

K returned in mere moments and reclaimed his place providing arms to hold me. I'm not sure whether I decided to let the birth happen, or whether the baby simply burst through my hesitations arising from my fear of tearing… There was a feeling of a gaping stretching yawn of my pelvis and vagina and an expulsion combined with lots of slippery limbs and a splash as the baby fell and was quickly caught… I went from standing to crouching to sitting back - half stumbling, half guided - onto the inflatable seat in the birth pool, and within moments I was handed the baby and was looking down into its face and it was red and scrunched up and crying, no, roaring on and on and on. And I had the strange feeling that this face and child was familiar to me in every way and that we knew each other intimately already and that of course I already loved it completely. Seeing my baby felt much more like a reunion than a meeting for the first time. I didn't feel love: I was love. And love pervaded every cell of me and of those around me and of this candlelit room and the warm water holding surrounding us and of the vast dark sky with stars through the window outside. Everything was awe and kindness: there was so much of it that it spread far beyond the bounds of what I would have previously considered to be the edges of 'me'. I allowed myself several long moments of breathing into its face before curiosity snuck a look at the genitals and discovered his boyhood. I realised I had known he was a boy already, somehow. "Look, K: C, then." I could feel K's arms encircling me from behind.

C was roaring and roaring and roaring and had been doing since he emerged. From being in a state of so much intensity and feeling the hugeness of the responsibility of birthing my baby, I now entered a state of no pain and so much relief and almost elation. Much as I wanted to rest now and just relax from here on, I was aware of the placenta still to birth, a final unknown obstacle I was to face and overcome before getting to clock off from all birthing-duties for the evening. C's cries were like a siren and it suddenly felt very intense being connected to him with the task of birthing the placenta still ahead of me. This moment was not a resting place: I needed to muster more action. A part of me felt that I had already given the birthing process every ounce of myself and I had nothing left to give. This was a worrying thought: I was aware of how much I *didn't* want to go to hospital at this stage.

I was supported to get out of the pool, the umbilical cord flapping snakily against my naked thighs… Hands held and supported both me and C connected together as we clambered wetly across the floorboards to the foot of the sofa. Towels were dabbed and draped to mop up bloody water now dripping in a line showing our course. A tupperware was produced and placed between my legs as I crouched and tried to bear down. I felt the energy of expectation upon me, and contracted a little with self-doubt and a self-imposed pressure to perform. My body in turn responded with… nothing. The element of time entered in for the first time since the birthing began. I knew that M would be worried if I didn't deliver in a timely manner… so I prayed.

What quickly became clear to me with a type of fierce certainty was that I needed silent, calm focus and to be alone for the placenta to be birthed fuss-free. I needed to be away from C's crying and others' gaze. I let them all know this… K cut the rubbery cord, white by now, tied it tightly with a double knot of thread. R, my homoeopath, had asked me to tell her when I first went into labour, and I had. She was therefore waiting up and at the end of the line for any advice or help if things felt 'stuck' or I needed extra support at any time. I decided to contact her now, and asked K [doula] to make the call, and to say that I needed help with this last phase. I heard them conferring softly outside the room on the landing, and then K came back with a little white pilule from my small homoeopathic pharmacy that she dropped onto my tongue.

I swayed with support to the bathroom, my legs still wobbly, sucking on the sugary pill. Things seemed to be beginning to take more form, and gathering into a feeling of coherence and confidence that I take this final step. I set the square tupperware into the toilet bowl, sat down on the seat, and breathed slowly, softly and steadily, keeping the clear intention in my body and mind of the placenta coming easily out. In a matter of minutes, it did just this: a large, soft expulsion. As soon as it left me, I was awash with many feelings: relief, freedom, elation, exhaustion, fullness, emptiness and a deep calm. I was aware that I had reached a new threshold: a place of safety. I felt I had made it through the birth successfully, avoiding being coerced, trapped, manipulated, disempowered, controlled, or wounded. I felt victorious and my heart full of joy.

I did want to go and be with C, but, knowing he would be safe and comfortable resting from the ordeal against his Daddy's chest, I wanted to spend time with M getting to know the placenta and umbilical cord. We spread it out in our large square basin and rinsed it off a little, and she showed me it's different features, what the tubes inside the cord were for, the pattern of networks, and some patches where there were changes in its texture: a telltale sign that it was starting to mature, what with C having taken his time to be ready for birth. It was beautiful, like nothing I'd ever seen, and it was mind-boggling that it had grown inside my body: this tree-like organ, a body in itself, connecting me to C and allowing for our most fundamental communion.

By now it was the middle of the night. I took a shower and then K, C and I rested together in our bed. I sipped warm herbal tea and cuddled with my family. K drained and dismantled the birth pool and then she and Mum did the washing up. They then both said a discreet goodbye and left our home cosy and spotless: the perfect nest for recovering and settling into being a family. I was exhausted, and soon agreed with K that I needed some time to sleep alone, so he held C to his bare chest all night while I slept through till dawn under the clean, crisp sheets of the guest room. **Naomi**

The day of labour, I was like running around, because I was intending to go to the Pyrenees to birth in the hot springs there, but instead what happened was (laughing) that I had gone to get some bits and bobs for the car to do the journey, and I'd gone to the butcher's, and then when I was in the butcher's, he even made a joke about not going into labour there (laughs). And, and I was like, "I'm going to the Pyrenees," like, der der der. I went out and then my car broke down...

and then I had to walk to my partner's yard and he'd run me a bath and it was a really hot day and so like, "I'm in the Pyrenees already." And our friend came over to help fix my car because he was at the time immobile because he had a severe sprain on his ankle. Then they went to fix the car, and then when they came back it was like certified that I was having really regular contractions and that I was in labour, but I was just deeply resisting because I wanted to be in the Pyrenees (laughs). But he'd even taken us round the supermarket as well, he was like, "Yes you're going to need this, you're going to need that." And he just intuitively picked up on all of it and I was still in super resistance, but fortunately my partner had already [prepared the] bath and so then I just went back into the bath for another like thirteen hours basically. I just resided and thought, I gave up and then, and then that was at the point she came anyway, was the giving up bit (laughs).

It was like so stereotypical of all my patterns, you're going through such arduous intensity and then I would pass out and I'd feel like I'm resting for half an hour. And then I'd wake up again feeling like, "Oh I'm so glad that I had the rest." And my partner then told me I was actually only asleep for like one minute at a time but I felt I'm really rested. And then when it came to the actual labour bit I just couldn't do it, I was like, "I give up, I'm just so tired." Like I went to the caravan because I was at the bath, I was in the bath at the back of his caravan and it was like over a fire and so he'd been tending the fire. And, yes I just kind of gave up. I was like, "Yes I'm over it", and then when I went to the caravan I just couldn't get comfortable and I was like "Ahh, what is going on?", demanding he tell me what's going on and he was like, "Nothing." But it felt so, it felt like you know that intense pressure pushing down, I was like must be a poo, but like, I must be having a poo, like what is going on? And then I needed to go back to the bath because it was so intense, the pain, outside of the water. So then I thought I'd hold back but he informs that it was nothing but (laughing) like just sheer, sheer mess going back there. But then as soon as I got back into the bath, then he could see the head and I was getting a bit stressed because everyone says that you should use gravity to help you in the birthing, but in the bath to get my body in the water I had to just be lying down and so I was a bit stressed but then, yes, as soon as he saw the head, it was like, oh no. I felt so vulnerable because I needed to make such a loud noise to just get her out and I'd realised that in the caravan, where I'd said "Oh I give up" I was pushing her out and sucking her back in. But then I just made this sound that was enough to get her out, and she just slid out. And it was so good and she had the cord round her neck a couple of times and we both got a bit flustered…he delivered her and then we were able to get the cord from round her neck … it was really, that bit was easy, her actually coming out, but the whole like getting to that point was challenging. And she was perfectly well… And then he moved me to the caravan to get a bit more privacy for the placenta. And the moment when we were in there the placenta came quite easy… It was really just because the baby started suckling quite soon and so it just came out quite easy. **Yony**

I'd been having gentle tightenings for a couple of weeks. I did a lot of walking. The house has this quite big garden, and then it backs onto the woods. So, I was just in the woods for a couple of weeks, really, just plodding, (laughs), waddling around, trying to see if, yes, just, just being with it. And then we were in the house one evening, and I noticed that my mucus plug had released and I thought, "Ooh, this is exciting." And I thought, "Okay, tonight's going to be the night." I think I was forty-one weeks, dead on at that point, yes, I'd been to the forty week appointment, and I knew that they were going to probably offer induction or a sweep or something. So, I was pretty armed, and I knew that I definitely didn't want any of that lot. And that was the last I'd heard, the last appointment I'd had… And so, we went into the bell tent after my plug had released, said goodnight and everything, went in, and I said to my husband, "Oh, I think it might be tonight, this is really exciting." And we were feeling really lovely, and we decided that we'd like to make love, because that's what we do. And (laughs) I went to climb on top of my husband, and my waters released at that point (laughs). So, it felt too hot inside, and suddenly, there was this big gush of water, and we thought, "Right, okay, maybe not then."

And so, it was very funny, but all of a sudden, I launched into labour, basically. It went from nought to a hundred very, very quickly, and I feel, with hindsight, that's, that's how I labour. That's, kind of, just what happens to me, all of a sudden.

It was November time, we'd got heating in there, we'd got makeshift toilet facilities in there, we were just in the garden, so, we could go inside as well, but I needed to evacuate everything, I needed to poo and wee and be sick all at the same time. And just felt really panicked by that, it was very intense, as birth can be, and I just remember feeling like I really needed to ground. So, I spent a lot of time just on the floor, you know, there was a very thin canvas between me and the earth outside. And I really, really liked that, I could just touch the ground. And yeah, my husband was sort of, bless him, trying to, trying to suggest positions I could get into and stuff, and I was just very fierce, like, "No," I just completely needed my space. So, we'd prepared for him to give me massage, and this beautiful playlist, and oils, and all of the rest of it, and I didn't want any of that. I wanted absolute silence, nobody come near me. And that was one of the reasons that I chose freebirth in the first place, was because I just know that I need space, and I need, and I only need somebody that I can absolutely trust to not come into that space and, and birth... I just need to be able to get on with it, because I knew that I could, I could do that... but yes, I just totally needed my own space during labour. And so, he kept the candles lit, he kept me warm and that was about it for eight hours. I was just doing my thing in a space, and my son was born at about twenty past nine in the morning. The daylight had come, and I was really... I remember being quite worried about the noise, about the neighbours, because I was in the garden, and there's houses all around, and I thought, "Oh, God, like, what if they can hear me." I don't think they did (laughs), I don't think they did, but, yes. So, he was born, and it was just incredible. My husband caught him, because I was on all fours, but sort of resting on the birthing ball. And yes, my husband caught baby, and that's amazing, and we just had about an hour then. I think he wasn't really interested in latching right away. I brought him up to my breast, and he was just transitioning into the world really, and that was fine. **Leonie**

Chapter 13: More labours and births

All the women who contributed their stories for this book spoke positively of their labour and freebirth, even when they were difficult or not as they expected.

Nothing really happened all day except kind of leaking. And then... as I got my daughter to bed, she was just under two and a half, that's when things started ramping up. So yes, H [doula] came over probably ten o'clock and they got the pool sorted. And I was feeling really positive. It was a beautiful, sunny evening, C was born on sixth June. And I just felt really, really peaceful, really positive. Felt I had the right team. I also had a birth photographer, who was a friend of mine, L, who was there. I felt really great. And my labour was very different to F's. I remember with F, it just felt like I didn't have to do anything, because it was just happening. But then with C's, my labour... if I was in hospital, it would have been described as inefficient. Is it inefficient? What do they say when you're not dilating efficiently or effectively? I can't think of the term. Anyway, it petered out quite a lot. I didn't contract as you would maybe... I wasn't the standard. And it was his position; he was in a really awkward position. And we now know after three births and similar stories, I have a tilted, twisted uterus. So this is why I can dilate brilliantly, but then I really struggle getting them out. So, because I had quite an intense time birthing F, when I was birthing... I was insisting through the whole pregnancy I was going to have this, sneeze and the baby would come out, kind of birth. And I had so many friends who'd had their second and that's basically what had happened. So I was geared up for my like, "Oh, there's the baby." And that wasn't how it was. Again, I was kind of quite angsty. I mean, internally though. And I had a cold; I couldn't breathe like I was supposed to breathe. And in my head I was kind of quite shouty and also very kind of verbal. And yes... I'd have a really, really overwhelmingly powerful contraction and, that would maybe last forty seconds, and I'd be like, "Wow." And then the next one would be a nothing, and then the third one would be a bit of something. But then the fourth one would be like a really big one and we were in a cycle of it never really settled into a really good rhythm. So it was really difficult to know whereabouts I was. If I'd have been my own doula, I wouldn't have known. Because it didn't seem settled. And it was like this right up until the end...

And there was a lot of walking up and down the stairs involved. And I think actually, there were points when I felt a bit too observed, because there were quite a few people there really. So H [doula] had said, "Why don't we just stay in the bedroom, and you have a walk up and down the stairs." So I did quite a lot of that. And then I got in the pool and I was in the pool for, it felt like a long time. And he was born at a few minutes to five, four fifty-seven or something... that's the thing with a freebirth – no-one's really looking at the time. And then someone, "Oh what time was it? Probably five minutes ago, who knows." And yes, it was really intense. I dilated and it didn't, he wasn't coming and I really felt, having had two experiences before, really intense one way, really not very efficient the other way. I really thought this third birth is going to be my easy birth, the classic hypnobirth it was going to be. And I've had to just come to terms with that fact that that's not how I birth my babies... it's a slog for me, I have to put in a lot of energy. And that's fine, but having been to some very beautiful, very peaceful births that happened within thirty minutes. One of my best friends had two babies; she had one on the toilet, one in the bath, with just me there. And I've accidentally not facilitated, but I've been at freebirths just because the babies have arrived before the midwives have. So I know that that can happen. But it's not going to be my story. So there was a lot of shouting. And I remember at one point, I was scared of the contractions, they were, I mean they weren't like C [first birth]'s, they were really... I was probably having one not too great one, but then a massive, intense one and a not so great one. And they weren't in a flow, but they were quite overwhelming...

H was like, "Come on. We maybe need to change your position." I'd been on my hands and knees for hours. I didn't want to get off my hands and knees; I was so scared to get out the water. She said, "I really think you need to go to the toilet, just have some time." And I was like, "Oh, I'm too scared to get out." And I kept feeling, and I couldn't feel anything. There was nothing there. And I was getting tired and I was worried that, I think I was more in my thinking brain than I was with C... I was thinking, "Is it going to be like C's? Do I need to be proactive?" So H said, "Come on. Let's get you into the toilet." So that's what I did. I went to the toilet and I sat down with the light off, and I held onto the sink. And then there was just this big whoof, and suddenly the baby came all the way down, right on top of my perineum. And I went from being like, "Oh this could be hours away" to being like, "Oh, oh, oh." Like trying to hold back like, "Not just yet" and I went hopping out of the bathroom. And I was like, "In the pool." And she was like, "Are you sure you want to?" And "Yep, yep. It's coming now. It's absolutely right there now and he's…" And then the rest of it was kind of stopping him like ploughing on through it. Trying to slow it down and just let it happen. It was really funny, that going to the toilet just being a game-changer for me really. There's a video of me... and somebody takes a picture and you can see his head's right here. And then he must come out and I sit back and just bring him up really slowly and sit back in the pool. And he's quite floppy compared to what both the other two were like. But fine… And it feels to me like thirty seconds after he was born, the door comes open, and in come C and F. Because they were sleeping on the ground floor, and F had woken, heard me shouting, woken C, saying, "I think Mum's having the baby." And the two of them had walked up all the stairs and so... And thank God they didn't walk in before he was born. They heard me shouting, so he wasn't born at that point. But it took them so long to walk all the way up, by the time they got there, he'd been born. But they'd have really thrown me off my track if they'd have turned up before he was out. But yes, there's this picture of me kind of going,… "they're in the room." It was really scary, having them both stood at the... And L going, "Oh, it's amazing. Your baby brother's just arrived." And C throws his nappy at me, I'm like, "Oh!" But they feel like they watched him being born, which for them's amazing really. **Cathy S**

Where women had several children they often compared their labours, all seeing the freebirth as progress compared with their previous experience.

Physically, my labour and birth with my second son was almost completely identical to the first. Emotionally it was a complete contrast because the calm of labour was never disrupted. I found my strength in knowing I could birth my baby alone. **Virginia**

My first was a planned home birth, turned breech at 36 weeks and my waters broke at 37 weeks. The fall out was reported in an AIMS journal... called "Do a caesarean and I will sue." [With second baby] I was the first woman not only to have an HBAC but an WBAC too in T [town]. I really did not trust hospitals and only told my husband to call for a midwife because the pain was so bad I wanted some help to deal with it. This baby was back to back and an hour after the lovely midwife arrived she was born.

We moved to S [area]; I had PTSD and had legal aid to pursue the assault and unnecessary C section. When I found I was pregnant again [third baby] I just didn't want to engage with the local hospital. I had already supported several women who went against their advice and had HBACs... I didn't trust them. Friends nagged me to find a midwife and at 27 weeks I made the phone call... only to be told I had to birth in the hospital... fortunately I met Mary Cronk [independent midwife], and penniless, we did a skills swop, she took me on. I had no idea I was in labour, too busy with a breast feeding support visit, but Mary's instinct made her call me, and she arrived ten minutes before E was born. Just her and me in the room. The birth was amazing.

With number four it was unlikely Mary could be with me, and I just had this inner feeling I didn't want anyone medical with me. I didn't want to be asked about my scar, to be monitored, have a VE... I just wanted to be left alone to labour in my own time, on my terms, uninterrupted.

Mary had to hand my care over to the NHS around 30ish weeks, may have been later... I met some lovely midwives, but they worked for the NHS, they had their protocols etc etc and I didn't want to deal with that institutional crap.

I had also reached the stage where not only was I 100% ready to take full responsibility for myself I had the confidence to tell my partner and my friends my plans. No midwives till after the birth. Friends would be in my home to look after my children and to film the birth.

My labour started around nine on Sunday night. Friends unexpectedly called and I happily chose not to tell them. I went to bed at midnight but the strength of the contractions kept me awake. By two I got up, enjoying every sensation, I danced with my baby, I could feel her moving down, it was beautiful. M phoned one friend to come over, then another, but I couldn't let him go to make any more calls. My eldest daughter joined us and sat quietly next to me as I roared I [baby] into the world…

Friends arrived with their son, it turned out it was frosty and their car was iced up. I's placenta slipped out and I just held my baby, elated, contented and feeling deeply loved by everyone present. I don't know who called the midwives or when. They were gentle, and I think they had sussed my plans anyway.

It was still [thought to be] illegal to knowingly attend a birth without midwives in those days, but my friends trusted in the birth process. I have always been aware of my Mum's influence in birth, she was very matter of fact, straight forward and down to earth. I had attended quite a few births as a doula before my fourth daughter, and... I almost feel that I was carrying the effects of supporting so many women to pursue their rightful choices in childbirth, against medical advice and protocols.

I know that when I chose to freebirth, I was wanting to break away from being a good girl and pleasing others/gaining their approval. I was so grateful to have had Mary care for me during that pregnancy because she was known in the community, and it was friends feeding back tidbits to her like "Caroline is really tired, doesn't seem her usual self" that would find Mary on my doorstep for a cuppa, long before her scheduled visit. I was not having any scans etc, but she had a knack of sensing when I really did need blood tests! I declined a scan when I measured a month ahead of guessed dates for a good four to five weeks, Mary used her Pinnard and hands and couldn't detect twins, but... I am sure I added to her grey hair.

Now I am going to share something I have never done before. I knew that I wanted to freebirth, but had felt worried about Mary's response, so when she had to hand me over to NHS care, it was a strange relief. I didn't want to upset her. The little girl wanting to please and be liked syndrome again. Again, we had no money, and M was very hard pushed with time to be able to offer skills swops, and so I also had a niggle in the back of my head for not being able to pay.

It was such a blessed relief though to labour knowing that no one was going to interrupt by asking to monitor the baby, check their position or ask any questions, to be honest.

In hindsight, I could have told Mary, or at least, told her that I wanted her to stay on the stairs or in the kitchen, and she would have been okay with that had she been well enough to attend. I did later show her the brief film of I's birth, and her sharp eyes pointed out that she had been back to back and turned on my perineum. **Caroline S**

Where women could compare other labours and births, they also considered the role of their children in their labour and some were very much involved.

He [partner] arrived and put up the pool. We'd already done practice runs – we knew it took 45 minutes to do that. So the pool was up. It was just as the pool was filling that the labour started to get a bit more intense and I started having to lean over, or kneel down on the floor actually, during contractions. So he was managing the taps and I was kneeling down with my head in his lap during contractions. But then I was getting up in between still and moving around. It was probably like that for about half an hour or something. And then my Mum had been to the shop and she decided to go and pick my daughters up from school early on her way back, which was a good idea. I'm glad she thought to do that. So they all came in, got changed out of their school uniforms. And I'd prepared them, thinking the labour was going to take quite a long time, so the plan was they were going to get into their onesies, bring their colouring books and some blankets and cushions and snuggle up in the corner of the room, so they could just observe and go to sleep if they wanted to, and they knew they were free to come and go as they pleased. As long as they were quiet. [To daughter]: So you got all your stuff ready, didn't you? And then, I think the labour was starting to get quite intense by then.

When the pool was filled... it was quite nice... I was lying there during contractions over the pool with my daughters rubbing my back and stroking my hair. So that was nice. And then the pool was filled up and I wanted to get in the pool straight away, but I had this TENS machine on me with all the wires clipped onto my trousers and I just couldn't get out of it so I kind of said, "Help!" And you all helped me get undressed, didn't you? So they got the TENS machine off me and everyone helped to get my clothes off, and I got into the pool and that was great. It just felt really nice to be in there. I don't know how long I was in there for – probably about 45 minutes all together. In between contractions I was giving instructions to everybody. I still felt quite... because I was in my own home, I felt really relaxed. I was able to easily go inward to focus on the contraction and then surface again and say, "Right, I need a bowl, I'm going to be sick," or "Please get me a drink of water," "I'm hot – I need a cold flannel." So in the end I had – L was there, my youngest daughter, with a glass of water and a straw for me to sip. My husband was there with the bowl. F [older daughter] was there with a cold cloth to mop my forehead. So in between contractions, I would just shout, "Bowl!" [Laughs] and retch a little bit and then I'd get a sip of water and then mop my brow. So that was nice, to be looked after.

I'm not quite sure what my Mum and the doula were doing at the time. I know now the doula was taking pictures because she took some lovely photos, which is a lovely thing to have. But I didn't really feel their presence very much. I just knew they were there in the background holding the space, so I could just be relaxed. So that was really nice. And then I think I was aware of my body internally in a way that I hadn't previously been, which was really interesting because I think, although I'd had home births before when I had my two girls, and I was very much going with the flow of what my body told me to do, I wasn't always... because there was a midwife present for the actual birth part, the pushing bit [in previous births]... I was kind of always waiting for them to tell me what to do. I was like, "I need to push now. Is that ok?" And wait for the midwife to tell me it was okay to push, and then I'd push. At the time I didn't realise, but now that was still kind of handing power to some other authority during that. So this time, I knew that I was the one who was in control of the situation, so I was much more focused on what was going on inside me. So that was quite interesting. It was probably the last 45 minutes of the labour that was quite intense, and I was on my knees, leaning forward over the side of the pool, because I always need to be upright. There was a point at which I was like, "Right, D [partner], you need to pop your swimming shorts on now and get in the pool to catch this baby because he's going to be here soon!" And I yelled to my Mum, this is probably time to call the midwives because I'm going to push the baby out. And I figured it would take them an hour to get there, so that was about the right amount of time. And then I did one big contraction... And pushed his head out in one. So that was good. And then it was really peaceful. I could feel his shoulders hard up inside my pelvis, against my hip bones. I could feel these two points of pressure inside me. It was interesting that through the whole pregnancy, the one thing I'd been worried about was a shoulder dystocia, like how would I handle that in a situation without a... And I'd quizzed the midwives about it because I've been at births where babies have been malpositioned and the midwives haven't actually done anything – they've just taken the woman to hospital and she's ended up with forceps or C section. And I didn't want that. I wanted to have a midwife who could handle that and help me have a natural delivery. And I wasn't confident that those midwives would do that for me. So I'd spent quite a bit of time reading about shoulder dystocia during pregnancy and different positions that you could get into if this happened. But actually during the labour, I didn't think of any of that, because you're just not in that headspace at all. But I think I'd had an instinct that something might not be quite right. Because he was quite a big baby – he was 9lb 9 – he wasn't humongous but the biggest of my babies. So I got his head out and I could feel his shoulders against my hip bones on the inside, and I felt him trying to... I was waiting for him to turn. I felt him kind of wriggle, wriggling his legs and everything to try and turn, but his shoulders didn't move. And I felt this next contraction building and my instinct was, I have to do something or else we're both going to get hurt. He has to move because there's a really powerful contraction coming. So I just cocked my leg like a dog as the contraction came, and that just made enough space for him to flip his shoulders round and then he came out with the next contraction into his Daddy's arms. So that was nice. And it was interesting that I was that aware of the inside of my body where I'd never really been aware of him inside my pelvis. My previous births I'd just been more focused on the burning sensations and not the inside of my body so much. And it was nice to know that I knew by instinct what I needed to do, because there was nobody else telling me what to do. I was the one who knew everything, although I knew I had other people there if I'd said I needed help. But none of them knew what was happening inside me. So yes his Daddy caught him. I turned over, lifted my leg over the cord and Daddy passed him straight onto me. And that was it. We had a little cry. And then we all had a cuddle. The girls were singing to him, weren't you? You sang some songs and we had a really peaceful beginning, and actually it was about two o'clock in the afternoon. What was it – 2.30? **Elena**

Sometimes, as previously mentioned, whether or not to call the midwife was left open and to be decided at the time but these families were well prepared and happy with that situation.

I felt my whole body just start to push. And I made like that mooing noise that people talk about. I was the cow, there it was – moo. And I was thinking, "I'm pushing. There's nothing I can do about it." I wasn't worried, I wasn't scared. But I just knew that there was nothing I could do. And I started pushing, and he got off the phone and he said, "Oh, she's [midwife] going to be about half an hour." And I remember thinking to myself, "She's not going to see this baby, she's not." So, as I started pushing, I had had an episiotomy with my first son. So I was very aware that I didn't really want any trauma to my perineum at all; I wanted it to be intact. And I'd had a great talk with my mother-in-law [a midwife] about how to preserve that. And I'd read a lot online about when to stop pushing. So I was very concerned that my body would take over and I would cause some damage. So with my fingers, I was feeling around, feeling what was happening to try and feel whether I was stretching – what was going on. I remember saying to S [partner], "Oh, the head's there but it's not coming. It's not coming yet." And he said, "Well give it time, give it time." So like, "Okay." But before I knew what was happening, I let myself push a bit more. I thought to myself, "Right. It's not there yet. I'm going to push. I'm going to push. And then in a minute there'll be something." So I kept pushing, and then there was a bit of a stinging, so I stopped and didn't push. And then I kept pushing again. And I kept thinking, "Is this the stinging that people are talking about? Is this the stinging?" Suddenly, after one big push, there was a lot of stinging, and I thought, "This is what they're talking about." And I looked my husband square in the eye and started blowing, I was like "Hoo, hoo. Hoo, hoo, hoo." And I remember thinking, looking him straight in the eye and thinking, "He knows what's happening. He knows that the baby's coming. He knows, he knows." And he was looking at me, and I was thinking, "Yes, we're doing this together. This is great." And all the time I was feeling and thinking you know, "That's the head." And to my surprise, having had like a four hour second stage with my first son, there was the head. And it was out. And the waters hadn't broken yet. So I said to my husband, I said, "Oh, we've got a baby in the bag. Isn't that supposed to be magical?" And he said, "What are you talking about, Cat? How can you know that?" And I said, "Well the head's out." And he looked at me and said, "Don't be ridiculous." And he'd been supporting me, holding my hand, you know, in front of me. Went round the back of the birth pool and said, "Oh, the head is out." Like this. He said, "Oh, I should probably phone the midwife again." And I said, "Well I'm going to carry on with this." I'm sure I wasn't doing it quite so matter of factly at the time. But I very definitely said, "I'm going to carry on with this." So again, I'm not really focusing on what he's doing. He's on the phone. I can hear him saying, "Well I don't think we need to call an ambulance right now. I think the baby's going to come out with the next push." And as he said that, I was pushing. Out came Z. I kind of leant backwards – he floated up to the surface. S put the phone down, peeled off the membranes from Z and as I pulled him out of the water he cried and was beautifully pink. And we both just went, "Oh!" S picked up the phone again and said, "Can you hear the crying? I think we're going to be okay." And the midwife obviously agreed and then she said, "I'll be there in about ten minutes." So, I sat back on the seat in the birth pool. Felt incredibly uncomfortable because I was still attached and I don't know, I didn't like it. So S helped me to get out, which he said was the most horrible part of it all, because holding a baby that's attached to me, also trying to get me out of the pool. So by the time that the midwife arrived, I was sat on the sofa, on lots of towels, all wrapped up in a towel with Z, just having a cuddle. And she came through the door and said, "Congratulations" obviously.

And then was very disappointed that she didn't get to tick it off as one of her home births that she attended...

We never have particularly planned to do it without support. Equally, I quite liked it. I quite liked being in my own home, on my own. I don't know whether if I'd had a midwife that I'd seen throughout and who'd come to the birth with me, I don't know if it would have been different. But I find it very difficult to imagine forming a relationship with anyone that's strong enough for them to come into that situation and to make me feel comfortable. It was me and my husband having a baby, and the midwife's there to check that medically everything's all right, but not really part of the actual birth.

I would never have had, what's it called, a wild birth. Where you plan not to have a midwife, or you don't even tell anybody, or anything like that. That would be a bit too much.

[Reflecting, three days after interview quoted above] I talked about Z's birth and how the midwives didn't attend because we didn't call them in time. And that made me reflect and think that perhaps on some level, I didn't want the midwives to be there at my second son's birth. I didn't feel that anything they could offer me was anything that I needed or wanted. And because the birth went so well, there was no point at which I thought, "I need someone to come and help." And again, listening to other women's stories... I go to a group on a Thursday morning with lots of women where we talk about our births, we talk about how we're getting on with our lives and our children – being Mums. Postnatal group - we talk about everything. And often, at the start of the group, people talk about their birth story. And someone came the other day and talked about, again the midwives forcing them to do this or that. That they went along with it, because they felt it was medically necessary, but perhaps it wasn't, and there were other options. And I listened to that story and thought to myself again, "Yes, maybe that's why I didn't feel compelled to call the midwives to come to Z's birth. And perhaps that's why I gave S the responsibility of calling the midwives, because it absolved me of any responsibility."... in my mind, as long as everything was going fine, there was no real reason to have anyone else there other than me and my husband. Because I thought we could probably get on with it okay. And we did, which was great. **Cat**

Some labours were fast and midwives unhelpful.

My husband's a frame drummer; he does these Middle Eastern frame drums. And I think maybe we made love and then we... oh no, we didn't... we just kind of like kissed a bit and we watched a comedy. We watched Groundhog Day, that was it. I remember we were in bed, laughing. And then they were getting more intense, I do a lot of dancing and belly dancing. So my husband got out the frame drums and I did a lot more standing up this time. So I was standing up, and I was holding onto the door, and I was just moving to the drums. And then it started... and then I was like, "Whoa, it's quite intense. I'll get into the water." Because I was upstairs at this stage. Went downstairs, got into the water. And literally I felt my cervix completely open in one fell swoop – just went whoom, and opened full. And because I'd been doing some like cervical massage, all round the area before. And so, and my husband had been... we'd been doing lots of work on massaging cervix... in our lovemaking. So had a really strong connection to my cervix, and I just felt it go. It was literally like whoom.

... so then I went straight into transition. But there was this part of me that couldn't quite believe it... so my mind kicked through, because my first birth was twenty-four hours from the first contraction. I was like, "Hold on a moment. I can't... this can't be that quick." So then, also because in both births, the transition for me was a bit where the adrenaline kicks in. And so I was like, "Oh..." And I think, I can't remember what happened, but I went upstairs to go to the toilet. Because I think it was that. I went upstairs and then I went into that real... my husband came in and I think I was in kind of like, "Oh my God, I don't want to give…" I always have this where I'm like, "I don't want to be doing this" Because it's the adrenaline, I want to run away from this. And then I went back down. And then, at that point, P [partner] was like, "I think I'll call S." Because that was my friend, so he called S. She came over. She came upstairs. And she was like... "I think she's almost going to give birth." This has only been a few hours from this point. So went back down into the pool... and then at that point they called the midwife just to say, "Oh, you know, this is the situation." And the midwife said, "She's about to give birth." I mean, I heard this later, afterwards. I was just in the pool at this point. And, "You need to bring her in." And my husband was like, "No, we're not going to do that. Okay, bye." And put down the phone. And then, and that was it: "So we can't get someone to you for at least an hour. You'll have to bring her in." And so it was like, "We're not bringing her in. So just bring someone when you're ready." But that was all part of the plan and they weren't going to be there. And then my husband got into the pool with me, and literally it was... it wasn't even like pushing... with F it was like push and the ring of fire, and then a couple of pushes and she was out. This one was just, I just felt one like wave. And this was the bit that went a bit... not pear shaped, but where my own mind got in the way. So I put my hand up to feel the head. And it was squidgy. It felt soft. And then I had in my brain, I had this moment of panic. I was like, "My insides are coming out." I stood up. "Argh." And my friend looked at me and said, "What is it?" And I don't know whether I actually said, "My insides are falling out" or something. And then it was literally one kind of... it was almost like an ejaculation and then I sat back in the water. One ejaculation and she came out. She was out. It was obviously not my insides; it was just that her head was a bit soft because... she came into the water, and it was just this one kind of lovely sweep, she came out. He picked her up and then he passed her straight to me. And then I got out of the water and I sat on the sofa. And this was all by candlelight and it was really nice. And then we just sat there and breastfed.

… so what I realised afterwards is that she got a bit of a shock from my shock. I had a bit of that moment of shock, and then she got shocked... so we took her to a cranial osteopath a week later and kind of got her back. Because she kind of, she didn't make much of a cry. She just went, "Wah" and then looked for the breast. And it was really amazing. It was just so... I think the whole thing took four, five hours, I think, from start to finish. But the last bit was super, super quick. Like there was... and that was the amazing thing – there wasn't even, I wouldn't call it pushing. It was just like whoomph, she was out. It was like one, two... it was like... and I've read about this, this kind of idea of it was almost like birth like ejaculation. And that's how it felt. **Rachel**

Some labours were long and the mother became downhearted but support from doulas, midwives and partners could make a lot of difference, even when the mother did not want midwives present.

I started having contractions on a Tuesday and I went for some reflexology on Tuesday lunchtime and... my due date was Wednesday, so it was the day before my due date. And I'd already started feeling like I was having some niggling feelings in the morning. My partner wanted to go out that morning and when he said he was going to go, I just burst into tears and said, "No, I really want you to stay with me today," So I think I kind of felt like it was imminent. So I went for the reflexology anyway, and then by the afternoon I was definitely having some really mild contractions and then they started, and I was sort of convinced of it in the evening. And I put on my TENS machine and then by Wednesday morning it was quite intense. She [doula] came over and it was very intense, so my contractions were definitely quite painful and lasting over a minute and coming really regularly. B [doula] felt the birth would be quite quick given how I was behaving and so she said if I wanted to get in the pool, use that pool and I was a bit scared to just get in the water in case it stopped everything. I think that was a hang-up from my first birth…although I loved the water, I was a bit scared of messing it up somehow. I think when you've had a birth that hasn't gone well, of course, you blame yourself because you think, "Oh, it's because I did this wrong, or I did that wrong." you just blame yourself. So, anyway, B, the doula, said, "We'll just be sensible about it. If it slows you down, then we'll get out, but I don't believe it will." So I got in and she was right; it didn't slow it down. And this must have been, sort of, midday…

So she [midwife] came over and she asked me if I was okay with her listening in to the baby. And then there was all the debate about that because I'd said I didn't really want it, according to the policy. But again when you're in labour, you're so vulnerable, and I think women, they naturally want to please people. That's a huge generalisation, but I don't know if that's accurate... You've got that double pressure of being a people pleaser and then also you could be putting your baby at risk not having someone listen. So I said, "Okay you can"... So we had, I had a couple of auscultations of the heart rate, but not, it certainly wasn't every fifteen minutes... so they were quite spaced out and they really did respect my privacy. I'd sort of hidden myself away in the bedroom and they only came in every now and then. And things started to slow down and there was clearly no baby, although everybody thought that it was imminent. And I didn't realise, but in the living room the second midwife had arrived and there was a student there, which I'd said was okay. But there were all those people congregating in the living room and all the resus equipment has been laid out on the dining table and everything, because they all thought that the birth was imminent. And I started thinking, "Oh, my God, this is going exactly the way my first labour went, why isn't the baby here yet, why is it, why has it slowed down?" So I'd started to think, "Maybe I should have an examination to see what's going on." And then it was suggested to me as well, and I said, "Okay, let's do it." I found that really hard because I'd had a really horrible midwife with my first birth at home and she'd done a vaginal examination and it was so painful and she tried to break my waters and things, with my consent, and that really hurt me. So the thought of someone doing a vaginal examination again, I was worried about how much it was going to hurt and what they were going to say and, and just thinking, "Oh, Jesus I'm going to have another emergency caesarean." I think I had put so much pressure on myself, especially as a doula. And people say things to you like, "Oh, doula's going to doula yourself and oh, you're so prepared, and isn't it so amazing how prepared you are and you're going to have such a great birth?" But I knew quite fully well that it didn't really matter that I was a doula or not, sometimes births just go one way and sometimes they go another way. And so anyway, I think I'd had this huge pressure that my birth really should be idyllic, and go quickly and everything was going to be fine, and it was clearly starting to not go that way. And I think I never really believed I was going to have this birth for my baby at home. I think as soon as my labour started, I felt really worried and I didn't have so much confidence. Which is interesting as well, because, you know, my job is to try and support other women to keep them going, keep their morale up and say all the right things to keep them in the right frame of mind. But I couldn't do it for myself and, and the mental challenge was definitely harder than the physical. Even with the pain of the contractions and basically the tiredness, the mental stuff was just really hard. So we did the vaginal exam and, and I was only three centimetres dilated, and so I just thought, "Oh, fucking hell" basically. But I didn't break down at that point, I just said, "Okay, well, that's good that we know that this is where we're at. Everyone go home, I want everyone to go home and just leave me on my own." And everyone was happy with that idea and everyone was a bit tired and hungry I think at that point… So everyone went home and B stayed with us. She went home about ten o'clock or something and then F, my other half, went to bed and I got back into the birth pool because it was the only place that I could feel really any relief or comfort. Because although the contractions were then starting to be quite spaced out, so they might be ten minutes apart, sometimes longer, sometimes shorter, when they did come they were quite intense. And with my morale quite low, and I was quite tired, the birth pool felt like the only place I could really deal with it. So I got into the birth pool and then I started to get quite annoyed because I thought, "Well, come on." Everyone said, "Well we're going home, let's have a rest, everyone needs to pace themselves" and I thought, "Well, that's all right for you to say, but I'm the one, I can't do that because I'm still having contractions." "Goodnight, all have a good sleep." And there I am in the bloody birth pool, and I was falling asleep in between my contractions and I thought I was going to drown at one point. Because I'd noticed that, I'd be sitting in the birth pool, but then suddenly my head would fall in the water or something, because I was just so tired and then I woke up my boyfriend, and I said, "Right, I'm going to call the midwife."

And so I called the midwife and I said, "You know what, I think let's just cut our losses…" And she said, "Have you tried listening to your hypnobirthing?" And I thought, "I'm going to throw this phone against the wall in a minute" (laughs). But I didn't do that, although she was right, I hadn't. I'm a hypnobirthing teacher for God's sake. So I hadn't listened to any tracks, I had just got myself into a really negative rut and thinking, "I'm not going to be able to do this and I'm going to have another two day… two, three day labour and then have a caesarean." And I was so, I was so dead after my last daughter was born, I found that really hard to recover from, very long labour and then a huge operation, so that was my fear. But I had another abdominal surgery a year ago, a mass removed from my abdominal muscle. And so it was another two nights stay in hospital and not being able to pick up my daughter. And I just thought, "I do not want another huge operation." But at eleven o'clock at night I was willing to give it all up (laughs). So I did what the midwife said. I got out of the pool, I put on my hypnobirthing track in my headphones in my ears and I leant, kneeled on the bed over some pillows and I really tried to focus on my breathing. And I just thought to myself, "Nobody else can give birth to this baby. Nobody else can help me actually." That's what I felt. I have to do this on my own. And I'd had those thoughts, for a long time during my pregnancy, and I think I've noticed especially first time Mums, they want the midwife there super early, because they feel like somehow the midwives are going to help them have the baby. And actually, rarely that's the case. It just sort of sets the clock ticking earlier, the sooner they get there. But the only person that can give birth is you, me, you know what I mean, so I just thought, I tried to really suck it up and I knew, I could feel the baby moving. I assumed it, I didn't know it was a girl then, she was fine, I was fine, I just needed to get out of my head.

So Thursday came around, the contractions seemed to have been slowed down even more, but that was quite good because I was able to get a bit of sleep and I was able to eat something. And so Thursday was just me and my fiancé F, and I sort of took it quite seriously on Thursday, in terms of giving it everything. So I made sure that I got some sleep whenever possible. I tried to eat little and often, even if it was just some biscuits or some bananas and cereal, I had some toast, just little things to give myself some energy and tried to drink lots of water. We went for a walk, we've got some woods at the back of our flat. We went for a walk in the woods, it was a nice sunny day and I did some spinning babies exercises and some mile circuits, which is another series of exercises to try and start a stalled labour. We had sex twice. It certainly wasn't enjoyable, but just, like, "Okay, just deposit the sperm near the cervix," and we'll see if it's going to try to speed things up a bit, and it did actually, it worked. And, and then I was texting B the doula and I was texting the midwife, just to say, "Things are still like this." In the morning, I had actually texted the midwife and said, "Can you come over and do an examination, I want to see if I've progressed?" And she said, "Well, given what you've said about the intensity or the frequency of your contractions, there's no point in me coming. Because you're only going to get more disheartened, so just stay where you are, just carry on," and that was the best thing really, actually. Because if she'd come and I was five centimetres or four centimetres, she'd have had to stay with me because that's the policy. So she was quite clever really in doing that and, of course, I wasn't thinking this at the time. I was just thinking, "Jesus Christ, come on, I want to know."... if I'd been my doula, I would have said what the midwife said. I would have said, "Come on, let's just keep doing what you're doing: rest, eat, go for a walk," all of that stuff. But again the fear and the doubt took over in my mind. And so when Thursday night came around, my mother-in-law brought our daughter back about six pm. When she came back, my contractions really picked up and I had two or three hours of really intense, frequent surges and then it all stopped again. But I felt really happy to have my daughter back, because I had really wanted her to be there. Although on Tuesday when my labour started, I wanted her to leave. I didn't know if I could cope with her and the contractions. But then when she did come back, I was very happy to see her and I was really glad she was there. And F went to bed, I got back into the birth pool, you know, to sleep, and we'd emptied the water and filled it up again by that point. And then I woke him up and I said, "Look, this is getting quite intense," and, and I was feeling most of the time my contractions had been low down, and at the front and then occasionally they'd be in the back. Because of my previous caesarean, I found it difficult sort of dealing with the contractions that were low down at the front, because, of course, that's where your scar is as well. And so I thought, "Well, how do I know...?" Well, of course, I know if that pain doesn't go away then that could be a sign that there's something going on with the scar. And it was, it wasn't always going away, but it certainly wasn't there constantly. But I wouldn't say that it went away between every contraction... and so that started playing on my mind as well. It's not just that I didn't have a good birth the first time, I had a caesarean. So thinking about all of that as well, just negative thoughts just really took over me and so I said, "Right, call B, I really, I don't want to do this on my own anymore because I've been doing it on my own since Wednesday, you know, evening, and now it's at midnight on Thursday."

And so he called B and she said, "Okay, I'm on my way." And she arrived half an hour later and just, for about five minutes before she arrived, I said, "Call her back and say, tell her to hurry up because I'm feeling like there could be a bit of pressure." I didn't, it wasn't that I was pushing, but it felt different and they were certainly quite intense. And, and when she came in I said, I said, "B, I think that I'm going to start pushing or I think I'm feeling pressure." And she said, "Okay, let's see what happens with your next contraction, then." And then the next contraction I started pushing. And I said, "Okay, let's just see." I thought, because I'm pushing, it could be two hours yet, or three hours before the baby arrives. But it felt really good to start pushing. And then, two more contractions and, it was really going well, so B could see the baby's head and so we said, "Okay, call the midwife, we can see the baby's head." So we called them and they started on their way, and... it was clear that she was going to be born quite quickly. So I said to F, I said, "Call an ambulance," because I didn't want to put my doula in a difficult situation. It was, it was more just like to protect everyone as a backup, because I knew that, at that point the midwives weren't going to make it. So I felt at that, in that, and this time I felt completely calm and I felt completely confident and I had complete clarity. I had no more doubt in my mind and I could just hear B behind me just saying, "Take it slowly, don't, don't rush." And then she came round to my face and she said, "It's okay, you're not going to have another caesarean." Because I'd said to her, that's what I really wanted her to say to me when we got to the point. And I knew that I wasn't going to have to have another caesarean. And it felt so good, the pushing part, I really enjoyed it and I listened, I was listening to what B was saying, in terms of, "Right, you know, just be, take it slowly." And, and she did say at one point, "Don't, don't push Katie, now, just, just breathe, just blow." Because it was clear she was going to come quite quickly, and then, her head came out and it didn't hurt. It felt really good and then I think my next contraction, I just went for it really and, and she came out and she was born in her sack and F caught her and tried to pass her through my legs. But it was so slippery, because she was in the sack. And I was, "Oh, look, I can't, I can't catch her, what's happening?" And B helped us, because there was a bit of floundering in the water. And I just put her on to my chest and she was clearly pink and looking fine, but I just kept saying, "Oh, my God, is she okay, is she okay?" And, and, you know, B said, "Of course, yes, she's absolutely fine, she's absolutely fine." And I just felt ecstatic. I felt, the fact that it had been three days in labour, I just felt so happy, like the happiest I've ever felt and couldn't believe that we'd done it... And in the end it happened exactly as I wanted it in my dreams. **Katie H**

And then at about seven o'clock I hit a bit of a wall and really needed my Mum. And I remember being in the living room crying that we had to get Mum back from wherever she was – she had to come back right now. So T phoned her and she was about 20 minutes away. And I think I was just feeling... like the thing that I lacked in freebirthing was that external reassurance of where I was in the process. I really wanted somebody to tell me where I was, how this was going. And I kept trying to find that, either find that knowledge within myself, or better still, get rid of wanting to know and just be on the journey. But I like answers, and I just couldn't shake that part of me that wanted answers. And didn't really trust that I knew the answers. So, and I kept thinking I don't feel, you know, O thought that it was this transition and I thought... I wanted it to be, but I really didn't think it was. I didn't think I was there yet, but at the same time it was all feeling a bit pushy. I don't know. And I think that really unsettled me. This - I don't know where I am. In this, you know, dark forest of labour, I don't know where... how far in I am. So Mum came back, kids came through and gave me a cuddle. And that was really nice. And then I took myself off into the bedroom on my own. Now, the others were born in the living room. But I felt like this one I want to be in the bedroom... But I like being really close to the ground when I'm labouring and when I'm birthing, I never wanted to be on a bed or on a surface; I want to be as close to the ground as possible. So I came into the bedroom on my own and it was basically dark. I think the curtains were closed and all the lights were off. Somebody got the other children to bed – I don't know who. But somebody did and they went to sleep. And then for... so it was about four hours between Mum getting home and H being born. And that, a lot of that period was really, it was really hard. I felt... well I felt completely lost is how I felt. I felt, I was scared, I felt unsettled, but so much stronger than unsettled – ungrounded, like I couldn't find my footing with anything. Yeah, it was like a spinning and lost. And I just believed that I couldn't do it. And I couldn't shake this feeling that I couldn't do it. I was standing up the whole time. But I got to a point where for the last couple of hours, I needed to give myself a good talking to. I went and had a banana and a cup of tea and just told myself that I could do this. And I didn't even feel like I could do that with this one, because that sense that I couldn't do it was so… was penetrating so deep I couldn't find a part of myself that did believe I could do it. And I just remember, like just crying. I don't think I was actually… there were tears but I was crying through every contraction that I couldn't do it. Saying, "I can't do this. I can't do this." to T, Mum one side and my head in T's lap. And I'd lie down in between. But I, if I was still lying down when the next contraction started, it was too painful. So I had to make sure I'd time it. I would have been terrible giving birth in hospital, because I cannot give birth lying down. I can't lie down and labour at all. I don't know how people manage it. It's so painful. Then, I think it must have been about ten o'clock, something changed. And I started telling myself out loud that I could do it. And I didn't believe it. But I knew that I couldn't stay in this forever, I couldn't… this baby was going to be born and I couldn't bear to keep feeling like this, this unbearable, quite dark, lost incapability. And I thought, "Well the only person who can get me out of this is me. So I'm going to start telling myself that I can do it." And in this we found this brilliant position. Like I love the way each labour brings its own positions. With each of them I've needed different things. And what I found was that I was on my knees, with my Mum with my left hand and T with my right hand, they would hold my hands and I leaned all the way back. So like my body was basically straight, but sort of 45 degree angle going back. Which was weird because I thought normally you want to be forward, why do I want to be backwards? But I was trusting this baby… she'd been, you know, she was on the right hand side where the other two had been on the left-hand side. She was not following the rules of what position to be in. And I knew she was doing that for a reason. But she knew what positions she needed, so whatever my body tells me to do in labour, I'm quite trusting of. Well it's more than that – you can't make me be in a different position. I just can't do it. So I had Mum and T on either side and I was pulling… they were holding me up and I was pulling on them. And I was crying to myself that I could do this. Saying out loud that I could do it. And the contractions were, they were really quite short.

…just before a baby's born, there's this particular smell that's all sweet and… I can't describe it, but it's absolutely unmistakeable. And T said at that point my tone of voice completely changed and it was like this sudden clarity that, "Right, okay, we are nearly there." Because my waters hadn't gone yet. I had no idea where I was… so as soon as I could smell that smell, I thought, "Right, okay, we are getting there." And it was just so reassuring. And then the next push, I felt her head come out of my womb. Which was completely mind blowing, because I had not felt anything like that with the first two… I felt her head emerge, like through my cervix, and it's still like… the memory of how incredible that was, it's still mind blowing. And then it went back in. But I thought, "No, this is it. We're here. We're there." And the next push she was halfway down. And then there was barely time to breathe... because it was so powerful and fascinating, like I can feel exactly where this baby is. And then it got to crowning and then I thought, "Oh this is the bit I've been dreading because this is going to really hurt." And her head just paused just gently, and then like effortlessly emerged. It didn't hurt at all. Still in a membrane. And I'm there kind of kneeling on the floor, holding her head and then I felt... and she didn't wait very long. I thought we'd have... like with M at that stage, we had a little chat, because there was a gap. But with H... I felt her turn back to... she turned left shoulder back and I could feel really clearly how her body turned back to the position she'd been in for months on that right-hand side of me. And then just out she came. And my waters went as the rest of her was being born. And just onto the floor in front of me. And her cord was slightly round her neck, it kind of went over her shoulder and then round and in. It didn't go all the way round the front. I just untangled her and picked her up. And I just said, "I did it. I did it. I can't believe I did it." Just over and over again for about ten minutes, was all I could say was, "I did it." And cried and cuddled. Beautiful pink, calm, alert little person. It took me ages to even check whether she was a boy or a girl. I just forgot. And I didn't need to check if she was okay because I just knew. And her eyes were open. She was so pink, it was weird. You know, she was not a normal colour for a baby that's just been born. But not a normal colour in a good way. And she was just so, so calm. And that wisdom that I'd felt all the way along. She was like, "I knew. I knew we could do this." **Beth**

Chapter 14: A mother's story and her doula's story

The mother's story

With my first I was already set on a home birth from the get go. As soon as I knew I was pregnant, I knew I was going to want a home birth. And the more I read about it, the more I thought, "Actually it's not beneficial for those midwives to be there in the first place." For physiological workings of the body, to have strangers there is actually not good for you. And so we discussed it with my partner back and forth and we did decide in the end to have midwives there. Definitely have a home birth still, but not a freebirth. So that was four years ago, almost four years ago. And yes, this time I was just like from the beginning I knew, "I can do this." You know... the midwives felt like a nuisance at my first; I didn't feel like I needed them at all. I didn't find them helpful. I actually found they were intruding. Anything negative I remember from my first birth was to do with what they did. So for me, it was quite clear that removing that factor was the way to go, absolutely. And that's exactly what happened...

I had thought out the space to be quiet and peaceful and they were going through lists of stuff that they needed and getting, I don't know, all sorts of medical things out. Although there was no reason to intervene, it was a very straightforward birth. It was maybe three hours of active labour, which is not bad for a first birth. They were very worried with both pregnancies that I'm advanced maternal age. I was 38 with my first and I'm almost 42 now. So they walked in with that in mind, "So this is a high risk woman." IVF pregnancies both of them...

[During her second labour] It was two hours, the active part... at 9.00 pm, my partner came, my ex-partner, we're separated, so he came to get H, my first born. It was comedy, because I was having quite strong contractions and we tried to hide it from him, because he's quite squeamish; I didn't want him to see that I'm in pain. And I tried to put his shoes on, to make it look normal. "We're going to Daddy's now. You know, everything's fine." And when I put his shoes on, I had a really strong contraction. And I was on all fours in the hallway, trying to pretend I'm putting his shoes on. And I ended up under that chair out there, because I was trying to hold on. I was actually giggling through the contraction, because it was such a weird situation. And H was like, "Mummy, what are you doing on the floor?" Because I was under the chair. And D [doula], you know, bless, she picked up on the whole thing, she said, "Mummy's just looking for something." And she put his shoes on. And he didn't notice a thing. But I constantly had contractions also during dinner. Every time I had one I got up and said, "La, la, la." And D involved him in a conversation. It was really, it was very funny. And actually, you know, that's good for oxytocin, right, it's just everything was just really relaxed.

And so he left at quarter past nine. And D and I just sort of barely made it up the stairs, because things were really happening at that point. And D is really hands off, right. And that's what we agreed. And she's been listening to my story for years now and our discussions about what kind of birth I want and she did it to a tee. She did it better than I could have asked for. Because during the sort of pushing stage, I got in the pool, D was behind me, so she wasn't, there was nobody in my space; it was just like from my perception. Obviously, I knew she was there, which was good, but there was nobody in front of me, that whole room that had been filled with bags at my first birth, and other people walking in and out, and everybody being hectic – it was just my bedroom. And there was nothing. Some women ask me, "So what's your birthing, you know, your set-up?" And I said, "I have a pool. I don't have any, you know, it's just my room." And that was like this normalcy really helped my body to relax, because it was like, "I'm just having a baby. You know, it's not a big deal, in a sense." For some reason, we never talked about the fan, but I wanted the water quite hot. So I was very hot. She must have seen that I'm sweating - I don't remember. But all the windows were open. The neighbours, I don't know if they were, they got the show of a lifetime, because I was very vocal, but in a sort of good way. And D, that's all she did in the final stages was doing the fan, sort of rhythmic. She said I was talking all the time and joking and saying funny things. And she said she never responded. I don't even remember that properly. But she completely left me in my space. And I have this wish that she would film the last part. And so that's when she just got in front of me. But I was not paying attention to that, it didn't interrupt my flow or anything. So we had the last few minutes on video. I still haven't managed to watch the full, because I get too emotional. Every time I start watching it, I have to stop it again.

So he was born. She gave me a towel. We were sitting in the water for a bit. Helped me out of the water at some point. And we were just sitting on the bed. And that, it was just like the most normal thing in the world, which I think it should be. There's no concerns, no. I just knew, if anybody had asked me at my first birth what I feel, you can feel literally baby's now coming down the birth canal. You feel everything, it's like textbook. I know not all births go that way, but many do, and the majority of them probably do if you let them. So this time it was beautiful, that I could actually just mentally focus on that. Okay, so he's there, and now he's there and now we're going to do this. And so even when he was crowning, I remembered my first birth, I was in panic, because I had been filled with all this fear. And yes, I think one of the midwives said last time, "And now, the last bit's going to be really sore." And I was just like, "Don't tell, let me feel it. It might not be. How do you know?" And this time I knew he was crowning – it is sore, but I knew he's going to be out in a minute. So, and on the video I look really relaxed, like I wasn't even, I don't think there was any noise even in the last, the last pushes. And that's exactly what I wanted. And I really believe that babies remember their birth experience as well. And that sort of quiet and calm, and he's been like this all along. Because my first is quite sort of fearful and sensitive – sensitive to noise and the birth we had will not have helped. Because there was just too much intrusion also towards the end. And they had planted that worry in my head... But this time I knew. I know what I feel. And I trust what I feel. So it was so calm after the birth. The placenta came off probably 15 minutes, 20 minutes after he was born. And D brought me the food we had agreed, my smoothie and some muesli bars and I don't know, I wanted a glass of Coke, which I never drink, but that's what I felt like having. And then the night was very strange, because my ex-partner wasn't here; he didn't want to be here. So it was just the two of us alone in the house. Which D now says she feels bad about. She feels like she should have stayed here. But for me, it was actually beautiful, because I was just looking at him all night. With hindsight the next day I thought I should have gotten some sleep. But I was just looking at him all night and it was just the two of us. And that's perfect. To me anyway. Like some people might want their partner there, but I didn't. **Carmen**

The doula's story

Carmen got in touch fairly early in her pregnancy to say that she was looking for support and definitely didn't want what she'd had last time. That she was planning to take more control of things and that she was in the middle of splitting from her partner and things were looking quite hard for her. And I was a bit concerned in the beginning that she was not, I don't know, that she wasn't really thinking through her decisions, that they were all quite reactionary. But then as time went on it seemed like she was thinking them through very well actually and this was her way of feeling safe and feeling that she had some control over things. Because being over forty and having an IVF baby it seemed like everybody had an opinion about what she should do. There were lots of shoulds; every time she met a midwife or consultant, everybody had a view on what should be done. And it usually included early induction, going into hospital to have her baby, lots of monitoring, growth scans, all this kind of thing, and she didn't want any of it. And she, from my perspective, built a pretty good relationship with one of the home birth midwives, and was up for meeting with her, having her to her house. And was pleasantly surprised by how different that felt to the community midwifery team she'd had last time and the opposition that they had given to a pool being in her bathroom or the stairs she had and all sorts of things. So this felt quite positive, and I was thinking even though she's talking about potentially doing it without midwives, maybe in the moment, on the day of the birth, she'll change her mind and opt to have the midwife there. So I didn't really know what she was thinking about it all.

But then as time got closer and those shoulds increased, every single time she went in for a bit of monitoring past thirty-eight weeks, they wanted to start monitoring her then. Every time she went in, she came out livid at the things that people were saying to her. It got so bad, I should probably pull up the texts to give you specific examples, because she'd send me texts with messages like, "Can you believe the doctor said this to me?" You know, "You may be taking the right decision but we'll see when we find out whether your baby lives or dies and you'll have to live with that consequence for the rest of your life, are you okay with that?" And she would say, "I just, I can't believe you're saying that to me." And then she'd call me afterwards, or text me afterwards, just so angry. So, I don't know, I suppose from my perspective, as somebody supporting her, it felt a little concerning how angry she was getting. I don't want somebody to choose to birth on their own because they're angry, but I also, I felt good for her that it was channelled into that sort of feeling over frightening her into doing the things that she didn't want to do, so it felt stronger. So we'd kind of talk it down from being angry into, well what do you want to do about it, do you want to see a different consultant next time? Do you want to go in for monitoring? Do you want to talk to your midwife about it? And she would find her way through to the next appointment the way that she wanted it. So she kept seeing different consultants, but every one of them was doing the same kind of thing.

So she got to forty weeks. She thought that things were starting at thirty-eight, that was when she started to get in touch frequently and say something's happening and then it didn't amount to anything. Or, oh something's happening again, it was probably wishful thinking or from her perspective it may have been that things would have happened had she not been so stressed, possibly. That's what was always in the air floating. So then, she got past forty weeks and of course then the midwives started to get involved in "We need to do something", even the ones that she'd put her faith in, like her midwife, started to say, "Well what about just a sweep?" And she lost faith in her at that point, a bit and started to say, "You know, I don't want that." "Oh well, you know, if you change your mind I can just come over and give you a wee sweep." And Carmen's an intelligent woman, you know, and she's very switched on to language and she was picking up on that stuff and saying, "I just don't like it, it all feels like bullying, why doesn't anybody trust me? Why doesn't anybody have faith in me and my body?" So I felt like my job was quite clear. It was just simply to have faith in her and her body and to listen and to trust what she was saying was right for her. So I fully got behind it at that point, I trust you. I know that what you are doing is right for you and I know my role, it's to get behind you and not have any opinions, just to simply get behind you, and it got a lot easier then, for me. Each time her midwife came to see her, she was saying to her, "You are going to call us, aren't you?" I think the midwife knew that it was quite likely she wasn't, and Carmen started to invite me to the times when she was coming over to her house, which was friendly enough. You know, everybody was fine with that, the midwife and I know one another, but she a couple of times said things like, "Well you two will phone me, won't you?" And I would just kind of look at Carmen and Carmen would say, "Yes, probably."

But then on the day that she eventually gave birth, that morning she had got in touch to say, "D I've had a wee bit of fresh blood in my pants" and I said, "Okay." And waited, you know, and she said, "I think it's, I think it's from my cervix because I've been having tightenings all night." And I said, "Okay what, what do you want to do?" And she said, "Do you think I should be concerned?" And I said, "Well, are you concerned?" And she said, "No, I'm not, I think it's from my cervix." I said, "Okay well, what do you want me to do, or is there anything I can do for you?" And she said "Well would you come to the hospital with me because I fancy just having a bit of CTG to check that the baby's well, not that it tells me that much but, you know." I forgot to say that over the weeks, the two weeks before that she had wanted to get away from all the CTG but one of the midwives had said to her, "You can have a cord scan to check that all's well with your placenta." And she was quite happy with that and she'd got one of those, but then following that one, they started to say, "We're not going to check your cord when we do a scan, when we do a CTG or a scan, we're not going to check the cord because that won't tell us anything." And she was like, "But the last time I was here, you did that and you said it was reassuring." And the doctor said, "Well it's only reassuring in that moment, anything can change." It was always that sort of crazy doublespeak that she was dealing with, where somebody would say, "Oh that's very reassuring but" and then bring in, "But your baby could still die." And she was saying, "But that's the tool you use to determine that all's well and you've used it and all is well, so are we not okay?" But there was always more to it so on that day when she said "I want to go in and have a bit of CTG, if all's well, I'm just going to get away from the hospital because I feel like things are happening. I'm over forty-two weeks pregnant, pretty sure something's going on. I think this is a sign that my cervix is changing." "Okay, I'm with you", so we went in and that was when the midwife got really quite breathless in her delivery. She started to talk to her like, "You understand that you're really taking a risk here", and she was talking really fast and breathing really shallow and I could feel Carmen getting pulled into this kind of debate. And then she asked, "Can I have my notes? I'm going to go." And then the midwife said, "No, you, you can't go until you have a word with the consultant." And Carmen said, "Can't?" And she said, "Oh I mean we'd rather you didn't." And Carmen said, "Well I don't really want to speak to a doctor today, thank you, you know, I'm pretty happy with the CTG here, all's well, I'm going to get going. I feel like this is what's going on with my cervix." And she said, "Okay I'll go and get your notes." And then she came back with the doctor because we know how this goes and so A arrived and he's very pleasant, he's very charming, but Carmen wasn't really in the mood for being charmed. So he tried his charm, he said something like, "Do you mind if I sit on this birth ball?" And she replied, most drily, "Well this is your building and your equipment so do what you like." And he said, "Oh, okay" and a bit disarmed, and then he said, "I'm very concerned about you and your baby." And she said, "Well we just did a CTG and all's well, so what evidence do you have to be concerned?" And he said, "Well the blood", and she said, "Well, it was literally a couple of tablespoons full and it hasn't continued and that was about two hours ago, so, I'm not concerned and my cervix has been tightening, or pulling, so it's probably my cervix." And he said, "We think you're having an antepartum haemorrhage and we'd really like you to stay here and start an induction process." And this is where I felt like I wanted to kind of bow at her feet a little bit because she said, "How will that help with the bleeding?" Touché. I had to stop myself laughing because it's so true and so few women ask these sorts of questions, how will your suggestion help with the thing that you're concerned about? And he said, "Well, it won't directly, but it means that we'll have you in the right place." And she said, "Well it's not the right place for me, doctor, you know, with all due respect, I'm going to head home now and trust me, if I'm bleeding any more, I'll be back, I'm not crazy, you know, I'm very sensible, grown up and I'll be back in if I'm bleeding more. But, can you just get me my notes now? We're going to go." And he was respectful enough and said, "Okay,

I'm sure you're right", kind of glancing over at me all the while. And then we left and she went home and had a lovely tea party with her son.

She started having some surges that afternoon, but she didn't let on to anyone, not even herself, she was just like, "I'm going to conceal all of this." And she got her three-year-old son back for the afternoon. It was a beautiful sunny day, it was Mother's Day, and she had this teddy bear's picnic with him outside. And she said later that she'd been playing football with him, she'd kicked the ball to him and he would like be the goalie or kick it back and sometimes when she was having a contraction she'd lean over and he would say, "Mum, why are you not kicking the ball back?" So they were trying to have this game, and that went on all afternoon, they had a beautiful time. And then she rang me later, about half past seven, eight o'clock and said, "Things are definitely happening now, I want you to come right now." It's quite rare for a woman to say, "right now", and knowing that she didn't have her partner there, I thought, okay, I'll go right now.

So I literally ran home from Tesco, got in my car, headed over, then found her to be in quite strong labour. And she was so together, she was saying things like, "You know last time, D, my labour started at, whatever it was, midnight" and she had her baby at five in the afternoon, she said, "This is like two pm in my last labour" and the baby was born three hours later. She was so right, in retrospect, that's how much later her baby was born. So I was saying, "Right, okay, well what shall we do? What would you like to do?" And she said, "Well I need to sort out for H [older child] to get back to G [his father]." "Have you called him?" "Yes, I've let him know, and he's going to come in an hour." And so she was feeding H and then whenever a contraction would come she'd disappear behind the kitchen worktop onto the floor and then compose herself and come back again and chat with H and me. And then G did show up, and even then Carmen was trying to put on her son's shoes, but she was crawling on the floor by this point. "How about I put his shoes on Carmen?" And G quickly took H and that was about half past nine. And then she said, as the door shut, "Uhhh", this kind of sound, she said, "What should I do now?" And I said, "How about we go upstairs?" Where everything was set up, you know, the pool and everything else, "How about we go upstairs and put a little bit of water in your pool" thinking, "We'd better hurry up."

And the pool was set up, she's got three shower heads into a wet room and the pool's in the wet room kind of wedged in with access from both sides and so I just got all the shower heads going. And she started taking photos of the pool getting filled and I found out later she had shared them with the yoga group (laughs).

She was thinking about letting others know. She said, "I'm finally in labour" to the yoga group with this picture of the pool filling. And then she said, "I think I need to lean forward." But she was having difficulty standing up, so I said, "Well how about you sit on the toilet?" So she came and sat backwards on the toilet and then came to standing and leaning on her bathroom windowsill, and that's pretty much where she stayed until the pool was filled, twenty minutes later, half an hour, and then threw off her clothes and got in the pool. And I don't know what guided me there but I knew that, there was one access in front of her, like looking directly at her from the other side of the pool that I could have chosen. Or there was the other side access which was kind of next to her, but behind her a little bit, over her right shoulder if you like. So I just sat down there and took out a fan because she was hot and I was just fanning her and she was just with her eyes closed and occasionally coaching herself (laughs) saying things like, "You know Carmen, you're doing really well." And I'd hear her coaching herself, I've been noticing this, that if we don't say anything, women coach themselves beautifully. It's quite astounding. And then at one point I recorded a couple of times her sound to let her hear later, because she sounded so strong and sure and confident. And I didn't have any doubt that she was fine and then she turned her head and she said, "You know, D, I'm really enjoying this." And I said, "I can see that" and then she continued and she started to say, "The baby's coming."

So I moved around to the other side, her eyes were firmly shut and then I began recording and she said, "I'm going to, I'm going to birth the baby now, the baby's moved down, I'm going to birth the baby now." And then she said, "With the next contraction, he's coming." And then yes she talked through it, just saying lovely things, the baby's head was born and then she said, "Oh that's the waters gone then." And she just told me this morning like weeks later, she said "I've just watched that birth video and I…" she said, "I noticed myself saying, "That's the baby's, oh that's the waters gone." She said, "I knew his head was out as well, but what I was saying was, there's the waters, you [health practitioners] were all wrong, my waters hadn't gone before, that's the waters now." She said, "I knew his head was out as well, but what I was saying was, "See, there's the waters." I said, "Oh I didn't know any of that, but I didn't feel the need to say anything to you" so I didn't say anything.

I don't think I've ever been at a birth where nobody said anything except the woman. Nobody said anything, nobody coached her, nobody well done-ed her, nobody delighted, nobody said anything or did anything. I just kept the fan going which seemed to be a rhythm that she was kind of anchoring on, just this fan, back and forth. And then she had her baby in her arms, she lifted him out of the pool so gently, it was the most moving thing. And I had a fleeting, it was like half a second of thinking, "Will the baby be okay?" And then a complete trusting feeling of, "It's all great." Almost even if he's not okay, because this is her choice, this is what she's chosen. Because of that conversation we'd had the day before where I asked her, "What if your baby doesn't make it? You're going against all the advice, what if your baby doesn't make it? Can we talk about that?" And she said, "Even if my baby doesn't make it, these are the right choices for me." And I said, "Okay, that's good." So, if we continue beyond that then, you know, she held her baby and was just so blissed out, holding him and loving him. There was a bit of concern when he was first born, I could see it, as she rubbed him vigorously, he didn't make any sound right away and she, you could see, was visibly relieved when he did, when he spluttered a little bit and then sneezed and then made a little cry, she was really relieved. And then settled into the relief of it all and the "Haaaah", that big sigh. And then stayed there maybe for ten minutes just pouring little bits of water over him, again, nobody spoke, well I didn't speak is what I mean. I didn't say anything, I just gazed on from the other side of the pool and expected nothing from her and then eventually she said, maybe after ten minutes, "I want to get out and go to the bed." And so dried her off and her bed was just like two metres away from the edge of the pool so she made it over there and then maybe a couple of minutes after that she said, "Here's the placenta coming." It was just so lacking in drama. And then the placenta was born and it's a good while after that before she said, "I think I'd like to cut the cord." So I went and found some scissors and, and she put on the cord tie and then cut the cord. And I went and put the placenta in the fridge and, then she had a shower while I held her baby and then got into bed all cosy and fresh with her son and, oh, just blissful.

I felt so, what's the word? I want to say vindicated, I don't know if that's quite the right word. I felt so proud of her, that she had taken her decisions and knew what was right for her, kind of sad that others couldn't have got behind it. Because I knew there would be consequences, somehow, I knew that somebody would have an issue with it. Whether it was her ex or her mother-in-law or the midwives who weren't called or the doctors or that somehow she would sort of have to pay, that somebody would insist on some kind of revenge, it felt like. And for that time, and I think she knew that too, because for that time, that night, when I said to her afterwards, "Come on, do you want to call a midwife now and just get a check and get everything finished?" Kind of put an end to all of this and get it wrapped up. She said, "Oh god no, I don't want to call anyone, I have to have this night with him on my own before all of that begins." "Okay" so a few hours after he was born, I left her on her own with her son, for the night, for well the few hours until morning.

And sure enough the next day they said they wouldn't come out to her when she called for a midwife. She called the home birth team and it was her midwife who said that they wouldn't come out because her son was now high risk due to the fact that he wasn't monitored in labour. That's a very concerning precedent if they want to start saying that, but, anyway she called me to tell me that and I said, "No, no, no, no, call them back" you know, or by that point G was there, her ex. I said "Ask G to call them and say that they have a duty to come out." And he could also call the clinical lead and explain what's going on and insist that somebody come out. And then after a couple of hours, her midwife did come out with, I think a senior midwife. She didn't remember much about her, but they stayed for two hours checking out her and the baby, seems like a very detailed check. And they determined that the baby had jaundice and needed immediate transfer for phototherapy which she did and her son was then separated from her to put under the lights which she was quite distressed by. And then the blood test came back that he didn't have severe jaundice after all. But they kept her in overnight and she came back the day after. She's still delighted with all the decisions she's taken, but she said that she just watched that video for the first time last night.

I think in her life of splitting from her partner and her mother recently dying and this taking charge of her birth has been quite pivotal for her. And for my part, it taught me a lot about following others' lead. I don't give advice anyway but I've not been in a situation where somebody's been so certain that this is right for them. Or in a situation where there's no partner present, it was just me and her, and her decisions, her choice to birth her baby in this way. I have worried in the past, supporting freebirth, that a midwife will show up and that I'll somehow be implicated in having practised midwifery or something. And I guess that's why I film, that's why I filmed hers, was to have evidence that I've not interfered in any way, I've not touched anything and that it's all her and the film makes that very clear. Not that anybody's ever asked to see it, but if they did, it would be clear enough that I wasn't a player in it. She didn't look at me, she didn't interact with me at all, she was on her own essentially, it would look like she was on her own. Yes. So I think that the initial reasons that she chose it were to stay away from the harm that she felt was caused to her during her first birth, but I think that what's come out of it is a lot of self-belief, which is really, timing-wise, it's pretty good for her in her single mothering of two children. **D,** doula

Chapter 15: A twin birth: a mother's story and her doula's story

This story of a twin freebirth, told by the mother and by her doula, is particularly interesting as both the mother and the doula are experienced midwives, though the doula is no longer registered as a midwife. They were both well informed and very aware of the NHS as a safety net should it be needed.

The mother's story

This is just two babies in there and that's just a variation of normal and that could have happened to anyone. So I had that decision to make really early on and I made that decision probably around 20 weeks, after the anomaly scan. Kind of felt reassured, felt like I didn't want to continue on with any growth scans or anything like that. And decided that I was going to trust, trust in the process and trust in the fact that I know my own body and if I wasn't happy with something I would seek help. So that's how it started. I started looking at alternative ways, and started looking around at freebirth, because there was no home birth service running at all. And that's been the case for a few months now and it's still suspended in my area due to the staffing situation. So if there were midwives available, I probably would have arranged to have a home birth, because I had a home birth for my first baby and that was a really positive experience. So that would have been the plan, but it just wasn't an option. So we decided as a partnership, me and my husband, that okay, if we got to 37 weeks then we would seriously consider just having them at home if everything else was good. If everything was normal, there was nothing that we felt was untowards or abnormal or any deviations from that. But I never actually disclosed that to my community midwife…

I had a few meetings with my doula and just talking as well about it and that only cemented the feeling, this kind of innate feeling that, "Actually I just want to have these babies at home, because I feel like it's a normal thing to do." Like before with a singleton and initially no different - they're not identical – they're non-identical, they have two different sacs, two different placentas, so they're just two different babies just sharing a womb.

It was two days before 37 weeks, it was a Saturday night, two o'clock in the morning and my waters went. And within five minutes contractions started and I ran a bath. And my husband was like, "So are we going in then?" Because the plan was that we would have to get to 37 weeks. And I said, "No, it's not happening. It's not happening. Because this baby's going to be here really soon." So by the time the bath was half full, I had a really strong urge to push and he was there in one push. He was really vigorously crying and it was just this really great experience, just to hold him and just have that really totally undisturbed time. By that time my Mum and my sister had arrived, because my husband had called them, and the doula. But E lived an hour and twenty minutes away so she had already set off. But it was just really nice to have this time with this baby with nobody mentioning, "Shall we go in?" So it was really weird. Everyone was just so happy that I'd had this baby.

Fine. So he was born in the bath. And then my husband lit the fire in the living room and we never got the birth pool operating... It was really weird that time between twin one and twin two because all your efforts and your energy is focused on this new baby and trying to care for him. But in the back of my mind I was thinking, my rational side was coming through and, "I've got to do this again at some point." And I think that's what probably contributed to the three hour gap between twin one and twin two, because I let that rational brain kick in and start thinking about that, it was weird. And M, he wouldn't latch at the breast. And I'd had this image in my head the whole pregnancy of first one will come – I will feed him, it will be sublime, it will be so lovely. And that will just help the second one come. Anyway, he wouldn't because he had this 90 percent tongue-tie and he was just poking around. So I was vigorously trying to express into his mouth like an hour and a half, which was quite challenging. And then I wasn't really having any contractions because I was focusing on that. And then the doula arrived, so E arrived and I gave the baby to my Mum to have skin-to-skin. Because my husband was supporting me, so my Mum sat in the corner in skin-to-skin with M, which was really lovely.

So she arrived and I felt the odd contraction starting up after I'd allowed M [twin one] to leave the centre of what was going on for me. I can't remember now what time they started back up again. But it was two and a half hours after the first one I think probably. And they were just mild, mild surges really. It was just messing about really. And I was saying, "I need to get this going. I need to get this going." And the whole time I was thinking, "Can I feel him move? Can I feel him move? I can still feel movement, so I'm happy." And then I was getting on my knees, I was standing up. I think in the back of my head I was happy to remain at home for that length of time because of the movement things. And after a while, I couldn't feel him move. And I was thinking, "Can I or can't I?" And I was starting to get really disheartened about it. And obviously I didn't tell anyone in the room at that time. I don't think I was in a rational state to be verbalising that with people. And also I think deep down in my head I knew this baby has to come out pretty soon, or I'm not actually sure what's going to happen. Even if I do make that decision to go in, I don't know if that's going to improve things. I think E, the doula, she could tell that that was going through my head, that things are starting to change – like the movement is starting to change. And we had these antenatal conversations earlier in the pregnancy and she had talked about using the rebozo and we went through some movements. So I knew what to expect if we were to use that in the labour. And it was always under the conditions that we would only intervene and use this if you are thinking about going into hospital anyway and you are going to make that change, that intervention, I may as well find you something while we wait. And that was kind of why she had suggested it because she knew that I was thinking about this as, "I'm going to have to do something now because I'm not sure if I can feel movement." I started to feel really disheartened about this. So she spoke about the rebozo and she said, "Well which one do you want me to do?" And I said, "Well the one where you shake my hips because I feel that's where things are going to really help." It's going to help the baby move down because these contractions were just kind of pootering about and he was still hanging about at the top. And I wasn't even sure if he was breech or cephalic anymore because he had been breech the whole time, twin two. And then after twin one had come, I thought, "Oh, has he turned?" Because I couldn't feel his head at the top. And when I examined myself and I thought I could feel a hard head. So she used the rebozo a couple of times, which geared up these huge contractions that were just roaring. And I just couldn't stop them. And within three, he had just dropped straight down and he was out. I was on hands and knees and E was watching from behind and she decided not to tell me that he was coming out breech, just not freak me out. And we just saw this bum and the legs kind of flop out. And then, at that point, I looked between my legs and I just saw these two little legs hanging down and a bit of umbilical cord. And I was like, "Oh. Okay. This is happening, he's actually coming out breech." And so then I felt his body come and then I could feel his head. And at that point I just had this little panic about getting his head out, just with the training and stuff that I've had, that if there's going to be an issue, it may well be with getting the head out, when you have a breech baby. And I just gave this almighty push and he just plopped out onto the floor and like two seconds later just heard this thud and that was the placenta just hitting the floor as well. And he was really shocked, he was really shocked. He was pale, he was floppy. He had a bit of a heart rate but he wasn't, certainly wasn't breathing and you know that look, that starry-eyed kind of look. So immediately I just picked him up, rubbed him and then just inflated his lungs and asked my husband to ring an ambulance, which he did. So by that time I'd done two rounds of inflation breaths, just puffing his lungs up and he gave me like a little cry, but wasn't really up for doing any of it himself. So I just was giving him some ventilation breaths as well and the ambulance crew were on the phone and they were starting at the very beginning. We were like, "We've done that, we've done that. Just send an ambulance please." But after a minute of just breathing for him, he suddenly was just pinked up and started moving around and looking around and just was more than happy to do everything for himself. And then just latched on straight away and had a feed. I think it took 18 minutes for the ambulance to come after we'd called them. So by that time he had come around and was feeding and my Mum was trying to clean up around us because there was towels everywhere, you know. In this really short three and a half hour labour I'd managed to use every towel in the house. I was too hot, I was too cold; too hot, too cold. So there were ice packets everywhere and then blankets strewn about the place and it was quite funny, to be honest. So then the ambulance crew arrived and made that decision to go into hospital to get checked over. So we went in and got checked over and stayed the night. That's how it happened really.

The paediatricians were really just confused about what had happened and why it had happened. So they wanted to do blood gases and because they were a couple of days early they wanted to do blood sugars. So we had like a run of them, having to get them out of the way. And so that took a while. We got the hearing screening done and the newborn check as well,... whatever you want to call it. So we stayed for all that basically, to get all the extra bits done and then went home the next day. It was probably the best experience I've ever had in my life, having a home, a twin home birth. Especially with the second one being breech. I never would have thought that I would ever be in that situation, to be honest. And I still struggle to figure out how I got to that place where I felt so at peace with everything that I was quite happy to just do it at home. And I would do it all over again, but I just think so many women have, society for one tells you that you can't give birth, you can't do it without help. So I'm really thankful that I stood by what I felt and had the courage and the support to do it. Especially from my family. Everyone in that birthing room did not bring their own judgement to the labour or the birth. My Mum, my sister and my husband and my doula completely supported me one hundred percent.

Nobody physically touched me the whole time. And that was probably the most important thing for me. Except for that rebozo, that magic scarf, which I'll forever be thankful for, because I just knew that he needed to come out and that scarf just set things off beautifully again. Honestly, I will forever be thankful to E and her magic scarf (laughs). **Yvonne**

The doula's story

Yvonne contacted me looking for doula support for her home birth; we had an initial conversation on the phone. I advised her to speak to other doulas because we always say that – don't choose the first person, you know. Shop around is always the advice. But Yvonne came back to me and said that she felt like I was the right person. And then we had a lot of contact by email and Whatsapp and we met up a couple of times to go through birth plans and make sure we were on the same page. So each of those visits was over two hours, so that we could go through all the plan and build that relationship not virtually, which is really important... everything that she said always just made sense to me, her decisions made sense, I just trusted her completely. I trusted her body autonomy, I trusted her decision-making for her and her baby...

She was pregnant with twins. I had supported a home birth of twins previously, that was supported by the NHS and the consultant midwife was on board and really helped support the lady with that. So although I hadn't seen many twin births actually, as in twin births as a midwife, I did get to see one as a doula. And how straightforward that can be when things are just left alone to be, as a physiological event. So when Yvonne phoned me and said that she was planning a twin home birth, I wasn't too fazed by the whole idea. However, she said that she wouldn't get any support from the NHS, because the home births were cancelled there. And we discussed other options like alongside midwifery units and there's nothing where she lives, her local hospital is quite close but there isn't any birth centre or alongside midwifery unit options there. So really, she felt her only option was home birth. She's had a home birth previously that was very straightforward. So she really felt stuck in a position where she wanted to have a home birth and wanted support from the midwives, being a midwife herself, but that support wasn't available. And she kind of threw the idea out there of she might have a home birth, she might have a freebirth, "Does that sound a bit crazy?" And I said, "No, if that's where you're going towards, then if that's what you want to do, that's fine. You can think on it." I mean, with Yvonne being a midwife herself, I knew that she wasn't taking this decision lightly, and knew the potential risks and had a full understanding of what twin births might mean at home. And so I knew that she was educated on the risks as well as on the benefits of all that. So I said I'd support her in whatever decision she decided to make, whether she went into hospital or decided to have her babies at home, or just waited to see how she felt at the time. So it wasn't a strict plan; it was more, "Let's see when these babies arrive. Let's see if any problems present themselves that may indicate a hospital birth as more sensible." And I would support her with a hospital birth. "Let's see when these babies arrive. Let's see how you feel when you're in labour. You know, you can change your mind at any time." She isn't far from the hospital. So we just felt our way through it. We made a plan for what would happen, her wishes around freebirth. And made a plan for a hospital birth that the midwives were shown. I think it was sent to their email. Yvonne didn't make the midwives aware that she was having, planning possibly to have a freebirth, because she didn't want to be judged on that. And also because she's a midwife and she works within the NHS trust that she's rejecting, I suppose. What that would mean for her not only with her own care, but also with her work, her future work with them. So we just kind of felt our way through it…

So I was travelling quite a bit to support her and there was no way to make that journey any faster because it's just a long way away. So I made the journey – they phoned me to say twin one had just slipped out in the bath… And it just happened so quick. And then I think she was thinking, "Okay, that was really easy. And baby's fine. So I don't want to be in the car on the way to hospital while baby number two comes out at two o'clock in the morning when it's freezing." Because it's January. So I continued my journey to her and when I arrived she was still in labour with baby number two. She was breastfeeding baby number one. And it was just such a lovely atmosphere. Everything was really calm, her partner was there, her Mum was there, her sister was there. The fire was blazing. It was just like so gorgeous. And so I just slipped into that space and said, "I'm here." And her partner reminded her that it was maybe coming up two hours and that was a bit of a threshold for her. But she said, "I don't want to talk about it. You know, I feel, I feel well. I feel baby moving, I feel the contractions are building. I don't want time discussed unless I feel I've got concerns." So we just continued, she fed baby for a while and then felt like she had to concentrate on this labour. So Granny had skin to skin, which was lovely. And we kind of danced together for a wee while, because I was a better height than her husband – he's very tall. So her arms round my neck was easier. She says, "I'm really sorry, but actually it's just more comfortable." So we swayed and danced for a wee while in the heat of the fire. And then we put some cold cloths on her. And she started to be a wee bit concerned about baby's movements, that baby was a wee bit quieter than it had been. So she started to tune into that a wee bit more. She self-examined herself a few times just to check if baby was coming down. She changed positions many times. And this was all maybe in about 20 minutes, half an hour, I could see that she was starting to get... she wasn't voicing those concerns, but she kept feeling her bump for baby's movements, she kept moving position... She was concerned that things weren't happening, but she wasn't maybe... she wasn't verbalising that, but she was... non-verbally showing signs that there were concerns. And I had kind of, "Do you feel baby moving more now?" And she said, "I think so." But I think he moved a wee bit she was... her non-verbal cues were telling me that she wasn't sure and she wasn't maybe so happy at that point. So I put some counter pressure on her back to ease discomfort. And then I suggested, "Do you want to try the rebozo?" Because I've got a rebozo in my bag. And she said, "Yes, I want to try that." And I said, "What position... what one do you want me to do?" Because we had demonstrated, we went through all these things antenatally. And she said, "Do the one where you shake my bottom" (laughs). So I did that for one contraction between contractions. You know, and with the next contraction it felt much stronger. And then to her, and sounded different. And then we did it again between contractions. And she really started to... she was trying to push before, but it had nothing behind... her body wasn't really assisting her with that. But then with the next contraction, she pushed baby out and baby was breech... I said, "Baby's coming now." And I saw the bag of waters and I thought, "That's fine." Baby's presenting part is right behind that bag of waters. And then the waters broke and two legs fell down. And I was like, "Okay. Baby is breech." And she had shown a wee bit of doubt. She was pretty convinced baby was head down, but had shown doubt with her self-examination that she was no longer sure of that. So I suppose that maybe wasn't too much of a surprise to me either. And then baby just unfolded in front of us. The arms were born and then she just... baby head delivered no bother. And she came, went closer to the ground and basically laid baby down with her body. And baby was a wee bit stunned by the birth, you know, not responsive, not breathing... very poor colour. But I had seen a breech before as a midwife, so I know that they're usually not in the best condition. When babies are born breech, they're a wee bit more compromised, take a wee bit of time just to pick up. So I wasn't too worried about that at all. And then we realised, we both realised the placenta had plopped out with baby. So when baby was born, the placenta came out immediately after baby. Although there had been no sign of bleeding, there was no bleeding at that point either, it was very strange. So we knew he was getting no support from the placenta anymore because it was out. So Mum instinctively rubbed baby down, felt for a heartbeat. Baby had a heartbeat – it was very slow. So she just started doing mouth-to-mouth. After a bit of stimulation and baby not being responsive, she started to give baby mouth-to-mouth and intermittently checked baby's heartbeat and rubbed the baby down and kept going through this motion of stimulating him. And she asked Dad to phone an ambulance, her birth partner, the baby's Dad phoned an ambulance. Everyone was in a bit of a panic in the background - the Mum and sister. Yvonne just kept breathing for her baby and she just kept checking and breathing and checking and breathing. And it felt like it went on forever. The call handler told Yvonne what to do but told her partner what should happen, but it was already being done. You know, he was being stimulated, he was... And then he just started to slowly come round. It felt like it went... we have no sense of timeline. But he just slowly started to come round and... colour picked up. He started to breathe, but still didn't have regular breaths, so Yvonne continued to support him. And by the time the ambulance arrived, which is ten, 15 minutes later, everything was fine. As usually happens, by the time they arrived he was pink, he was breathing, his tone was great, he was feeding. The minute the baby could breathe, he was on the breast, like it obviously helped his support and recovery, because he just wanted to latch on immediately, the minute he was kind of with us really. So the ambulance came. They were all fine and respectful and all was okay. But Yvonne decided to transfer in, just to get her babies checked over, particularly twin two. So we all transferred in and the babies got checks and everything. And everything seemed fine. In fact, the baby that had the problems was baby number one, because he really struggled to feed and had the tongue-tie and ended up... well they both ended up jaundiced, but because his feeding was more poor... they both had jaundice checks and things like that over the next week or so. But it was actually twin one that had a bit more input, I suppose, with the hospital and checks because of his feeding. So that's my side of the story.

...It was scary when baby was born and... as time went on, he was very slow to respond and you've not got any support... so I just supported Yvonne to do what she wanted to do. I knew that she had the skills, she knew what she was doing, so I was just supporting her in a nice, calm manner to do what she had to do. Because everyone else was obviously very upset. Yvonne and her family had had a bereavement – her Dad had passed away during this pregnancy. And I think it happened in Yvonne's house with ambulance staff, but they couldn't revive him. So obviously, for the wider family that were there that was all very traumatic, and bringing back these memories of Yvonne's Dad. So Yvonne was completely in the moment instinctually; she wasn't obviously in that head space, but I think everyone else maybe was. So, but... I didn't have all that on board, so I was able to just be there for Yvonne and just stay close by and stay calm for her, so that she could stay calm. So overall, [I feel] pretty positive about the whole thing, but yes, bit of a scary one that we maybe didn't see coming. But you know, that is birth, it's so unpredictable. I don't think Yvonne... she doesn't regret her decision certainly to freebirth and feels it was the right thing for her and the babies. And we know that hospitals can be helpful and can save Mums and babies, but sometimes they do more harm than good. **E**, doula

Chapter 16: A premature twin birth and the death of a baby

Before I experienced labour and birth first-hand I had only witnessed industrial, medicalised birth. The hysterical movie and TV representation of a woman's screaming, futile efforts; labouring urgently, pushing unbearably, with the frantic assistance of uniformed professionals.

The much-loved Monty Python sketch of a labouring woman who asks what she should do is told, "Nothing my dear, you're not qualified!" is no longer funny because it was and continues to be true.

I would soothe myself from the moral injury, sustained as a student midwife by watching births on YouTube: births that were the wondrous, spiritual, majestic event that every woman deserves hers to be.

By the time I was a teenager (late 90's-early 00's) I expressed bafflement at the fact that people went to the hospital to give birth. I found the clinical, disempowered environment, far from one's own creature comforts and where the bed is the central focus, a terrible way to facilitate childbirth.

I thought back to my wild pregnancy and short unassisted home birth of premature (nine weeks early) "undiagnosed" twins. I'd opted out of receiving mainstream care because maternity services had reported me, on account of my birth choices and other concerns of theirs, to multiple agencies in the borough where I live. I was hounded mercilessly throughout my pregnancy by Children's Services whose support I declined. My move to Jamaica whilst 26 weeks pregnant was a direct result of my fear that they would attempt to take my child from me at birth. I had to flee to an unknown place away from my support network of family and friends to avert this from happening.

I feel a lot of things about the hours and days following my birth: part sad, part jubilant.

I laboured alone - just me and my baby, O (I'd been happy with this name for both a boy or a girl and settled firmly on it by my second trimester) – nobody attended as was my wish. I know myself and know that when I'm in pain I want to be alone, in a dark, comfy place to endure it.

That meant no well-meaning friends, no midwife with one eye on the clock, no paid doula, no matriarchal Mummy or Grandma urging me to do things her way, giving her superior advice based on her own distant, misremembered births.

I knew from my training that birth is a delicate thing, the hormones required are shy and need dark spaces, feeling unobserved. Labours that are progressing entirely smoothly can stall after a car ride to the hospital, with dire consequences. You might scoff that I'm being dramatic but a labour stalled could mean an otherwise unnecessary surgery for Mums who had desperately wanted a physiological birth and could have had one. Safety of the baby is not, as the more misogynistic people declare, the only desired outcome.

In my case if I hadn't opted for wild pregnancy there's only a few clinicians in London who wouldn't have had their concerns about a premature twin who presented feet first. So it was better that they didn't know. After six hours of labouring through the night I felt the sensation of crowning but it felt ever so small and not the extreme stretching I'd anticipated so I, on all fours on the bed, reached a hand around to feel the presenting part. I think I must have gasped. After feeling only tiny softness, my first thought was uterine prolapse and I was momentarily terrified before realising that surely if I were experiencing uterine prolapse I would be in agony and I wasn't.

Exploring further I found tiny toes, "Oh. Exhale. It's a footling breech." I could handle a footling breech. On the next expulsive surge O's whole body was out, dangling by his head. On the next expulsive surge which was maybe a minute later? It's a bit of a blur – his head came with such a teeny length of cord that I was incapacitated, confined on my hands and knees on the edge of the bed with my newborn hanging three inches between my legs. For the first few minutes of life I thought O was dead and that that figured because I'd not felt kicking throughout my non-descript, highly ordinary pregnancy, only what I called gurglings. I called them gurglings or rumblings because they weren't clearly legs kicking but a bum poked up here a bony knee or elbow here and there. The movements were sporadic at 31 weeks without any discernible pattern. From what I could tell by peering through the arch of my legs, he was grey and hadn't cried or made any sound yet. I reached through my legs and rubbed him vigorously. I located my phone (mercifully close as I'm a typical millennial who sleeps with their device) and sent a voice note to my next door neighbour very matter-of-factly stating that the baby was born but he was dead. A few minutes later he spat something up and seemed to croak. Okay, and we're back. O is alive. I somehow managed to waddle to the door. Did he cry? I don't at all remember in my exhaustion.

The neighbour arrived (my dear friend) and did what I couldn't do for myself, torniqueting and cutting the cord that kept O and I so closely attached. She cooed over me and what I thought was my one infant son. She had a friend from Canada on the phone for a second opinion/advice/guidance and this faceless voice brought in the worry about a retained placenta and, being so thoroughly immersed in babyland I found her voice and input an irritation. I had invited my neighbour in, not this other woman. I began to take on some of her concern about the placenta and fearfully tried some light cord traction.

It now seems absurd that I failed to realise there was one more baby to come for 50 minutes as O dangled on a tiny bit of cord. But after a quick trip to the bathroom and seeing myself in the mirror the tell-tale signs of a knee and a bum was there. In my delirium I was terrified, thinking I had to do another six hours of labour again for this next one but my acknowledgement that there was another to come seemed to herald his arrival – The second born had the good sense to come head first and with one expulsive force (again no pushing, it's involuntary akin to when you have diarrhoea or a bout of vomiting) he was here, followed almost simultaneously by their placenta. I had one placenta, two cords and I believe two amnion sacs. I was planning a lotus birth so was pleased that one of my sons could still enjoy this gentle way of arriving earth side. My friend and my sons and I sat on the bed for five hours, laughing about their entry, overjoyed by the sudden good news of twin boys. We guessed at their respective characters and the little gurgling the second-born seemed to make almost immediately post-birth we found adorable but then suddenly worrying. My friend who was not up to speed with my plan to lotus birth suggested we cut the cord now as it was difficult to manoeuvre him with a large placenta attached and the bag that my Auntie had made to carry it in was not really fit for purpose.

I surrendered my fervent wish to have a lotus birth. It suddenly became less important than the convenience of me being able to take both twins out for breakfast to be congratulated and to display my miraculous surprise. Once the cord was cut Twin two started to deteriorate, looking a little blue grey and using accessory muscles to breathe. Panic set in as I tried to remember the steps of neonatal resuscitation and arrange how to get him to a hospital. After a few minutes of resuscitation, I felt Twin two go floppy and this is when I believe his soul left his body. I told my friend, "he's gone, he's gone" but my friend and the local new Mum that she'd called on the phone said, "No, No keep trying" and I obeyed. He went grey and floppy and died in my arms at home but my friend and the random people that she called made me persist in resuscitating him against my better judgement.

He was five hours old when we began to seek medical care. We went by taxi to a clinic who just looked horrified but didn't help; we then went to another clinic but their resuscitation technique was worse than mine as was the ambulance when we finally got him in an ambulance (they had no premature or neonate masks so couldn't administer oxygen).

The doctors worked on his lifeless body for two days. I felt awful that I resented him. I couldn't accept that he had got through all that gestation only to die. I didn't understand why he didn't want to remain with me, his chosen Mummy and his cherished brother for a lifetime.

When R, my second born twin was dying, being worked on by loads of professionals shoving their hands into his incubator to stroke/soothe? him and I was invited to do the same. I felt annoyed at him for not being stronger, for taking himself away from O and I, for forcing us into the medical system but when he finally died I felt so sad and I asked his tiny grey body why, why had his soul wanted this brief incarnation but he didn't answer, his spirit was long gone.

If a midwife would have been there I suspect they would have noticed Twin two's poor state right away and he would have survived.

It's very hard to talk and think about. So grateful to have my one little boy at least. **Reign**

Chapter 17: A stillbirth

I had my freebirth but it wasn't with the outcome hoped, as baby was stillborn. Nothing to do with actual freebirthing though, as baby had died at least two to three days before the birth they said in hospital but I didn't realise as I thought I still felt some movements.

In 2017 with my first I had a very traumatic hospital birth… [with her second she was booked for a home birth but the midwife insisted on transferring her to hospital] if my partner would have understood what I said to him about calling the midwives I don't think I would have called them till after birth and it would have been wonderful. Baby was 4.070g latched on straight away…whole labour was four and a half hours from my waters breaking. [In both these labours she felt bullied and unheard.]

My third last birth. After my previous experiences I said I'm having a home birth. I declined consultant care, I declined any measurements: no weight, height, BMI, no bump measurements, no scans (they still booked them for me even though I said no, but I cancelled). I only agreed to listening with Pinard. I would not give anyone a chance to make up a problem. And I joined the freebirthing group. Unfortunately, as this pregnancy was unplanned, my partner didn't want the baby and said he will leave me if I go ahead with it till I was about eight months and then he decided he'll stay but still didn't want the baby. So all this pregnancy time was very hard for me as all the way I was alone with no family here and not really having any friends or just anyone to help a little bit emotionally or physically with everything going on and with two little kids and starting to homeschool the five year old one because of racism and bullying in school. It was very hard and lonely. So I struggled to connect with my baby on the level I did the previous one. I still wanted her, still loved her but I didn't listen in as much as I should have. But she was making this pregnancy much easier than previous two as with my first I had the morning sickness all the way through and second time most of pregnancy but this time only at the start. I did have bad SPD through all my pregnancies.

…On 22nd of April I started having some painful contractions. That was a few days before 37 weeks so I was worried I'll go into labour and no one will come out if I need them. I was very stressed that day as still had a lot to sort out before the baby comes and me doing everything on my own. Next day my plug went. I was having painfulish tightenings ever since. In the end of last week I wasn't exactly happy with the movement. I was a bit worried but kept thinking that with the girls it reduced significantly as well. I also didn't want them to start having a go at me for not wanting an ultrasound and only allowing to listen with Pinard. Especially after I read on one of these groups where Mum went to A&E because of reduced movements and because of having children and partner with her she was treated horrible. I didn't have it in me to have someone else treat me like that and because of my previous experience I wouldn't expect anything else.

So on Saturday because all day I was waiting on some movements and only felt once her bum move or slip down and was worried I said to her to just come. It doesn't matter that everything isn't ready but I just want her in my arms safe. So around 6pm, possibly before, I had a strong contraction. Contractions were very irregular once an hour or twice but I knew my labour had started. It wasn't what I expected as I thought it will be quick after my previous. But was very slow and long and painful, completely different from my previous. In the start I was trying to have some sleep after I prepared the bathroom and set everything ready. I made sure kids go to bed on time. I tried to sleep till two or three o'clock, I'm not too sure but couldn't really as they [contractions] were painful even though still so irregular and slow. So I went to bathroom and emptied my bowels. Then I was labouring on toilet including sitting other way around with pillow on the top and wasn't too bad for a while. I also had put on some labour meditation play list on Spotify and I really liked it. I lit a candle and opened the blinds so I have a little light from outside even though it was dark outside it was making it lighter inside. Then I laboured on my birthing ball leaning on it with bum up, then I run the bath but after I got in it, I hated the feeling of the warm water on my stomach and me, so quickly got out as felt sick from the warmness and the smell of candle so put it out, I didn't want a smelly one in first place but I didn't have any other ones on hand. It was getting lighter outside. This labour really was different, the pain was different and I kept trying to connect with the baby but couldn't. With previous one it felt like she's trying to crawl down the birth canal but this one wasn't, she just wasn't moving down like that. And it kept being slow process. I was standing and holding on to sink and windowsill and kept circulating my hips like in all my labours and saying yes when I felt like no and just kept saying "come" and try to stay open. I thought I might be transitioning. Then I took my pillow and got on my bath mat where I put towel over me as I was naked and a bit cold as had had window open because of candle smell and heat but I closed it as didn't want baby to be cold. I put the kids' disposable bedsheet on the mat. And leaned over it while hugging my pillow and pushing head in the side of the bath when having contractions so I wouldn't slip away. It wasn't the most comfortable way but also not the worst. So I had a feel between my legs and there was the sack just there ready to pop or come out. After a bit I felt like I need to push just a little bit and the waters went. There was some meconium and water was a little bit brown but again nothing major not smelly, lumpy or green. So I carried on mooing in my pillow hoping no one hears me (I had my two daughters and stepdaughter in the next room). Then I could feel something coming out so put my hand under and was trying to be lower so she doesn't fall and I can catch her. Then with next contractions I wasn't pushing anything because I just wanted my body to do it. So for a little while nothing happened and then my body started pushing a bit. It didn't push whole body out in one go it was quite few contractions. Then she came out and I caught her.

She wasn't breathing so I straight away started trying to help her. I put my mouth over her mouth and nose and was trying to gently blow in, it didn't seem to be working so I rubbed her a bit with a towel but nothing while talking to her then tried to blow a bit more. Then I opened the door and shouted to my partner to call an ambulance saying baby was born and not breathing. So he straight away did and it seemed like ages for them to come. He stayed on the phone and told me to do light chest presses and blowing after I placed her on the towel on the floor. When they came, after not a long while of trying to resuscitate her they wanted to cut the cord and I said, "No," I said, "She needs that blood and oxygen" and they said no she had everything and when I said no again the young paramedic said to me, "Trust me we went to uni for this stuff." As if I was stupid and didn't know anything. To which I simply replied that I done a lot of learning about it as well. Then I looked at the cord as it was still full of blood and the woman said to me, "Look it's not pulsing" and then I saw the knot. I was trying to loosen it and said look there's a knot and it's all still full of blood. But no one cared that I said I'm coming with and she can stay attached. She was cut off taken in the first ambulance. Then after I cleaned my arms and legs in the bath a bit they let me go to the third ambulance with placenta still in me, I had quickly put a nappy on myself. And my partner gave me a dressing gown. When I got to hospital they kept bothering me about birthing placenta and injection and I said that I don't want the injection and these hadn't been normal circumstances so how could I birth the placenta and I don't care about their made up hour and they were throwing risks of infection and retained placenta to me to which I replied that injection increases the risk for it. I declined the check and just kept asking about my baby, they said she was in the other hospital, I was in maternity one so why wasn't she? Doctor said that they thought we were both there and they just came from there because they wanted to check me. Then just kept bugging me about the placenta like broken record while all I wanted was to be with my baby and know what's happening.

Then a woman came and said that she was born dead. I just burst out crying. I did have a bad feeling because why was it taking so long for them to tell me what's going on. They said to try to birth the placenta and they'll get her ready and put us in the room together. I was having contractions all the time through this but this pressure feeling for some reason I was putting down to needing a poo but then I let it go in the toilet and placenta came out. The true knot was still there. No ultrasound would have shown it. How could I save her if there only was the before where she's fine and after where it's too late?

I was trying to protect her from everything so she would have no birth trauma. I carried her right to the end through all the hardness and everything. I wanted her all the way and even after birthing her alone, I am left alone. I really birthed her alone because she wasn't there anymore, that's why it was slow and painful in different way because it was just my body doing the work because my baby's soul was gone, that's why I couldn't connect to her during labour. I wasted the time I had her in me being sad about things what were happening around me and being so alone that I didn't appreciate that she was making me not alone. Now I have no baby, no, no kicks, nothing. I can't imagine what I would do if I didn't have my other two daughters. So as empowering birth is supposed to be, I don't feel empowered. I feel like I failed. I failed her. I will never have her.

I named her L which means little fairy... She's magical and will always stay little. And she's so very beautiful and perfect.

The only thing I would add is, after speaking to the police and trying to understand the times as I wasn't looking at the clock, my third birth was only a bit over two hours in the bathroom. But probably because I was alone and she wasn't with me helping, it seemed long and slow. I was shocked when I realised that it wasn't long at all. But all of it seemed so slow. My partner and police told me the ambulance came quick as well. In my head everything seemed to last forever. **Silva**

Section 5: After the Birth and Wider Issues

The mothers in this book had very different experiences after the birth of their babies. Whaterevr followed, all felt positive about their freebirth. The response of NHS staff and other services could very much influence their postnatal experiences.

For some, the time after birth was a settled and magical time in their own homes with family surrounding them. They were able to get to know their new baby, supported by family and close friends or doulas. For some women and families the birth of their baby and the love and joy that flowed from this was marred by poor or negative responses from maternity or other services.

For a few families, the involvement of services – especially Social Services was devastating and caused ongoing hurt, guilt and trauma which was difficult to recover from. The families did their best to cope with these intrusions to protect their babies and other children. All drew strength from their freebirth and their own wisdom, knowledge and intuition, enhanced by their decision to take birth into their own hands. NHS staff and Social Services can, however, be intimidating and coercive.

Engagement with these authorities demonstrated firsthand to the women a number of things: the power invested in these organisations, as well as judgemental attitudes which dictate an approach designed to protect the organisations and those working for them, rather than the individual mothers and families.

Whatever happened, all the women felt that they had grown from their experience of freebirthing, and that this stood them in good stead following the birth of their baby.

Chapter 18: After the birth: joy and compliance

Most of the mothers were overjoyed after birth and appreciated being at home in the period immediately after their freebirth.

When he came out, I laughed and laughed. Overcome by a kind of ecstasy and happiness I can't begin to explain. A bit like being on drugs, but with a clarity, a pause, a sweet rise of awe at the moment you straddle two realms and pull your baby from the water and lift him to your chest…

Then we hunkered down and stared at G and his dark hair and dark eyes and familiar smell, and it was almost just like any other day. A sense of home welled up around me, and I was thankful to be in my bed, surrounded by my people – now five bodies, instead of four. **Kendal**

All very straightforward, and just the biggest high of our lives, it was amazing. **Leonie, third freebirth**

I would say it's the most influential and amazing experience I've ever had in my life, yes. **Nicole**

It was bloody amazing. I couldn't stop from telling anyone who'd listen. **Reign**

I had the freedom, it really happened as I thought and it was really magical and special and… And it was real… it was very good, yes. And you really feel powerful and it really makes you high, you really feel like in connection with all the universe. And it is something that goes higher. **Bea**

I'm really, really, really pleased I did [freebirth] (laughs) because, not only the actual birth itself, but after the birth was so nice to not have anyone else there, not be hurried to deliver the placenta, and I took two hours and that was a really nice time, bonding with my baby and with my partner and it was lovely, that was really lovely, yes. **Rosalie**

Physically, my labour and birth with my second son was almost completely identical to the first. Emotionally it was a complete contrast because the calm of labour was never disrupted. I found my strength in knowing I could birth my baby alone. **Virginia**

It was amazing and I'm so glad that I didn't give up. The recovery, it's just chalk and cheese, like worlds apart from what happened last time. I only started crying in week two when I started to feel a bit tired, because I was getting woken up every hour, whereas with my first daughter I cried every day for probably months. Whereas this time, I just felt ecstatic; I felt like I could do anything. **Katie H**

And it was lovely, and I stayed in bed for the next week and got waited on hand and foot, which was something I'd never experienced before and was brilliant. It definitely helped me have a good start. And I had a placenta smoothie straight after the birth. I had actually six over the first three days. I didn't have the experience that I'd had with my previous three babies of day three, having these massive painful breasts as my milk came in, and spending the whole day crying, and the baby crying because the breasts were too big to get latched on properly. The previous three had had that like clockwork on the third day, and I'd been expecting it. But I had the placenta smoothies, my milk came in within 12 hours and I didn't have any mood swings at all. I didn't have that crying for a whole day, which was really nice. And R's been a really peaceful baby and very happy, and I think it's a lot to do with how he was born. And he seems to recognise all the people that were there – even my doula friend, who he doesn't see very often, but he's always got a big smile for her when he sees her which is really nice. And it was nice for us as a family to all be there together. My son, who's 15, didn't want to be present at the birth, because it's a bit gross (laughs). But he was very happy to come home from school and have a little brother to cuddle up with. So that was a nice surprise for him when he got home. But yes, it was good. It went basically just as we planned it. I think if I was to do it again, I would be even more confident to do it with even less assistance. **Elena**

… and shortly after [the birth] the placenta came, I think it was like eight minutes, which it was really the most amazing and relieving feeling… it was the most relieving sensation ever. And that's a part of it. You know, your body created this organ too, and to feel that move, like there was something about that. All of it was incredible, but there was something about the placenta that was just… I don't know how to explain it, it was just so relieving. So, yes that's another thing that was just so powerful in a weird way - I didn't expect the placenta to be so strong a feeling like that. And we did again, staying in line with the natural process, we did a delayed cord ceremony and we held… I think he was attached to the cord for maybe two and a half hours. We just took him in and left the vernix on him. And once the cord was completely white and limp and wrinkled, we did a burn ceremony with it. And yes, burned the cord to separate the placenta… it was very important for me, because I did some research on it. And I also talked to a woman who had given birth… she did a home birth herself. She was telling me about the… and all my friends who've gone through birth had been telling me about the hormone drop; how your body just… how you have these weird thoughts and these emotional moments with birth and then having to also take care of baby at the same time. And how you often feel disconnected and everything, so I didn't want to go through that. And this woman had explained to me that she was doing smoothies afterwards with her afterbirth. And so I wanted to be sure to do that. And I didn't do it every day, but most days, and it made a huge difference. I mean, I don't know what it's like without it… that made a big difference to my ability to manage and to become more into myself and everything. **Nicole**

Although I don't know because I've not been in hospital but I remember waking up weeks afterwards and just thinking it was great and looking at my baby and how wonderful it was, instead of waking up and thinking all my stitches are sore or whatever might have happened differently but never mind I've got my baby now. It was all positive, it wasn't a sort of never mind about the birth, I've got my baby now, it was just kind of a really happy feeling all round instead of being something that I wanted to forget about. So, it was good. **Sarah-Anne**

… and as soon as she was born, I [partner's mother] and A [older child] came into the room and they saw the baby. And then me and J [partner] went to sleep and breastfed from half past eight until twelve o'clock, we just slept and cuddled. And then at that point, afterwards called the midwives and the placenta still hadn't come out. But it's because I had been lying on my side or lying on my back and just breastfeeding the baby to me and knew how important that was. So I called the hospital and said, "Oh you're thirty-nine weeks. How can we help you, Jessica?" And I was like, "Oh I've just had baby." And they were like, "Oh my god, you poor thing!" And she was like, "Are you one of those…?" And I was like, "No, it's fine, don't worry." She was like, "Are you one of those freebirthers?" And I was like, "No, no, I was planning on having a home birth." And she was like, "Okay." And then she was… I said, "The only thing is, the placenta hasn't come out." And she was like, "well just squat down and give it a wee push and it should come out." And that was really all the information I would have needed last time really, instead of the sort of panic that was around this. This woman was just confidently, "Sit down and give it a squat." Placenta came out, and then the midwives arrived sort of around one o'clock, after she was born at about eight. And I have to mention, actually, that they were not very happy. **Jessica**

I swear it was the most mind blowing thing I have ever done in my life. It was the most empowering thing even talking about it now, I get chills, it was so perfect. It was everything and so much more. Everything that I've ever even dreamed of. It was that dream birth, do you know what I mean. And from there… I actually went back into the pool and just lay with her then. And within five minutes my wee boy and my Mammy came through the door. And L was just over, rubbing her head, kissing me, you know. And it's like, "Your baby sister." And it was just beautiful, it was so beautiful. And then I was able to go into the bathroom again and I just put the container in there and I sat on the toilet just to deliver, so it took about an hour and forty minutes for the placenta to come. So I then stayed in the pool a good while and then I sat on the toilet for a while until it came. And like I had L feeding on my left breast and L was on my right. And he's just wiping her, you know, he's just rubbing her wee head and all. And it was just so beautiful, it was absolutely amazing. **Christina**

Some women spoke of their freebirth as healing previous trauma.

For myself as a birthing woman, I really needed that freebirth, that's really kind of healed my experience. **Carmen**

Just as they had done during pregnancy, some women spoke of their awareness that the NHS was there as a safety net if needed after the birth.

So to be at home in my own space this time, gosh yes, it makes me quite emotional thinking about it. This time it was such a beautiful experience in comparison. I got wrapped up in my towels and got on my sofa. There was a lot of blood and I think again that was quite frightening for T [partner] because he didn't know if there was something terribly wrong. But we kept checking in with our contingency plan and we knew that at any point we could call an ambulance if there was something medically wrong. And that I could also change my mind and decide to go into hospital and get some help. **Emma**.

Different midwives responded very differently when called after a freebirth and their response had a considerable impact on the new mother's experience. For some this wasn't too disruptive or distressing, some were even pleasantly surprised that the midwives were positive.

… just sat and fed, it was just really beautiful. And then about an hour later, the midwife turned up. It was so funny. They basically got this woman out of retirement to come. I don't know what was going on... and then the irony is, they could have got this woman who was in the town... who was an independent midwife, who was there who could have come. But instead, they got this very old-school woman that came out. And she came in and it was all candlelit, and she turned the lights on and she said, "well you've been a very naughty girl, haven't you?" (laughs). And because I was in this completely ecstatic state, I just found it all very funny. And then I just said to my husband, "Look, give her a cup of tea and get her out of here as soon as you can." And then, I think at this point I hadn't given birth to the placenta. So I'd just been sitting, feeding and chilling. And so she got me squatting over the thing, and I did that. And that was all fine. Then my friend made me... we'd already decided to make a smoothie out of some of the placenta, so I had like a placenta smoothie. I think this woman thought I was completely crazy. And then she was a bit sort of, she was like, "You need to do this. And you need to do that. And de, de, de." I mean what was quite good – I went upstairs and she gave me a little examination. Which, look, I was grateful for because I didn't know... I didn't think I'd torn, and I'd had no tears or anything or any problems. And everything was fine. And then she went. I think maybe someone else came as well. I think... but I can't remember. Yeah, I think there was another person there that came, but it was all very short; they kind of just told me off and then checked me out, then left. Because I think because of the politics of what happened before, I think they all knew that I'd deliberately not called them, and they were all a bit pissed. Well I wouldn't say all, but this woman certainly was. And obviously I knew that there was an underbelly of upset with me from some quarters... But it was fine, because it didn't... I just found it really funny, because I was just there in that very ecstatic place. And also because I am a pretty resilient person. I mean... to me it was just like, "well that's her stuff and…" you know, and I was grateful, it's good to have a professional to check that everything's okay. So I was happy with that.
Rachel

Well, actually they were really quite nice, it actually shocked me a bit [midwives were called by paramedics after the birth where there had been no antenatal contact with maternity services]. It actually shocked me because they were really lovely and I probably told them a bit too much truth, that you know, I guess someone within that profession, it kind of goes against it. But there was one midwife that just was so supportive of me and all my decisions and they even said at the end of their visit like, they asked do I need any further medical attention and I said no, "I don't want it, I don't need any." And they agreed, you've done it this far without us, why would you need us. And they were really pleasant and because Social Services then started to get involved, then one of the midwives would come out with them and she was just super supportive and just informed us that ultimately, Social Services runs on consent and so if I don't consent to it, then I don't have to. Because they'd all said how healthy the baby was and, and me and how well she was feeding and so they didn't have any actual health concerns for either of us. So that was really nice to actually be supported by them. **Yony**

And then he wouldn't breastfeed and it had got to about five, six o'clock and we decided that we'd call the midwife out to check that he didn't have anything that he shouldn't have within his throat, or something that we weren't aware of. So they came out and had a look and said it was a quick birth so he's probably not expelled enough fluid out of his lungs, and when he does begin to feed it will probably float up and it'll come out. Which it did. She went home. We let her weigh him. We also weighed the placenta on the scale, which I don't think she was too pleased with! (laughs). So we did that too. We didn't take any paperwork that she offered or anything. So quite a quick visit. And we all went to bed. It was just very nice and easy and everything I'd wanted the birth to be really. **Laura**

I wanted to do a gentle separation and maybe leave the placenta attached for a few hours and burn it off rather than cut the cord. That had been my plan. But then we were in the pool for a while. The midwives were very good, because it was the two ladies that I'd met during my antenatal appointments, so I knew them, and they were really respectful of the atmosphere when they came in. They were talking in low voices and not rustling plastic bags too much, because they didn't need to get very much of their kit out. So we were in the pool probably for about 20 minutes or something, and then we decided to get out so we could get dried off and I felt like the placenta was on its way out. So I stood up and I had a colander with a metal bowl from the kitchen to catch the placenta, so I had someone hold that under me, and I gave a little push, thinking the placenta was about to be born, but all that came out was blood, and it was quite a lot of blood. We all went, ah, maybe that's not so good. So at that moment, one of the midwives went to get the syntometrine but the cord had already stopped pulsing by that point, so the other midwives suggested we cut the cord and I just agreed, because if I am bleeding there's no point in faffing about. So we cut the cord and I got out and actually, I felt fine. I was standing up for a couple of minutes, I didn't feel light-headed or anything. There was no more blood and the placenta itself came within a few more minutes. So it was all OK. But I wonder if they hadn't been there that soon then I maybe would have… I don't know… them just being there kind of medicalised it and made it potentially scary, just for a couple of moments. So I think if I was to do it again, I would make sure there wasn't anyone there till we'd got past that stuff. But then if I had been bleeding, it would have been good to have them there. I don't know. We would have handled it… But it was fine. They were generally really nice. They did only what they needed to do in the room and then they went through to the other end of the house to do their paperwork and stuff, so they weren't disturbing us. My doula made me a lovely bath with bath salts and rose petals in it and that kind of stuff, so Daddy and the girls snuggled up in bed and sang songs to the baby, didn't you, while I had a bath and got cleaned up, and then I just got into bed. And then I had some nice soup that my Mum had made and lots of chocolate energy balls that we'd made earlier, even though I hadn't got round to making the cake. **Elena**

But for some women negative attitudes and comments from midwives after their freebirths were unpleasant, disruptive and sometimes deeply invasive.

I remember feeling quite invaded by their presence, actually. It wasn't the same kind of, like, celebratory thing. It felt kind of, like, I wish I hadn't bothered, kind of thing. But also it was good to just have them come and do those checks. **Alice**

… then she had said to me, "you could have just asked for a home birth" and she was saying, "actually what you had done was quite illegal" but she just sort of said, "I am just letting you know, I am not going to write anything down but you know if anything had gone wrong and you had not taken appropriate [action] you know you could have actually been prosecuted" and that was quite a heavy thing to say. **Polly**

Looking back, I think that after the birth is when I found it difficult to assert myself with the NHS and felt a lot of pressure to accept their services. There was an expectation for me to accept the services they offered and follow their advice and when I didn't do this, or if I challenged this I felt judged by them. For example, I'd had a tear when giving birth, however, I decided not to have stitches and the impression I got was this decision was seen as neglectful and shameful. I was put under pressure by different people to have the stitches because it was recommended. I didn't have them and I was and still am happy with my choice – my body has healed well. But it did shake my confidence at a time when I needed support and kindness the most. **Emma**

And sure enough the next day they said they wouldn't come out to her when she called for a midwife. She called the home birth team and it was [her midwife] said that they wouldn't come out because her son was now high risk due to the fact that he wasn't monitored in labour… then after a couple of hours, she did come out with, I think a senior midwife. She didn't remember much about her, but they stayed for two hours checking out her and the baby, seems like a very detailed check. And they determined that the baby had jaundice and needed immediate transfer for phototherapy which she did and her son was then separated from her to put under the lights which she was quite distressed by. And then the blood test came back that he didn't have severe jaundice after all. But they kept her in overnight and she came back the day after. **D, doula,** describing the midwives' visit to Carmen a few hours after her freebirth (see chapter 14).

A community midwife came out – someone who I didn't know because my community midwife wasn't available. She came to our home to do her checks and ask me lots of questions which felt quite invasive to be honest. Looking back I would have liked to have asked them to wait longer until I was ready. But I didn't feel confident to say no. I felt much more judged after the birth, but it may also be that I was also more resilient to their judgement before giving birth. When my baby was tucked up inside of me I didn't need as much support from others. But afterwards I felt that both of us were vulnerable. **Emma**

Yes, we called before the placenta came. They were a bit put out I think but of course at that point it seemed quite unusual but it was the one particular midwife who I'd just felt, I cannot really put my finger on it, but just felt I didn't really want her to be there at the birth. There was that one particular midwife who came the next morning... maybe she felt a bit awkward in that sort of situation but by then, she kind of made out that we were incredibly lucky and that it could also have been dangerous. But I mean I did say to her at the time that it was just a quick birth and that that could happen and I didn't feel confident enough to give her the impression that we had decided not to ring. Yes, I think she was okay. She wasn't happy with the way we'd tied the cord so she put a little clip on and she said you had the placenta, because we had the placenta in a stainless steel bowl... It was lovely but maybe it was just really lucky but I felt like it was just what I'd dreamed that it could be and it really felt quite almost meditative and sort of just kind of... not too many people, sort of calm. It was good. **Sarah-Anne**

Lack of resources for midwifery services had an impact on some women's experience. Sarah W had a freebirth while their phone call to the triage service for a midwife to attend her home birth went unanswered for 45 minutes. After the birth two ambulance crews arrived and she was admitted to hospital.

And I think if I hadn't had to go to hospital sort of an hour after he'd been born, I would have appreciated the process a lot more. Because you kind of lose out. My blood pressure was really high and they said my stitches were quite complicated. They were quite close to my urethra. So they wanted to have some decent lighting. So yes, so I got the home birth, but not the really nice chilled bit afterwards... we had to stay in overnight. It stayed high, but then the hospital was so hideous and awful, they just left me on a gurney after I'd been stitched, with a constant blood pressure machine on. And then kind of wondering why my blood pressure was staying high. As soon as I got checked into the ward... because I just said, "If you're going to keep me in overnight, I want to rest." My blood pressure went straight down afterwards, so I don't know. And I don't know how much blood pressure goes up naturally because you're giving birth and perhaps doing it without pain relief, and I don't know how much is a natural amount to go up. **Sarah W**

The restrictions around Covid made the situation even more difficult for mothers and doulas.

The hearing test also, which couldn't be done at home; it needed to be done in the hospital. And we didn't want to go to hospital. We had absolutely no concerns about his hearing. But because it was part of their service to offer they were insisting it happened. I felt as though I was choosing between neglecting his hearing and the safety of his life in case we went into hospital and he caught Covid-19. We chose not to have the hearing tests in the end. **Emma**

There was one [birth] I was recently involved in where the woman has signed the agreement to keep the peace [abide by Covid restrictions at a home birth to have only one birth partner]. She certainly wasn't agreeing to only having one person there and she was definitely going to have myself and her husband, and her daughter was asleep in another room. And the birth went so smoothly and so quickly, and she didn't even look like she was in labour, not active labour. And then there came a point where it was clear she was about to birth her baby, but it was quite sudden, I think even for her, she didn't expect it. Whereas, suddenly she looked at her partner and I and said, "The baby's coming down." And I may have said something like, "Great," and that was it, or, "Yes great, and just get ready to pick your baby up." And so she did. She birthed her baby and we were all a bit surprised, and then we called the midwife, who arrived and was very, very cross that there was an additional person there. And I was instructed to stay in the other room. And then I heard a rumour that she was very cross, because I had facilitated this freebirth as she saw it. **D**, doula

The postnatal interaction is one where the midwife potentially has great power. While some acted with sensitivity, some abused that power and others acted as they felt they must, with an approach steeped in risk and routine. For some women, having a midwife come into their special after-birth space and make impactful decisions that could not easily be challenged or resisted had devastating short-term and long-term consequences.

It was great. It was a really great experience. And then after we'd given birth, it didn't turn so great because there was then the involvement of the hospital that soured it. But the actual birth experience itself was fantastic... longer than I expected it to be... I don't know why I thought it would be over in minutes. I didn't expect to be in labour for 25 hours. But a couple of hours after I'd given birth, I rang delivery suite to tell them I'd given birth. Their reaction was one of horror, that I'd given birth at home without a midwife present. And then when the midwife came – the community midwife who was on call for home births – came to the house, she was totally out of her depth. She was really horrified by what we'd done, to the extent that she was very shouty and saying that we'd put everybody's life at risk, that it was a child protection issue, that I could have died, A could have died, and she was really horrendous. She made up the name of a paediatrician at the LGI and said that this paediatrician needed to see us immediately, otherwise things would escalate. And then we went to the LGI, which in hindsight, I should never have done. I'd just given birth, A was only a couple of hours old. We got in the car and went to the LGI because this midwife said that if we didn't then things would escalate, and we assumed that she meant Social Services. We got to the LGI and this paediatrician didn't exist, and she'd basically made up a story to get us in, so that we could then be interrogated by three different doctors about why we'd decided to freebirth. Luckily the supervisor of midwives, who was on call, also came down, and she was really fantastic actually, and was the calm in the storm of all of the other craziness from the other staff that were on, and luckily wasn't horrified and she actually tried to be a bit more like, "these guys need to go home. There's nothing wrong with A, there's nothing wrong with the mother, she's not ill, the baby is clearly in good health, feeding is established…" So we eventually went back home to start what should have been an undisturbed process. She was really good afterwards, because I made a very long and formal complaint about that particular midwife who saw us after birth, and she was involved in that complaint and was very good at helping me resolve that problem. But apart from that bit, the actual birth experience itself was fantastic and I wouldn't have done it any other way, except I wouldn't have phoned the midwives afterwards, in hindsight, and I wouldn't have gone into hospital on her instruction. I would have asked to speak with the supervisor of midwives rather than go on her say. I didn't know that then. I didn't know anything about that system at the time. We felt bullied into going in and so we did, because we didn't want our baby to be taken away from us and we didn't want any problems to occur. So we did what we felt we were bullied into doing. But in hindsight I wouldn't have done that, but obviously hindsight is a wonderful thing.

We were frightened and we had this tiny baby and we were like, what's next? We were interrogated, essentially, by three different doctors, all sort of checking our story, as though we'd done something wrong. I had actually printed out the Royal College of Midwives' documents on freebirth and that it was not illegal. I actually had them with me so I somehow had remembered to take them to the hospital with me and said, "look we haven't done anything illegal. You're saying that we have, but we haven't." And I remember the supervisor of midwives saying, "Look, you haven't done anything illegal, it's perfectly fine, and we need to try and get you home." And she was really fantastic and we're very grateful that she was there. And she continued to be fantastic afterwards when I complained about it and in the support she provided – continued to provide in the years afterwards when we were exploring freebirth with the MSLC. So she was like a blessing really. But the other staff were not so hot. **Lindsay**

The next morning, after a leisurely breakfast in bed brought by Mum, I had a facetime with B so that she could show me how to breastfeed. C did a lot of crying, and we decided to have a go again later, when he was in a more peaceful mood. We decided to call the midwife and fill her in that the birth had occurred. I no longer felt vulnerable to fear-mongering or being unempowered. I now considered myself to have traversed incredible terrain without the processes considered essential by her. I felt proud and simply curious as to what her response would be, and what if any after-care she might consider necessary at this stage.

After being in touch with her by phone and setting up a visit, I was amazed that my sense of accomplishment felt diminished. She seemed cross towards me, as if she believed me to be deviant and the birth a transgression that was most puzzling and irritating to her. Although she didn't say so, I *felt* her thinking, "Why didn't she want our support? How fussy she is, and so ungrateful." The negativity I felt in her presence continued. **Naomi**

Carmen compared her experience after two births. After her first birth, at home with NHS midwives:

… then the other thing was to assess my tear afterwards. Neither of them felt confident to do so, which was frustrating. They said, "Yes, we suggest we transfer you to hospital because of that." Obviously very frustrating; you've just given birth at home. There was no bleeding. Again, I think my doula at the time… she was my backup, so we didn't know each other as well. And she was still in training. So I feel like she wasn't feeling confident to sort of advocate against what they were saying. And then they said, "Yes, we're going to call an ambulance now and transfer you to hospital." I know now that I could have insisted, and that's what I did with my second. Or just stood my ground and say, "I'll go in the next day, because I'm not bleeding, I'm not in pain. I'm happy, I don't want to go to hospital at 1 a.m. thank you." But sure thing, within, I don't know, you don't have any sense of time, but after a very short time I had four ambulance staff standing on my landing and looking at me while I was like naked on the bed, nursing my baby. And it was just a horrible. They could have managed the situation a different way. There was four men as well. I mean, I don't have hang ups about the man seeing me naked, but you know, if you go for IVF, you've done it all. But it was just completely off. "But they have to be here because they need to assess the situation." And I was just like, "Nobody's dying here. We're just transferring me to hospital. There's no need for you to stand there and invade my privacy." It was my bedroom. And then I said, "Can I have a shower?" Because I felt like really… I don't want to go to a public space without… and they denied me a shower. And then I just, again, it was just my survival instinct kicking in and I just said to them, "Okay, I'll just go for a quick pee." And of course, I went to have a shower. And then I heard them bitching. Sorry to use the word, but bitching outside the shower room door. "Now she's having a shower." She called me a smartypants. And again, just lucky for them that I was too tired to have a conversation right there. But it was a two minute shower. And it was their decision to call an ambulance. "These people are busy" she was saying, "We have to go, you know. We don't have time."… And then they took us into hospital. Obviously the sinking feeling of like walking through those doors; I didn't want to be there. And it took a very long time. I think we went in at 11.00 and they saw us at 1.00. And during that time they withheld food and drink from me because I might need a general anaesthetic… And there was no reason to believe that I was going to need a general anaesthetic. So again, while I was there I felt completely out of control. There were constantly people coming in and out, but not really talking to us. And it took a long time for us to be seen, which I understand, public health service and so on. But it ruined the whole experience. I was tired, I just wanted to get to bed. Eat something, drink something, go to bed. And then instead I was then talked into having stitches at 1.00 a.m. And I found out this year that they weren't actually necessary. I saw it in my file. The doctor at the time said it's a second or third degree tear. But in my notes it says first or second. And that's also what it felt like. I know I'm not trained to assess myself, but it didn't feel like a third degree tear and the stitches weren't far enough to suggest that… and I had a lot of problems with those stitches. It was horrible. The stitches were worse than giving birth.

[After the freebirth of her second child] I recovered much more quickly from this birth, even though I'm four years on and I'm geriatric. So, but I was much better. And also when we went in for phototherapy, one of the consultants came over to assess my tear. And I decided to not have it stitched, and that was another – outrageous to them. They sent three different people in to convince me that I should have it stitched, because I'm going to regret that for the rest of my life. And I'm not regretting it, because I healed just fine. But that was another, you know, where I just felt, "Okay, now I've had my freebirth." "So he was born before arrival." And I said, "Yes we never called anybody." You know, I just kind of rubbed it into their faces, like, "Yes, we just decided not to call anyone." And that was some of the consultants that had been talking to me for weeks about how dangerous all of this is. And one of them even said, "And here we are after all, in a hospital with your baby." **Carmen**

Many women lied about their freebirth. For some this was to avoid "being bullied."

We had discussed what we will say, but because of other friends who had had bad experiences of being bullied when they decided to have a freebirth and told the midwives, we decided to not say anything. And just pretend it was a BBA, Birth Before Arrival. It's weird that you have to lie in order to be treated with more respect or to make sure you're treated respectfully… But that's what we decided to do. Because with a new baby and a toddler, you really don't want to have to fight anything (laughs). We just wanted to have our baby moon, so he called them and said, "The baby arrived so quick." **ST,** herself a midwife

Once the baby was born, the parents were responsible not just for the baby but for establishing the baby's relationship with the state. Some professionals made this process very smooth. In other professional encounters the shadow of state power was felt by the parents if "child protection issues" and "things escalating" to Social Services were mentioned (see chapter 20). Registering the baby was also a situation where the assistance of a health professional was needed, and an example of where a lack of professional support led to significant stress.

Oh, there was a funny thing… we suddenly realised on the day that he was born… if we've got to register his birth, how do we go about proving that he is ours? R said, how does that work? Because obviously with F, you normally have a thing from the midwives you take. So R actually phoned the doctor down in… our local doctor, a lovely doctor. The only time I've ever seen them is when I've been pregnant and wanted a letter to prove I'm pregnant for this maternity thing that R did. But they are lovely. And he said… I remember him coming out for F's birth and he was great, coming up all that way – our track's over a mile long. We're quite a way out! He said, "oh, oh, em, oh, I don't know actually. What do we do?" (Laughs). No-one knew what to do. It was so funny! Anyway, he came out and we thought he was just going to bring the form… to say that he is ours and… but he thought we wanted him to come out for a health check. Which was fine. He looked at O. Then afterwards we were like, do we get anything to take to…? And he goes, "oh, er, well, er…" We were like, well that's why we wanted you to come up here! (Laughs) because we didn't want him to have a health check particularly. Anyway, so we still didn't really know what to do. He said, "I'll have a word with the people down at the surgery and see what I do with that. I don't know actually. I don't know what I'm supposed to give you for that." Because normally it's from a midwife. Anyway, after some backwards and forwards, R picked up something from the doctor. Oh, that's right, he wrote a letter and we had to take it to the register office. She then phoned the doctor when we were there and he said, yes, that's right. **Peggy**

I do just want to mention a piece of administration that took just over a month to square away. It involved daily calls, and I was shunted from one department or office to another with nobody who seemed equipped or willing to help. It seems from my conversation with S [midwife] that because I didn't invite her to the scene within 24 hours of the birth, she couldn't issue C with his NHS number, and she couldn't tell me how I would go about getting one either. Nobody seemed to know. The hospital thought it was the midwife's responsibility, and the midwife said try the hospital office staff. I heard the same thing again and again from the various administrative staff-members at the hospital: "Normally, if a baby isn't born at the hospital, it is their midwife who issues the NHS number." Again and again to different people I explained that no NHS midwife had been present at the birth, and that she hadn't visited until the following evening and so wouldn't issue the number. "Was I foreign?" I was asked. "Did I have settlement status, or was there an issue with this?" "Had I had my baby abroad?" Nobody seemed to have heard of a scenario like mine before and my answers to their limited lines of questioning seemed not to yield any results. I went round in circles speaking to different people for several weeks before I was signposted to a government health and social care agency whose authority seemed to be above others I'd spoken to thus far. By this time, I was growing increasingly anxious that C didn't have an NHS number and that this was evidently very strange and unheard of, but without any obvious remedy. I finally got through to a woman called W who was covering for someone else who was on holiday. She was the first person who seemed genuinely curious and surprised by my situation and determined to help me if she could. I decided not to let go of our connection. After several more weeks of calls and emails back and forth with W and the women covering for her while she was on holiday, and while she in turn corresponded with various people, C at last received his NHS number. Although this whole process was an extremely frustrating faff, it also very much interested me that there was evidently absolutely no well-trodden bureaucratic path for those people like me who chose not to invite a midwife 'in the system' to be present at their birth. And although retelling my story so many times to different admin workers was boring, there was also a part of me that was quite proud to announce my situation to so many office-working women all over Sheffield and the U.K. Perhaps in some very small way my words were making small shifts in the minds of all these women about what is possible for us when we choose to step outside the normal way of things. **Naomi**

Chapter 19: Problems

Some women encountered problems in labour, during or after the birth. They were prepared for them and able to deal with them or seek appropriate help. Often they were so well attuned to their bodies that they moved so as to facilitate the birth in circumstances which would have necessitated medical intervention if they had birthed within maternity services. Some commented that they were able to listen deeply to their bodies and babies because no one else was there interfering or telling them what to do.

As his head passed through, it felt slow and pulled me wide open in my vulnerability. Everything remained stationary. I touched him and arched my body to look down as he partially emerged in the water. Time seemed to move in slow motion. I anticipated another contraction, my body postponed, pausing in those exhausted moments. My mind kicked in and I knew I couldn't birth him completely in the position I had adopted. I felt him move, as though he was trying to push forward. Something about this sensation bestowed peace upon me. It washed over, enclosing my body, as I knew exactly what I needed to do. I became attuned, synchronised with the process. I tried not to resist the next contraction, pushed a little and felt him wriggle again. I had to move. Laid on my side in the dim light of our bathroom, I summoned the strength to utter that I needed to get up. He could not be born until I was standing. D [partner] helped me to my feet. I felt incredible, grounded, intuitive, knowing – an embodiment of strength. With the next contraction, he came in one swift movement. I called to D to get ready to catch, worried he would slip into the water. My hands never left his body as D helped me grasp him in my arms. I lifted him to my chest and with eyes closed, he looked peaceful – perfection, contentment. **Melissa**

I got his head out and I could feel his shoulders against my hip bones on the inside, and I felt him trying to… I was waiting for him to turn. I felt him kind of wriggle, wriggling his legs and everything to try and turn, but his shoulders didn't move. And I felt this next contraction building and my instinct was, I have to do something or else we're both going to get hurt. He has to move because there's a really powerful contraction coming. So I just cocked my leg like a dog as the contraction came, and that just made enough space for him to flip his shoulders round and then he came out with the next contraction into his Daddy's arms. So that was nice. And it was interesting that I was that aware of the inside of my body where I'd never really been aware of him inside my pelvis. My previous births I'd just been more focused on the burning sensations and not the inside of my body so much. And it was nice to know that I knew by instinct what I needed to do, because there was nobody else telling me what to do. **Elena**

And then all of a sudden, just after half two, my water broke and all the contractions were on top of each other and I could feel my stomach tightening. Oh my God! This is coming on! This time I just remember it being really like a really heavy weight bearing down. When I was pushing, I felt... I felt down, but I could feel his nose facing towards me, so I knew he was back to back. And then right next to his ear... I couldn't work out what was wrong with his ear. It was taking ages to push and then after a little bit I realised it was fingers and he had his hand next to his ear. I was like, he's really stuck – what am I going to do? I just remember thinking, in my head I was thinking I need to turn over. My others I've birthed kneeling up with my hands over the side of a birth pool. And this time I was kind of rolling on my back and lifting my legs over and round, and I kept doing that until he pushed his way out. **Laura**

So I had planned to deliver him in the pool, but so every time I got into the pool everything stopped. I was just so relaxed. I just was lying in the pool, having the surges and labour was not... I was just too relaxed. Every single time I got in, just nothing happened. So I had to get out. And I was walking the stairs a lot, because my waters hadn't fully released. And I knew that probably needed to happen for the labour to progress. So me and my husband went up and down, up and down the stairs which definitely helped, it was hard at the time, but it definitely helped the labour progress. And that's what C my doula said to try - like it's crazy, because you know, if I had been at the hospital, or even with midwives here at home, they would have been starting to talk about maybe transferring and emergency section, stuff like that because I wasn't progressing on their time scale, even though I was on my own baby's time scale. I wasn't going by their boxes and their guidelines and all that. I just knew I needed to do the stairs, I was just taking it at my own pace, where do I want to go now – I want to go to the stair. I did the stairs a lot and then the waters were starting to release, and then I could feel things ramping up a wee bit then. And I decided then, although I wanted to be in the pool, I wanted to be in the bathroom. I wanted all the lights out. So I felt like I was going into a cave, you know, like instinct when you want to be in the dark, small space. And just me and my husband, and I just sat on the toilet for about an hour and a half. And we were breathing through it and he was making me laugh and stuff. It was lovely. And then C came up towards the end and she thought, just from the noises I was making and things, that it was close. So she called my Mammy up. Within 15 minutes and I could feel baby's head. I just knelt down beside the bath, birthed baby into Daddy's arms and baby cried straight away. And skin to skin and it was just beautiful, yes, it was lovely. And my first birth was lovely too, but as I say, the end almost... I feel a bit of animosity came in towards the end, because phoning the ambulance and saying the heart rate was dropping and stuff and forcing me to push Z out, rather than breathe out, like the way I did this time. So I just loved that part of it, that I was only just following my body and I trust it and yes, it just was beautiful afterwards. We went into the pool and just had a few hours there, skin to skin. And it was lovely. **Holly**

He wasn't back to back, but he was, kind of, favouring my right hand side. And so, I could feel that it was a bit more grungy, like, he was having to turn a bit, it was painful. My first two labours and births weren't what I would describe as painful. I mean, I was laughing in my second one, but this was sore. But I knew nothing was wrong, it was just the position that we'd both got into, you know, my pelvis was perhaps slightly more wonky, because I'd been holding children on one side a little bit more. It was just something that our bodies sort of needed to figure out. And I just felt really reassured that it wasn't anything wrong, and it wasn't. I did have to gather myself. **Leonie**, third freebirth

I knew I had a low laying placenta, I was prepared to die, ultimately, in case I had birthed the placenta before baby. And so my friend had prepared us with a few tinctures to help pass the placenta and to stop haemorrhaging... it was at the front of my body whereas the baby was behind it... my doula friend showed me how to feel what position baby was in... when we were trying to hear for the baby's heartbeat, we thought that that was the baby's and put the stethoscope [on] it and then it was very clear that that was the placenta... And she allowed me to know the difference between what the placenta feels like and what the baby felt like... I didn't... [bleed], maybe a couple of times, but that was actually probably more that I was overdoing it a bit and it was more towards the end actually that I started to spot... I thought that actually I was going to lose the baby because I'd been spotting a bit. And, sometimes if I was doing too much or a bit stressed out then it would go into spotting. But then I would just have to rest really, and it was okay... because she'd said, you have the power of just willing it [placenta] to move and to ask them all to cooperate, then that's what happened. I just kept asking for us all to get in position and the placenta kind of came up and round a bit. And then... the baby did start to engage, she started to engage like about two days before labour, so it actually was very obvious that she would soon come... [after the birth]... then another ten minutes or so the placenta came out really easy. It was really just because the baby started suckling quite soon and so it just came out quite easy. **Yony**

It was just as well that we had made preparations as the placenta didn't come for hours and hours despite all our best efforts, having a pee, squatting, having a little tug on the cord, baby on breast. My partner made an incredibly strong brew of ground ivy which I sipped while he went to muck out the cows. Suddenly I let out a huge moan as my womb contracted and expelled the placenta. How happy we were! We had envisioned the wagging tongues and fingers... if we had had to go to hospital and now we had done it! Birthed our baby our way! **Caroline B**

Sometimes, after being born, the baby needed help which the mother gave.

She had lots of mucous. I remember instinctively sucking on her nostrils and spitting into the water, which I hadn't done with the others. **Hannah**, after her third home birth and second freebirth

And she came with a very tight cord around her neck, because I had a very long cord. At first, she was a little floppy so I just stimulated her a bit and spoke to her and blew into her face, and she immediately picked up... I sucked from her nose a bit. **Michaela**

On a few occasions the doula helped.

I wouldn't attempt it, definitely would not, without a doula, because I've seen these couple of things that we would have just freaked out... He had the cord around his neck twice, and she flipped him in the water to unravel it... And then when she put him on me, she wanted him to breathe audibly and he was just being quite quiet, he was still getting oxygen from his cord, but she asked me to rub him really vigorously till he made a little noise. And there was a bit of a tense moment where I just kept on doing that, and until it actually happened, it was a little bit scary, and then he did. And also she asked me, which I would not have known, to suck the mucus from his nose and suck some of that water out, and spit it out and do that; I did that a few times. **Rosalie**

Many women had a backup plan in case they encountered problems and did go to hospital when this happened.

Although last time didn't go quite to plan, because I had to be transferred to hospital. I had a placental abruption and I had got up in the middle of the night. I had kind of felt a bit niggly all – he was 15 days over – and I had felt a bit niggly the evening before and then in the middle of the night I had got up and I thought that this was things happening and I decided, although I didn't really feel like I wanted to go in the bath, I decided to run a bath cause that's what I had done previously and when I got into the bath it just there... turned pink and we had phoned... I had to shout on my husband and he came down and he phoned [independent midwife] to see what she thought, but the plan that we had in place was that she wasn't going to be able to come until after the placenta was delivered and so she said that she couldn't obviously come out but it sounded like I needed to go to the hospital to get checked out, so my husband had phoned an ambulance and they came out and I was really scared to go to the hospital but I spoke to IM on the phone again and she reassured me and so we went in and we were in literally sort of five minutes and he was born so he was really close to coming while we were still at home but perhaps it was just that there was obviously that problem and when the placenta was delivered there was a large blood clot attached to it and so then I lost almost a litre of blood while I was in the hospital so I had to stay in for a while and sort fluids out and things, but he was fine and I was fine afterwards, so it's just... I suppose just one of those things that can happen, but it would maybe make me think... I don't know if it would make me think twice about having unassisted again. I think it would make me think about the care I had beforehand and the care that I was going to put in place for afterwards more than anything... **C** had planned a freebirth for this birth after two previous freebirths and two NHS home births and a first baby in hospital.

Many women said they would know if something was wrong and this was certainly the case for Hannah who had previously had a freebirth.

I'm one of four as well. S [partner]'s one of five. So with my fourth, we had a really, really tough time after about, was it for two years we'd been together? We lost the first pregnancy at around Christmas. That was actually just before C, who was my doula, had her fifth baby and I was there for her birth. That was okay. When I got pregnant, for some reason it just didn't feel right and I kind of knew that it wasn't, something wasn't quite right. The next one, miscarriage, was much harder, because I did have some of the symptoms of pregnancy and then they just stopped. And we were actually up in Edinburgh and I said I actually want to have a scan, which was funny, because I didn't scan at all with O [previous freebirth]. And the baby had gone pretty much around that time of me, thinking, "something's not right," because I was nine weeks and the baby measured about… so really in that time, the baby had stopped growing. That was pretty awful and I carried that baby a long time before spontaneously miscarrying, so it was maybe three or four weeks even. But interestingly, all this stuff that you read when women have a miscarriage and they say, "It's a missed miscarriage," and I'd started to think that your body will at some point let go. It's just sometimes emotionally you hold on for a little bit longer because you need to before you're ready to let go. That seemed to resonate with me anyway. So then there was that baby and that was in April I miscarried, and then I got pregnant again, in October, November time.

Twins, and I just knew straight away it was twins. Again, over Christmas, I kind of thought, I should be feeling some kind of, apart from being really tired and feeling very sick. But then I started to feel very much better, much quicker, but I was about eight or nine weeks, I thought, "this doesn't feel right." So I decided to get a scan and lo and behold, two sacks and yeah, they were maybe about seven, eight weeks, the babies. So they'd gone again at a similar time to me feeling they'd gone, and that was miserable. We were having a loft conversion at the time and had workmen in and there was no space to grieve. **Hannah**

In Hannah's next pregnancy:

I had lots of scans this pregnancy because I felt that emotionally I needed it. And maybe about nine weeks, we were going up to Glasgow and I thought, "Being away from home and being nine weeks and this is often when they'd gone before, I feel I need to know before going, that everything's okay. Because I don't want to go away again and have another loss." And there was a little heartbeat, strong as ever just, "I'm here, I'm okay, you switch off, you go on holiday." And we took, we decided to have the NIPT [non-invasive prenatal testing] test then, just because I'd had loads of miscarriages. I've got a sister who's got disabilities and I wanted to know and be prepared if that was going to be the case. And that all came back and clear and, yes, twelve weeks and I'm still pregnant and I felt pregnant and a bit in disbelief. But feeling good, and the pregnancy was great, really, really, good. **Hannah,** she went on to freebirth.

After a long and painful labour, Darelle decided she needed the gas and air which would have been available for an NHS home birth, which she had in fact booked as a precaution, even though she was planning to freebirth.

I was using TENS machine and I was finding I was struggling then, I was struggling with the pain then, it was really painful. But I did hypnobirthing…and I didn't find it helpful for me. I think that's actually because I'm ADHD and I just think that…my mind works differently… So I was like, wait half an hour, wait an hour, see what happens and then.

So he'd [partner] done that, so I'd asked, I'd mentioned it a couple of times, but I hadn't really said fully like yes, call them. But then I was like no, I think I need to call them. So he phoned triage and they were basically like, the home birth service isn't running.

So, then they were like can you drive in? And I was like I cannot go in the car, I cannot. I was absolutely, I was at this point where I was completely involuntarily vocalising, I couldn't, I was in loads of pain. And they [contractions] were quite close together. I was in the bath and the bath was not really helping me enough. With hindsight I wonder if the birth pool would have helped but I think I just needed a bit of extra, I think I just wanted the pain relief. Once I got to the hospital and had gas and air, I was much better…

We were on the phone to this call handler [ambulance control]… for about half an hour before I say to A [partner], "Can you ask how much longer it's going be." And they were very like hedgy, they didn't want to say, "Oh the ambulance service is very busy." Okay, but do you know like have you got a time frame? And then they said about an hour and a half. And I was like, I cannot wait an hour and a half, and we'd already been on the phone with them for half an hour. And I was like, is that an hour and a half from now or an hour? I don't know, and obviously that's their estimate, isn't it. So I was like, "Nope, nope, nope, we've got to drive in, we've got to drive in." So we cancelled the ambulance because I was like, "I cannot wait, I can't, I can't cope that much longer." Because I was just trying to get through until they arrived. I think at that point my main plan was just get gas and air when they arrive and then see where I go from there. Because I might not have transferred, I might have just been like, let's just see where I am. Especially because I think by the time, if, if I'd have waited for them, probably would have had the baby at home.

We got in, eventually, and then A had to wait at the reception while I went through on my own. And then they took me to a room and then A joined me straight away, so that was fine.… when they examined me they were like, "Oh she's fully dilated." By that point I was fully out of it though, I was like involuntarily pushing and everything. The baby was born at five fifty a.m. So I think the thing that I found most difficult really was the fact that if I'd just had somebody to come out to me, I would have been fine, wouldn't have needed obviously to go in.

It was a nightmare getting out of hospital, I had to harass them… I'm disappointed I didn't manage to birth at home. But I don't know if it was for the best, because if I'd had that kind of little weird episode with my breathing [after the birth] at home, A definitely would have called an ambulance, he a hundred percent would have called an ambulance. So I guess I liked what one of the other ladies called it, 'free laboured' (laughs), I like that.
Darelle

A few women spoke of admissions to hospital after the birth that were distressing and sometimes deeply traumatic. In some but not all cases these could have been avoided.

And, and on the third day I took another look at myself, and I realised that my cervix base had prolapsed. It had actually fallen out, it was literally just hanging down next to the clitoris. It was completely painless. And I washed my hands and pushed it back into its place... And then a trainee midwife came out, and she was also pregnant, I remember and she was in her summer dress. Showing off her bump. She said, "Look, I just can't tell whether you're hurt or not. I think you need to go to S [hospital]. This was like the post traumatic stress inducing thing. Because that was the hospital where they cut me [previous caesarean]. And so it was the first time I'd been back there. And it was the third day so that's when all your hormones kind of start isn't it and... that's when the baby blues can set in. And it was for me, because that was the day my daughter got back... I thought I was going to have to be sewn up... And they were giving me scare stories like, "Oh, you've left it too late, so you'll have already started healing in the wrong place," and they were going to have to correct that. And after keeping me waiting for about three hours, like... crying, laughing and being in a very altered psychological state... almost in this waiting, in this kind of examination room. They finally came in, looked at me, well, didn't look at me, you know, that's the only internal examination I had... in the whole pregnancy, I think. She said, "Oh, you're absolutely fine," and then, a finger up the bloody back passage. And, "Oh, you're fine there as well," and then a snooty kind of condescending, "If you ever have more children, we strongly advise that you get yourself some assistance next time." **Rose**

I feel guilty about how we ended up there [in hospital] because if we hadn't seen that midwife (a stand-in for our regular one) we wouldn't have been referred in. If I had opted out of seeing a midwife altogether, which I did after G's birth, I'd have watched this cold carefully and by the next morning, seen it improve. We wouldn't have spent three nights in a hospital, with F having needles stuck repeatedly in his arms, given two different kinds of antibiotics (and for no reason, since they cannot help a cold at all), and being checked and prodded every two hours. He wouldn't have had a lumbar puncture. The conclusion of it all being that unfortunately, just as I assumed, he had a cold. Two colds actually, at once.

But I did see a midwife, and I did follow her advice. I didn't feel able not to, or even know if I wanted to refuse it. After all, regardless of what I thought I knew, what if it was serious and I was wrong? What if I was mistaken and actually the symptoms of a cold were really the symptoms of something more serious?

And here is where it gets murky for me. Because the doctors and nurses who came and went and tested and prodded, all did so with the best of intentions. They were running at worst case scenario, because that's what they do. That's what they have to do. They see the worst cases and they work on the safe side of everything being potentially, high risk. But these people don't know me, or my ability to know my own child, my perception of him or his health, my own concerns. They don't understand why I might not want him, at five days old, to have a needle put in his spine, to test him for the very worst case scenario when he displayed absolutely no signs or symptoms for that scenario.

They don't see that there is also a risk to having those things done – a risk to the healing that needs to take place after birth, to the time and space and safety of place women need to bond with their babies. To feel okay. To go up, instead of down, where the hellish fog of postpartum depression can easily swallow women whole.

But there I was, in the hospital, feeling torn apart, weeping, protective, and unsure. Bleeding and heaving with aches through my body, feeding non-stop, and unsure. The very system that I stay far away from in birth and pregnancy is the one I ended up being consumed by during those days. And maybe it was my fault for agreeing to things in the first place, or for not refusing, or even knowing if I could refuse, the tests they felt were necessary. Maybe it's not, because what kind of sanity does a woman whose body has just opened up, have? What kind of decision beyond panic and fear can a mother holding her infant make, when someone suggests "sudden decline" or "infection risks" or a whole host of other things which aren't applicable, but could be, maybe, if things took a turn for the worst?

And if I hadn't had that midwife in my home, who was nervous, and who made a judgement call my own midwife would not have, if I hadn't seen a midwife during my pregnancy because of the bleeding that came in the first few weeks and taught me in the most visceral way that our bodies are wild and unknowable, if those things had been different, I'd have had no strangers in my home, as I had chosen with my birth, and I'd have watched my baby get a cold and lose that cold in the safety of his own bed.

I hate that he had a canula in his hand, that his whole, tiny forearm was wrapped tightly and strapped to a board, that he had so many invasive things happen to his new, perfect body so soon after he was born. That there is a half hour of his life I don't know about – taken by strangers and strapped to a bed when they attempted twice, unsuccessfully, to do a lumbar puncture. I hate that every time I suggested that it seemed like it was just a cold, that there were no actual reasons to think otherwise, I was made to feel as if I couldn't possibly know anything, being just the mother and not the doctor. I hate how much it spoilt that precious time after you give birth, which I never got back, and which I am still grieving for now.

And it makes me even more resolute in my decisions not to partake in that system, because I don't believe it does the best it can do for many women, and because trauma is not the exception in women's birth stories, but the norm.

And I am also grateful that during those days that were achingly hard, I had friends who showed up over and over again, who stayed late, who brought me dinner and toothbrushes and snacks and hairbrushes. Who sat with me and made me laugh, who took my kids after school, or drove them home. Who knew, even when I said I was fine, that I was not fine, and who got angry when I couldn't get angry. Those things were a saving grace, and kept me together.

The silver lining, and it has been important for me to find one, is that I have those people in my life, and that I learnt again, in a less than ideal way, how precious that space after birth is. How much it should be protected, and how the same principles I apply to birth have to be extended into the days and weeks after birth too.

And maybe I should have made a different decision, and maybe the system should be better, and maybe I will always feel guilty, but I also did the best I could do with what I had in that moment. In that moment what I needed was support - people who listened to me, trusted my instincts and understood us as individuals, and that didn't happen. It couldn't, because that's not how it's set up, which is exactly why people like me turn away from it and towards other people, other resources, and ourselves.

Maybe I will feel differently in time, when I have processed everything more, and the rawness has smoothed away into just a thing that happened. An event, after an amazing birth. When my regular midwife visited me later, she inferred that she wouldn't have sent me in to hospital but then said, placatingly, "Well, you have been lucky so far though, haven't you?'

At the very least, this has been a lesson learnt, that I can bring with me to my support of other women. Maybe the bruise of it will fade and I will be able to enjoy the story of my birth without the sadness of what happened after. What happens to us when we are pregnant, when we birth, when we are caring for our newborns - these are the things that stay with us and that we carry always, that are far heavier for us to bear than we anticipate. We have every right to expect the best, to want more than just to be sometimes lucky, and to stay away from anyone who doesn't hold those same hopes for us. I knew that before, and I know it better now. **Kendal**

Things were kind of all right really for a while. But I did in the end, this is a kind of a sad ending, because I did end up with a really, really severe postnatal mental health, you know. And I ended up, I ended up in the Mother and Baby Unit for quite a long time. I'm only really just coming to terms with it all now, because I lost the first year of my baby's life. Oh, and I wanted to avoid hospital and interventions, and I ended up being fed anti-psychotics, which go straight through to the milk. As they wanted me to stop breastfeeding, so they could put me on more drugs… They wanted me to leave the baby with the staff during the night. So that I could supposedly get some rest. But then obviously all the other babies seemed to be all right with this. Whereas, my baby, I'd let her go, get my head down, feeling not very relaxed because I wasn't with her and then I would hear her screaming the place down. And I'd just get up out of my bed, and go and find her, because what else are you going to do?… And, and I'd find her, and they weren't even carrying her, they'd strapped her into a pushchair. And wheeling her around the ward, and I was just, like, "Look, this is not all right."…

[Rose had gone to Morocco to the baby's father]

I went into a postnatal psychosis. Somehow flew back to the UK when the baby was three months old. And within twenty-four hours of arriving, I'd been sectioned. And literally, I was very confused. I hadn't changed my clothes… and was separated from my older daughter for a month. And the only reason I got out was because they were threatening to put her into foster care, so that my treatment could kind of continue. And I was just, like, "No way." So I ordered, it was like, I said, "Look, the section's up, you can't keep me here any longer." And because I wouldn't harm, because I wasn't posing a threat to myself or anyone else they said that was okay. Even though I could have been, I could have harmed myself. I wouldn't have harmed anyone else. I was, yes, I was deeply suicidal, but this isn't really the birth story. But the postnatal bit is actually part of the birth story still, isn't it. It's all connected somehow. And the things that happen in the birth can really trigger these events that happen after the birth. But for me, they said, "Oh, you must have had a traumatic birth," and I said, "Well, no I didn't actually, I had the best birth I could have asked for." However, you know, and then you think, "Oh, but the first birth was a traumatic C section. **Rose**

Sarah knew, from previous experience, that her baby could be premature and would therefore be likely to need special care in a neonatal unit.

My birth journey hasn't always been easy with my first four children all being premature, the fourth due to hospital error. It took a lot of faith in my body's ability when the decision was made to home birth our fifth. My husband and I decided we would happily stay at home from 36 weeks and fought hard to get support from the hospital to do so. Having midwives and doctors in and out the room, interfering with the birth process and not allowing me to go on to birth as I want were the deciding factors of a home birth and the freebirth...

Once again he [partner] instinctively knew what I needed and brought I [baby] earth side onto my chest. We quickly kept her warm, skin to skin, towels, blankets but as she was 36 weeks and one day, I was glad to have midwives on the way. For the second time I experienced the fetal ejection reflex. Allowing your body to do what it needs is truly moving and I know that I was able to fully give into the natural process because I was in a calm protected environment that my husband created... I came home from NICU on day nine and she has been showered in love by her five siblings and us. **Sarah M**

Lunar suffered a classic obstetric emergency, rapidly called NHS emergency services and was grateful for her emergency caesarean section, while still glad she had planned to freebirth and would do so again.

After six weeks of increasing prodromal labour and lots of seemingly false starts (plug lost, bloody show had, contractions regular and strong day after day and on personal inspection cervix a good three fingers dilated), the day finally came (41 weeks and three days), I woke in the early hours aware of the subtle change in the contractions and slipped quietly out of bed to use the bathroom. This cemented the feeling that today would be the day, I had the biggest smile on my face as I climbed back into bed, snuggled against my husband and whispered in his ear "today we will meet our baby my love" he squeezed me tighter and breathed out an adorable "yaaaaay." I managed to rest like this curled together for a few hours, then was hit by a real need to be upright and moving. We quietly moved downstairs, the rest of the house still snoring in their beds, low lamp light and rhythmic music, I swayed gently, my husband and I smiling at each other, things rapidly got stronger and closer together and we sent a message to our doula S asking her to make her way to us, then suddenly with the very next contraction I felt a wonderful gush of warmth as my waters broke, we laughed together "baby is definitely coming now" another message to S and everything so damn perfect, I felt so in control, sooo happy and in touch with my body, it was divine.

Then the next contraction hit it seemed to begin to rise and then suddenly turn back on itself, coupled with a strange slippery sensation inside me, my first thought as I reached down, was that I would feel a foot in my vagina and that baby had turned breech, but no, I felt a warm rubbery loop beneath my fingers and the words "oh shit" escaped my lips, I immediately laid down on the day bed and began piling pillows under my hips, the next words out of my mouth were "sweetheart, message S and C (my midwife) and call an ambulance now" he swiftly followed my instructions, he could see the loop of cord and knew that our freebirth was now over and we were in a race to get to the hospital and to safeguard our baby.

It wasn't long before the first response vehicle arrived, I had moved into a head down position with hips arched high as I could manage and could feel baby moving now up against my ribs and the cord pulsed gently inside my vagina which was comforting, water still ran down my legs at intervals and I could feel my heart pounding. The thing I remember most at this point was that as soon as I realised the cord had prolapsed I could feel my body go on shut down, I assume compliments of the adrenaline now coursing through me, the contractions only moments before that had been so strong and earth rendering, now completely ceased, the only surges I felt were the lightest of tension pulling upwards, almost like an anti-contraction. As I had these I felt the cord being pulled back in, curling/coiling back into the warmth of my vagina, where there had been a significant loop now there was perhaps half this outside me.

Very quickly two more ambulances arrived (not sure why we needed so many? haha) and we quickly boarded one assuming once more the head down hips up position, I held on for grim death on the most horrendous journey I have ever had, we were really speeding along, siren blarring, my husband and one of the paramedics held my middle and legs and I had a vice grip on the head rest trying to keep upright as we sped along, it really felt like my shoulders and arms were being ripped out of the joints and my back was on fire having been arched in this position now for so long, every bump and turn jarred me to the core and my mind was racing. So calm on the outside, two voices in my head, one cool as anything, the one I let speak, the other in the background crying for the loss of the perfect moment and my freebirth, so fearful for the little life inside me, who I sooo desperately now just wanted to rip out and make safe, hurt deeply to leave my two year old son for the very first time ever in his life, feeling torn in two, worried on what would happen next, how I'd recover from what I knew was coming.

Finally we arrived at the hospital and I was rushed directly into theatre, my poor husband running beside me, his voice shouting to let him through, pushing past people, how he couldn't leave me, not now, being an imminent category one emergency caesarean with general anaesthetic, he wasn't allowed to be in theatre, but he knew how much I feared the hospital after my last birth, the trauma I carried a very real and painful scar for us both and he clung to the gurney, I turned my head to him, a mess of sweat and hair and called out "its okay my love, don't worry, I will see you soon." My midwife C reassuring him, she would be with me, her little cold hand in mine, I could tell he was sooo torn up but let himself be escorted out, my doula, S just outside waiting for him, at least I knew he is not alone for the agonising wait ahead.

The next part is a blur of activity, my birthing necklace being removed, me having to carefully move between the gurney and operating tables, all the while keeping position, the mask being pressed to my face, being told to breathe deep, C checking baby's position (yes I was fully dilated and baby would likely have been born in the next contraction or two into my husband's loving hands if the cord hadn't fallen first, oh the irony). C listening to baby's heartbeat, so strong and unmoved by the whole event, little fighter inside me, bless him. Then laid flat, heart and mind racing, I feel them painting my belly, the man at my head shouting "she's not out yet hold on" me screaming in my head, "wait, wait, I'm still here, don't cut yet", then the world turning inside out and blackness.

They open me up at 8:08am and baby is born at 8:09am, apparently one of the quickest c section births they have ever seen - he is ready to be born and impatient to see the world. He is perfect, top Apgar scores, he is quickly checked over and taken for skin to skin with my husband, who has been pacing like a trapped/caged animal in the waiting room, my doula S trying to calm/reassure him to little avail. Holding his son helps him regain a little of himself again, the rest floods back as soon as he is back by my side.

I don't know how much time has passed in all this, it seems like forever and yet also a blink of an eye. Finally I am coming round, feeling very out of it, seeing my little boy for the first time and trying to kiss him, not understanding why I can't, still wearing the oxygen mask haha. Apparently I am beaming/glowing and totally in love through the fog of coming to, I remember it like a hazy half dream, saying "OMG I loooove him sooo much and he is sooooooooo beautiful" high as a kite still, hahaha.

My time in hospital was thankfully short, I MADE myself do all the stuff they insisted on (stop all pain drugs, get up and out of bed, urinate unassisted and eat and keep it down) and walked out of the hospital that next day, in agony yes, but bloody determined. My time in there was made so much better by S and J, my doula dream team. They stayed with me when my husband had to leave to see to our then two year old. They took turns to keep me company, hold space for me so that the hospital felt less triggering and I could sleep feeling more safe and they were my heroes who rescued my placenta, hahaha. J even photographed and weighed it for me on request and then very kindly printed it and made me some amazing pills, yes I do soooo love placentas! I will always have a very special place in my heart for these two ladies.

My birth story is sooo far removed from what I so wanted it to be, my birth plan thrown to the wayside at the final moment, but I did have an amazing free labour which I wouldn't change for anything and I did what I had to, to save my precious little one from possible harm, there was no way to foresee this happening, I didn't have increased water volume, which appears to be the only real risk factor (the chances of a cord prolapse are very low, I think like one in 500 - 1000 births), just a case of the worst of luck, marking the sacrifices we make as mothers for our babies, it enforces ever more how knowledge is power and I know for me it was a life saver. Another scar added to this strong body of mine, one I will wear proudly for always.

I think as a freebirther it is important to see that sometimes things don't go to plan, that emergencies can arise with no warning, even when you are doing everything just as nature intended. That is why educating yourself and fully grasping your commitment to take full responsibility for your choices and actions is so important. I know that the same month this happened to me another lady who was home birthing also had a prolapsed cord, she was encouraged to quickly push baby out by the midwives in attendance, then they rushed to the hospital. That baby had to go to NICU and was very unwell indeed, with suspected brain damage. I don't know the full ongoing story I am afraid, but it just shows what can happen when you make one simple decision/choice. My intuition totally told me not to push or encourage him to come, the very opposite in fact and I told the ambulance driver that when he said I could push if I needed to. And yes the C section was very hard recovery, but he is a very clever healthy happy two year old now and I can't say what would have happened if I had chosen differently. I still want my freebirth, will have to see if Mother Nature blesses me again, as I am coming to the end of my birthing days now sadly at 41. Have had two wonderful home births, one terrible hospital induction, that put me off for life, then the amazing freebirth labour with an ECS [emergency caesarean section] finish, been an exciting and varied birthing journey that has taught me so much. **Lunar**

Several women knew enough to wisely ignore some professional advice.

When I'd rung up at lunchtime, she'd said, "Whatever you do, don't fill up the pool." And I was like, "Well you told me that last time. I'm definitely filling the pool because I didn't get to use it hardly at all last time." So my partner filled up the pool and I was in and out of that, and it was really lovely, listening to Bob Marley and being in and out of the pool. So my waters broke about half past three and I jumped into my lovely pool. And so... just before my waters broke, I said, "It's really getting serious now.".. so I said, "Well let's ring the triage team again." And we ended up being on hold for 45 minutes.

And this is how we ended up having a freebirth. So at the point at which I jumped into the pool and my waters broke, it was like, "Oh there's a head here." So after 45 minutes, I said, "B, I think you probably need to switch over to an ambulance." Because that's what they tell you to do. So this is the bit of planning for a freebirth that I guess I wish I'd have done. Because they tell you when you do anything, they say, "If the baby's coming and you're on your own, you must ring an ambulance." So we rung the ambulance crew and they helped B to deliver it, to catch him. But fortunately we had enough knowledge to not do things like get an old pair of shoe laces, which they still tell you to do, which is crazy... Yes, to get some shoe laces out of a pair of shoes. And B [partner] was like, "No, no, it's fine, we're comfortable and we don't need to... we don't need to do that." Which was really good. **Sarah W**

… so they [midwifery triage] said, "Right okay, call an ambulance then if you can't drive in." Like I couldn't go in the car, so I, so we called an ambulance and we were on the phone to them, oh gosh, the call handler, (sharp exhale), "Get a clean piece of string and a safety pin." "Tell her she has to get out the bath, she needs to lie on her back." So I'm just there like, "No," and then she was just so insistent that I had to get out the bath, I can't give birth in the bath. **Darelle**

Chapter 20: Referral to Social Services

The thing most frequently reported to have "gone wrong" with freebirthing was the involvement of Social Services, with their power to take children away from their parents. Cases where children were removed from their parents after a freebirth have been reported in the AIMS Journal, which some of these mothers read, and in the wider press. Many women feared the power of Social Services in this regard. One woman who contributed her story to this book later had her baby taken into the care of the local authority and the baby remains there as we go to press. Her story is not updated here in case this could have a negative impact on her attempts to regain care of her baby.

My biggest fear with freebirthing was not that I or my baby would die (that wasn't something I feared at all for the record) but that as a less than mainstream choice, someone somewhere would decide that we were "obviously" bad people and should be reported to Social Services. I am well aware of my rights and of the law, but I am also well aware that many people who think they know better are not. Whether it was luck, our approach, or something else, we were treated respectfully and kindly during our interactions with the NHS this time, which is wonderful, but it does sadden me that I had to feel so protective and act so carefully and guardedly to achieve this, a normal, natural, unhindered birth on my own terms. I would have loved to have been open about our decision to freebirth but felt the risk to our family was too great. **Claire**

So I didn't say, "I intend to freebirth." Because I was scared of what they might do, because they do fucking report you. Sorry. But they do. And so the only thing I could do is not tell them. Which is a dreadful basis for a relationship. **Beth**

Sometimes this was a threat. The threat of referral to Social Services led to one mother being sent to hospital unnecessarily after a freebirth.

We felt bullied into going in [to hospital] and so we did, because we didn't want our baby to be taken away from us and we didn't want any problems to occur. So we did what we felt we were bullied into doing. But in hindsight I wouldn't have done that, but obviously hindsight is a wonderful thing. **Lindsay**

This threat could be used to pressure women to use health services.

So we had a really good experience and it was a family experience. When we decided not to have a health visitor come in, they threatened us… with Social Services, but that was the only bad experience we had… our midwife called them and told them that we are normal and that we are really looking after our kids. **Michaela**

Registering the birth could be a problem after freebirthing and registrars sometimes referred women to Social Services. Midwives could help resolve this situation.

She was five days old... we had gone to register her and then were told that we couldn't register her because they had no official paperwork, so I had to get in touch with my midwife... but she came out that day, she could make sure the paperwork was filled out and she sent the paperwork down, or she put it into the council building that was nearest to her and then she came to visit that afternoon because she was told that somebody had to come and visit... by Social Services, somebody had to come and visit to make sure that the baby was alright because I had done something really wrong. Because when N was registered and the fact that the registrar had to ask for information, Social Services were alerted... which again is something that makes you worry about whether it is actually a legal thing to do because Social Services will say to you that it isn't and that you should have somebody there and that you've done something really wrong by not having antenatal care and stuff, even though it's all supposed to be a choice. **C**

And we didn't call the midwife at all, and that felt really good, just having that total space again just to get on with it. If there was an issue, we would have called somebody. And I'd read about the sort of legal obligations of what we'd need to do after birth. So, I'd pre-prepared the address of the local Child Health Department, and I'd pre-prepared a letter and a photocopy of it, so, we'd got everything just I hadn't put the details in, obviously, because we hadn't had the baby yet, but ready to say he was there, the witness was the father, he was born at this time. We didn't weigh my second or third child ever. We've never had them weighed, so I didn't put the weight down. What else? The address, I think, the date of birth, that sort of thing. And so we sent that off within, I think it's thirty-six hours, you need to do that, and obviously that's what the midwife would have done; that's what they do if they attend. So, we'd done that paperwork, and that was fine, and we were just having a really, yes, just a blissful time, and undisturbed for the first couple of weeks. And then it was when I came to register him for the birth certificate, because we'd chosen to do that as well. I think my husband had been with my eldest, and I went by myself with I, our second child. And we didn't have a car at that point, so it was a bit of a pain, I had to get on a bus or something for like an hour, it was quite a long way, and it was summer, and I just two weeks ago had a baby or three weeks at a push, but it was quite early, I think because we just wanted to get that done, and with hindsight, yes, we did that very differently the third time... and all was good until I went into the room, and, basically, and she said, the registrar said, "Oh, hang on, we don't have him on the system." And I explained a bit about, "Well, I freebirthed, I didn't have a midwife in attendance, so I sent off the documentation myself." I just gave her some context, and her body language immediately tensed up, she just didn't know what to make of it really. And again, I keep talking about hindsight, is the useful thing, but with hindsight, I would have sent the letter by recorded delivery, and I would have called up to check that it had arrived. And coincidentally, we did get an NHS number through the post a couple of days after that appointment. But the registrar referred me to Social Services at that point.

She said, "Look, I can't go ahead with the appointment, you're going to have to sort this out." And she didn't tell me at the time that she was making a referral, so, she just said that she cancelled it, I'll need to rebook it, and you know, I then needed an hour and a half bus journey home. It was really, really stressful. But then I got a phone call a few days later from a social worker, just explaining that I'd had this referral from this registrar lady. And actually, it was a really pleasant conversation, it was only about, I don't know, twenty minutes long or something. And I just explained and that thankfully, I'd written that email to the Head of Midwifery, and she said, "Oh, this, you know, this looks like it's got nothing, you know, I can throw this out immediately, there's nothing to carry forward," and that was that. So, I made another appointment and registered him.

I don't like confrontation. I thought I'd been really careful, I thought I'd done everything that I needed to do. And then the registrar of all people was where we came unstuck. And it's been really useful, a lot of the women and families that I support, I do say, "Just make sure that your letter's arrived, (laughs) and definitely follow it up." So, that's been a useful experience, but it was stressful at the time. **Leonie**

Some women were referred to Social Services by midwives without their knowledge. This was experienced as threatening and traumatic. Melissa wrote about this specifically and equated her experiences of rape with those resulting from the actions of midwives and social workers in this respect.

My son was born at home in the company of my husband, our twenty-three month old daughter and our doula. I had planned and chosen not to invite midwives to the birth. During my normal, healthy pregnancy I sought antenatal care with an NHS midwife. I decided to opt out of care at approximately thirty weeks gestation and at this point I discussed my plans for an unassisted birth with the Supervisor of Midwives. Ticking all her duty of care boxes, she also reinforced her appearance of support when she reiterated the Nursing and Midwifery Council's guidance regarding health care professional's role in supporting freebirth.

It was to my surprise when two weeks later I received a letter from Social Care informing me that an appointment had been made at my home where a social worker was due to visit, offering an assessment to determine if there was anything they could do to 'help our family'. Taken aback, I responded, politely declining their appointment, backed with my knowledge of medical guidelines and my understanding of Human Rights Law, which both supported my choices.

I filed the incident to the back of my mind when I did not receive a response and two weeks after I sent the letter to their office, my son was born in our bath. Everything was just as I had planned it and after his peaceful arrival into the world we quickly took to bed, where we remained sleeping and breastfeeding for seven blissful days.

It was on the evening of the seventh day that I received a phone call from a social worker who believed I was still pregnant. She insisted she come to my home the next day to discuss my birth plans and I again declined. I was in two minds about whether I should inform her of my son's birth but as her tone evidently became more rude and condescending, I decided against the idea. I felt pressured by her demands and told her

I was going to hang up the telephone.

Feeling slightly anxious about the incident, I called AIMS the following morning who kindly offered advice regarding how to move forward in our contact with Social Care. I was pleased that I found reassurance in AIMS chair Beverley Beech as that afternoon two social workers arrived unannounced at my home. As my heart raced, I caught my breath and opened the door, my newborn son fast asleep in the sling I was wearing. They queried the details of my son's birth and requested entry to the house. I asked to see the referral notes first, which they did not have at the time. We agreed that if they brought the original referral paperwork, we would speak with them.

Just less than an hour later they returned with the appropriate documents. Feeling scared, I was too upset to speak again and so asked my husband to take the lead. He remained on the doorstep for the duration of the fifty minute conversation, recording the details to protect our position. During the exchange, Social Care relayed to us that since their prior visit 'head office' had made the decision to escalate our case under the Child Protection Act, Section 47, meaning they believed our daughter and son to be at risk of significant harm. An outline of the procedures was verbalised by the social workers but as we still had zero evidence as to why we were under investigation, there was little response we could offer at this point. We eventually turned the social workers away and instructed them that we would be in touch once we had read and understood the initial referral.

Upon reading the original document, I was shocked to find that the referral had been made by a local midwife who I had not met before, countersigned by the Supervisor of Midwives. The reason for referral was written as, 'plans to self-deliver at home without medical assistance.' I was upset to see this justification; as well as going against the NMC code, referring me to social care for my birth choices is in breach of my Human Right to choose how and where I do so.

For the rest of the afternoon my family struggled to focus on anything other than the intrusion from Social Care. We still felt unsure about our position and the reason for their involvement was unclear. As we rallied to find more information about our legal position we were shocked to receive a third visit from the same social workers, this time escorted by two uniformed police officers. After they knocked on our door at seven in the evening, I looked out of the window in horror. Their presence was threatening and panic filled me as I visualised my two year old daughter and seven day old baby being taken from me. I was overcome with emotion and again asked my husband to speak with them. The social worker insisted that she see our baby and me as part of a welfare check; reluctantly, I came to the door. I did not feel in a position to rationally discuss the situation and the conversation rapidly became heated. I retreated, taking my son upstairs while my husband allowed the social workers and police officers into our home.

The next hour passed slowly as I listened to the social worker question my husband over our parenting choices, backed by the officer's insistence that if we submitted to their requests the resolution would be easy. We still remained in the dark as to why an investigation had been followed up and nobody was forthcoming with information. She referenced our minimal engagement with health visiting services and the false accusation that we were not registered with a GP. Neither of these statements were in any way related to our plans for an unassisted birth, nor are they legal requirements. We failed to see how any of the information correlated.

Upon their departure, our family was left exhausted and shaken. The next day we took our son to the GP, to try and gain some breathing space with Social Care's demands. The appointment was another trying challenge and upon our return home, we received a visit from two midwives, including the Supervisor of Midwives, who were sent by Social Care.

The duration of the midwives visit was the lowest point of the experience. They carried out checks and procedures that I had not consented to and I felt questioned and judged in my choices. My son cried as they measured and weighed him. I felt helpless. After they left I was numb. I exchanged messages with my doula, telling her how empty I felt, robbed of my free will. I felt violated by their actions and they had no interest. Despite the repeated script that they were concerned for the welfare of our children, they seemingly had absolutely no understanding of the negative impact they were having upon our lives.

The days and months that followed were full of difficulties as I struggled to come to terms with what had happened. After the case was closed I launched myself into multiple complaints procedures; spending hours at a time composing long, drawn out letters, going over every detail; which I had taken care to document throughout the ordeal. Social Care were reluctant to engage with my concerns and refused to take any responsibility over their heavy handed approach.

Meanwhile, an independent investigation was carried out against the midwives. By 'independent' the Local Supervising Authority of Midwives for the East Midlands meant works outside of my NHS County. The investigator assigned to the case was brought from the NHS in Leicester and concluded that the midwives adhered to policy throughout my care, although some recommendations for improvement in the standards and clarity in referral procedures were to be made to the hospital.

At D hospital, after taking my case to the Maternity Services Liaison Committee meeting, I held a one-to-one appointment with the Head of Midwifery. Although she remained conscientious of my emotions, her underlying tone remained loyal to the interpretation of the written regulations of the trust and she informed me that if I were to plan an unassisted birth again, she would not hesitate in contacting Social Care. I was disappointed by this response and her attitude frightened me more than offering any insight into my unfortunate circumstances. I expected to find the Head of Midwifery in prime position, upholding physiological birth and facilitating services which enabled women to make fully informed choices; instead she was actively restricting their freedoms.

Through the months of reliving the event, going backwards and forwards over conversations and letters, was not getting me anywhere. I was no further at peace with what I felt had been taken from me unnecessarily. I was fighting a system that was so entrenched in its own beliefs, so invested in its own protection, that it could not see the damage it was causing. Just as I had been on a journey through pregnancy to understand the choices that I felt were best for my son's birth, it was now time for me to take responsibility for my own emotions. Despite the injustice I shouldered, that would never reach a conclusion, I had to hold myself accountable for the way I felt about what had taken place.

This was a moment of liberation. In the freeing of my own limitations, I found new clarity. However, a new period of reflection quickly emerged to push my boundaries further. As I reconsidered many of my views with fresh perspective, an old feeling haunted me. This sensation resisted change as my internal anger held me back. What my experience with Social Care had conjured up was the reminiscence of previous struggles in life with power and authority.

I was brought up by a domineering single mother who battled with mental health issues. Into my teenage years I suffered with low self-worth, I turned to alcohol, I became very confused, miserable and began to self-harm. I made friends with large groups where openness and breaking the rules was embraced. I entered into a string of abusive relationships over an eight year period. This mostly involved emotional and mental abuse but numerous encounters also included rape. I found this particularly difficult to process, internalising all of the pain to the point of denial.

The world around me reinforced my suffering. As I struggled to even comprehend the true meaning of retaining the right to decline or consent, the messages I received about being a woman assured me that I was desirable as long as I looked just the right way to be deemed attractive. Complicit with the requirements, I struggled to find my own voice and I rarely spoke about my true opinions. I felt oppressed and I rebelled, placing myself in difficult positions that were to leave me traumatised.

My experiences of rape affected me on a level much deeper than I ever anticipated. For years, I was unable to verbalise that I had been raped and this became a very demeaning frame of mind to feel trapped within. I found it difficult to neatly define my rape and constantly questioned, perhaps I deserved it? Maybe I was asking for it? I came to believe it was normal, punishing myself with guilt and scrutiny. I spiralled into a vicious circle of self-destructive thoughts and behaviour. It was during this time that I unexpectedly fell pregnant for the first time and the birth brought a gift.

After a quiet, unquestioning pregnancy my daughter was born with relative ease, in water at hospital. I went in with very little information other than the many perpetuated myths and negative stories that are relayed frequently between the media and well intentioned relatives. There was a huge amount of luck regarding the circumstances, such as the midwife in attendance but what it returned to me was a belief in myself. Birth had been a healing passage for all of the trauma I had allowed into my life. It was a reclamation of my true self and almost immediately after my daughter's arrival, my life began to change. I found the voice that I had quelled through the disguise of others' perceptions and expectations. As I swept back the layers of all I had held on to in order to protect myself, I found true power in my honesty. I felt compelled to seek out more knowledge, soaking up information about the history of birth, its wider societal and cultural context as well as an understanding of the biology and physiology which gave me the tools to find answers. It opened my eyes to a completely new paradigm shift that supported my own self-discovery. When I became pregnant for a second time, I trusted myself, I trusted birth.

There is often an assumption when a woman considers unassisted birth that she has perhaps encountered a negative experience, therefore feels as though she has little choice. I responded to these comments by explaining that my decision to freebirth related to my first birth as much as its connection to any of my prior experiences. I felt absolute positivity; my choices were not made out of fear.

Perhaps spending years of my life lying to myself to protect a system that marginalised its victims left me questioning its value but at the time, this did not enter my conscious thought relating to my birth choices. Such unapologetic structures of injustice are mirrored throughout models of public service. Dictated by policy with protection of its benefactors at the heart; yet we so frequently place our trust and our responsibilities in their hands. As far as I was concerned, I was free to make decisions that I felt to be in the interest of my baby and myself and nobody else retained the power to remove that from me. Unfortunately, this belief was called into jeopardy at the whim of a third party.

When the Social Care's witch hunt came to an end and they were satisfied with the information that they coerced us into sharing, we felt persecuted. Although this was not a surprise attack by a stranger in a dark alley, the feelings of shame, disgust and anger were all present. Such fear mongering generalisations about the reality of rape and rapists protects perpetrators of violence, supported by a culture of victim blaming. They took our right to autonomy, our right to freedom and placed the blame firmly with us as a family, asserting that they were only doing their job; our claim to our Human Right of dignity was worthless. Stripped of choice, our power was forcibly removed behind a facade of constructed myths that control who we think we are.

Our society has already succeeded in the division of humanity; class, race, religion, lifestyle, gender and now we find ourselves pairing physical versus mental. Our duality creates fear, all or nothing, life or death. While these opposing extremes make it easy for us to prescribe labels, such black and white thinking eliminates the grey area of balance and crucially, choice. Breaking down these self-constructed barriers is a tool we possess in overcoming such damaging structures. It's not revolutionary to recognise that rape is not about sex, it is about power and control. Systematic abuse is no different, leaving the same imprint of trauma on both the body and the mind… My midwife referred me to Social Services for opting out… it culminated in a violation of my rights and privacy…

it profoundly affected my transition to motherhood leaving a lingering imprint and I was, more than ever, grateful for my wonderful birth to keep me grounded. **Melissa**, following the birth of her second baby, first freebirth

This experience had a long lasting impact on Melissa and was an issue for her in her next pregnancy.

With my third baby, I was naturally somewhat hesitant about engaging with the NHS again. There was no doubt in my mind that planning a second freebirth was the right choice for us and our needs. However, I was concerned about once again being penalised for those decisions.

Initially, I did not want to engage at all but I was concerned about being flagged as a concealed pregnancy and so I decided to book in purely as a box ticking exercise. I was very nervous about what type of midwife I may meet. At my first appointment I was relieved to meet an open midwife. She met my needs with great respect and understanding, to the point where we had a very open and honest conversation about freebirth. Her approach was refreshing, before she knew anything about me she presented ultrasound scans as a choice, reinforcing that I could decline - which I did and had intended to do. This attitude of choice was a breath of fresh air. However, she was not my midwife and was only covering that day. Our brief appointment eased my nerves somewhat and she assured me that 'my' midwife was an understanding midwife too. I requested my next appointment at home and she accommodated that.

My next appointment took place at my home. In attendance with my midwife was the SoM and my husband accompanied me. As with our previous care, we intended to decline further appointments with the NHS and inform of our decision to freebirth. Again, I was anxious and tentative in my approach but again it was met with great respect and understanding. Both midwives listened to what we had to say, did not question our views, I did not feel like she was trying to just get her paperwork done and she appeared to be open minded in her approach. It really helped me eliminate the worry about Social Services that had plagued me for so long and I was able to fully connect with my pregnancy and moving forward into birth as a third time mother. My third pregnancy was intense with great reflection. I engaged in a lot of yoga, swimming, drawing, journaling and finding an inner space to be nurtured and as a source of understanding and knowledge. This kind of internal journey is, for me, crucial to the birth experience.

Nothing could have changed my mind about birthing unassisted except the occurrence of a genuine, serious medical issue. In this hypothetical scenario I would readdress my options and choose what was most appropriate for me and my circumstances at that time. **Melissa**

Moggie was referred to Social Services because she told the midwives that she birthed with only her son present.

They sent me a Social Worker. He was nice but it was really awkward because you know

I had to stick to that lie and that was terrible – I hated that, thinking I hope T [older child] is not going to be around when he comes and visits and says that actually we had friends here. It was quite stressful that because I told the midwives that I was alone with him when I was giving birth to J [because she thought freebirth was illegal and sought to protect her friends who were present].

They were worried about T – they thought it was quite traumatic for T. I tried to be as like truthful as possible about what happened during the birth as I was just screaming my head off, you know I could understand listening to this story you would think that "maybe that little boy needs sort of like extra talking to and stuff." The Social Worker did not actually see T that much, so it was good. **Moggie**

One mother whose first freebirth story is in this book, recently had her second freebirth. She received a letter from Social Services just as the book went to press. The letter informed her that, after investigation, the case against her family would be taken no further. She was shaken to receive this letter as she did not know there was a referral to Social Services, or who made the referral, or who did the investigation. The letter made her fearful of the power of health professionals and concerned that this fear and stress could lessen her supply of breastmilk.

For two women, referral to Social Services was such a threat that they could not continue to live where they were.

Well we had a bit of a drama because someone thought they heard someone getting murdered and so they called the police and the paramedics. Apparently I was screaming "Help me." So about ten, fifteen minutes after she'd been birthed, then we had police coming round to the bath and they got really distressed because of the bloodied water and they were trying to get me out of the bath. But I was adamant that I needed to birth my placenta and that they leave me alone until then. And my partner was really great at keeping them at bay. And then he moved me to the caravan to get a bit more privacy for the placenta. And the moment when we were in there the placenta came quite easy...

Well, they [police] wouldn't believe my partner when he was saying I didn't want any further medical intervention. And so they demanded that a paramedic was to see me. And, and so he permitted this one female paramedic to see me.

Well ultimately, I had to consent, I had to sign a form to say I consented to no further medical intervention. It [knowledge of her rights] was due to When Push Comes To Shove [doula website], them sharing, ultimately our rights and language, how to use it. So then when they were attempting to get us to go, I just knew that I didn't actually have to go and so I just said what I knew. And she [paramedic] actually said I was really well informed... like she thought that that was okay, because I was well informed, then she felt that that was acceptable. And so yes, that was pretty good, so they left us, left us to it, but did send out midwives later on that day to check over the baby.

Well, actually they were really quite nice, it actually shocked me a bit (laughing). It actually shocked me because they were really lovely and I probably told them a bit too much truth, I guess someone within that profession, it kind of goes against it. But there was one midwife that just was like so supportive of me and all my decisions and, and they even said at the end of their visit, they asked, "do I need any further medical attention," and I said, "no, I don't want it, I don't need any." And [they] agreed, "you've done it this far without us, why would you need us?" And they were really pleasant and because Social Services then started to get involved, then one of the midwives would come out with them and she was just super supportive and just informed us, that ultimately, Social Services, it runs on consent and so if I just, don't consent to it, then I don't have to. Because they'd all said how healthy the baby was and me and how well she was feeding and so they didn't have any actual health concerns for either of us. So that was really nice to actually be supported by them.

[Social Services] attempted to keep visiting. They attempted, and I just kept asking what their reasons for their concerns were, and they were unable to provide it. They kept saying it was the health of me and the baby and at the time I was observing a forty-day confinement period. And so then I just had to, I just had to say to them that if you're not willing to respect my forty-day confinement, I believe that you're acting from prejudice and then we'll have to escalate the issue further. And from that then the case was closed and that was fine.

But then the health visitor reported me for not meaningfully engaging with the health visitor because I didn't feel it was necessary.

Well we're still in the process of figuring that out. Because they're saying that they need to come back out for a visit, but they're not actually telling me that I've been re-referred and the case has been reopened due to the health visitor. And they told me that the health visitor had concerns of: one, me not meaningfully engaging with her and the health visitor service; two, me not registering the birth of the baby; and three, me not registering the baby at a doctor's. And then they have concerns about our environment. So we live off-grid and at the time I was at my partner's place. He lives on a yard, out the back of a farm, or it was once a farm… and that's where the birth was, in the bath at the back there. And he's got some free-roaming animals that he set free that people abandoned there which are like pigs and, and chickens… they wanted to keep visiting there but the people at the farm there, they actually don't really like… so it was always a ticking time bomb for us to leave and so now I've left from there so I know that my current circumstance doesn't actually meet their requirements. I'm still attempting to keep them at bay. So it's just about how we're living really… Ideally, I would rather not [register the birth]… I'd rather attempt to avoid that but I am aware that there's loads of legislation changed during Covid, which has made it more challenging. And especially as Social Services are really, really trying to get involved. **Yony**

Children's Services hounded me mercilessly and my move to Jamaica whilst 26 weeks pregnant was a direct result of my fear that they would attempt to take my child from me at birth. I had to flee to an unknown place away from my support network of family and friends to avert this from happening.

Children's Services should be supporting mothers but instead they didn't listen to my thoughts on the mental health condition I have managed and have personal experience of. They labelled my lack of interest in pharmaceutical drugs as a "dangerous lack of insight." They poo-pooed the work I was doing with my private integrative therapist and said that my not wanting to remain under a chronically underfunded and understaffed mental health service as proof that I was uncooperative and hostile towards professionals.

They didn't care that I had hired a doula, ignoring her reasonable declaration that home birth was safe and that I'd be more likely to have an undisturbed healthy birth at home as I wished without midwives who had already explained they would be duty bound to auscultate every 15 minutes. **Reign**

After the freebirth of her 6th child, J and her family experienced prolonged distress from the action and inaction of Social Services. The ensuing court case resolved the issue, though feedback to the family was lacking.

I understood it was a legal obligation to register the birth of my baby but experienced difficulties reaching the correct department. In an attempt to promptly resolve the situation I contacted local postnatal services to seek assistance. To my disappointment nobody provided any help, instead I was informed by a health visitor that I would be reported to Children's Services. I challenged this action as unjustified stating my decision to freebirth was a legitimate choice, but was unable to resolve the disagreement. This reaction caused me distress but despite feeling ambivalent I wanted to act in good faith and demonstrate understanding of my newborn's human right to access healthcare. I agreed to an initial visit from a midwife despite my initial desire to decline. The attending midwife appeared knowledgeable and respectful of my choices, even attempting to assist with registering the birth by prompting my reluctant GP to take action where I had previously failed. She confirmed the health and well-being of both myself and newborn and informed me she was to attend a meeting arranged by Social Services, assuring me she would advocate that the initial referral was unjustified. Unfortunately this was not to be the end of the matter, the situation was now beyond my comprehension, there appeared to be no respect for my rights to accept or refuse treatment and believed I wasn't being treated with dignity and compassion. I couldn't understand why professionals would administer such pressure without recognition of the detrimental effects that could ensue.

I was overwhelmed and clearly having difficulty articulating the legitimacy of my personal choices. I thought it wise to seek assistance before engaging in any further action so reached out to N founder of When Push Comes To Shove who in turn put me in contact with The Autonomy Hotline and Beverley Beech, all of which were familiar with freebirth. The love and assistance that was to follow far exceeded my expectations, they reinforced my emotional strength and resiliency enabling me to think clearly and act rationally to the changeable situation, whilst continuing to care for my newborn and other children effectively. I was provided with all the help I needed to successfully register my child's birth as well as ongoing guidance and assistance to act according to my moral intuition.

When the designated social worker (SW) informed me of their intentions to investigate, I again attempted to reaffirm the legality of freebirthing and my understanding that it should not warrant their interference. It was alluded to that a Greater Manchester Policy considered me to have had a 'Concealed Pregnancy' obliging them to act. I was unfamiliar with this document and my questions regarding its origin and legitimacy were not answered satisfactorily. I remained confused how a pregnancy openly recognised by all friends and family could meet such a definition. I felt legally, morally and ethically obliged to maintain privacy on behalf of my family and requested written details of their accusation and concerns including copies of all relevant documents so I could perform my own due diligence before consenting to any further action.

The SW happily provided her email address to which I sent written confirmation of my requests including a SAR (subject access request) for documents. Four weeks passed without response so I issued a follow up email to query the matter offering further clarity on my expectations and highlighting the implied legal obligations of a SAR. The SW coincidently made contact the same day but denied receiving my emails. To avoid unnecessary confrontation I once again sent copies of my previous emails and SAR, this time ensuring confirmation of receipt. I was frustrated that I would probably have to accept further delay, but felt I had to bear some responsibility for not obtaining proof of receipt in the first instance. Interactions remained sporadic and my requests were left unanswered, I became increasingly concerned I was not receiving fair treatment, blind obedience appeared to be expected rather than a working partnership based on mutual respect.

I put my concerns in writing and sent them to the director of Children's Services and my local MPs in the hope they could assist to no avail. I was however informed that Social Services would not be able to respond to my SAR and was provided details of an alternative department to issue my request, which I acted upon immediately. Children's Services continued to be uncooperative, exerting further pressure to conform to their visitation requests including an unannounced visit to my home escorted by two uniformed officers in a marked vehicle. I did not appreciate this public display at my private residence as it unnecessarily created anxiety in my children and provoked my neighbours attention to the situation. Again I engaged to reaffirm my willingness to comply on receipt of written confirmation of the situation and following a short conversation all parties left peacefully. I was left with the impression we were in agreement and I would shortly receive written details as requested. The situation was extremely stressful. Nonetheless I continued to respond promptly to all correspondence and remained willing to cooperate. Throughout the whole process I continually sought out information and guidance and again I'm very thankful for all the help and assistance provided by AIMS, Birthrights, Family Rights Group, G and M.

Despite all my efforts to engage with Social Services, 10 weeks after initial contact me and my partner were abruptly served with a court summons for a Child Assessment Order with possible escalation to a Child Protection Order for all our children, scheduled to take place less than 24 hours later at Family Court. We were taken aback by this choice of action especially since on multiple occasions we had indicated we would agree to the proposed assessment once provided with the reasons for it and evidence supporting it. The paperwork and disclosure issued with the summons provided the first insight into Children's Services concerns outside of their initial accusation, none of which had been brought to our attention previously. I cannot say I agreed with their recollection of events and was quite alarmed by the selectivity of the documented details both past and present including the opinions of professionals I had encountered. Throughout the whole process I had attempted to be respectful and mindful of the perceptions of others however, it didn't appear to have been reciprocated. The accusations were focused on the children being unknown to health and education and lacked perspective. We had been given no opportunity to discuss the reasoning behind our choices nor opportunity to address or rectify any arising concerns amicably. We increasingly believed we were being subjected to an unsolicited personal attack breaching our human rights to live outside of societal norms.

As a breastfeeding mother it was not practical for me to attend court personally so my partner bore this responsibility. Thankfully despite the short notice we managed to acquire legal counsel on a direct access basis which proved invaluable in ensuring fair representation and procedure was adhered to. I provided a written statement addressing disclosure which was filed during pre-hearing discussions and included documentation to refute anything I considered misinformation. I was provided remote access in order to be able to participate in discussion and decision making outside the courtroom.

As what was a dispute had now been escalated into a situation we considered unhealthy for the children and a threat to the stability of the family, we agreed if the Court indicated the criteria for the making of an Order was met, we would not actively oppose the assessment and child protection medicals. We also readily agreed to a virtual meeting taking place at Court between the children, the social worker and the Guardian, from which no concerns were raised. The Court highlighted its discontent that the Local Authority had not dealt with their concerns in a more consensual way and without recourse to the Court and ordered the minutes from all strategy meetings be provided to us within three working days. A child assessment order in accordance with s. 43 of the Children Act 1989 was granted in respect of all the children. We were obliged to make them available for assessment at the family home by a home education officer, social worker and the court appointed guardian. We also had to attend a child protection medical at a local hospital.

The home education officer, Children's guardian and doctor all assured us on conclusion of their visit/assessment that they had no cause for concern and were satisfied we were fulfilling our parental responsibility and our children's needs were indeed being met. Following conclusion of the assessment period we have not received any further correspondence from Social Services and to date have never received any form of written documentation related to the details of the case. Very recently we did receive documents from our SAR request, five calendar months after confirmation from the correct department, it is from this documentation that we are now aware the case has been closed.

In hindsight I am deeply saddened by the scrutiny and stress my family has had to endure but I am overwhelming proud of my partner and beautiful children for remaining undeterred and upbeat throughout this unwelcome intrusion into our lives. I do not regret any of my choices and I am eternally grateful to all those who helped me. **J**

Chapter 21: The impact of the freebirth on the mother

All the women we spoke to were positive about the impact of the freebirth on them, even if the birth didn't go to plan, if their feelings were complex, or if they had difficult interactions with health practitioners.

It was lovely but maybe it was just really lucky but I felt like it was just what I'd dreamed that it could be and it really felt quite almost meditative… not too many people, sort of calm. It was good. **Sarah-Anne**

Liberating, yes and empowering, and humanising. I don't think I've realised how much of a human I was until this, it awoke all, well, all the animal parts. It awoke everything. **Katuš**

So I decided to do it myself and it was really a wonderful experience. It was really special and informed me a lot about how it is… I would want to give my daughters the idea about what we need to birth. Because we don't need very much at all. Except like your partner, your love, you know. **Jessica**

At the time I felt very empowered that we had done it ourselves… **Moggie**

… you feel powerful after the birth when it goes in the right way. So extremely powerful and elated. I was almost slightly manic, because I was just so excited. I was more excited about having survived the birth than I was having the baby, and that's dreadful, isn't it, but that's the way it was. **Rose**

I had a really easy breastfeeding journey. I had no problems breastfeeding. I had an incredible bond with my son. I was in really good health. I remember the day after giving birth feeling happy to go out for a walk. I was really joyful. I had no… sort of the baby blues that people talk about… me and partner felt really strong, that we'd done it together. It was like we've done this - we can do anything. It was such an amazing experience for us to do that together as a couple. When we listened to other people's birth stories and people who've birthed in different ways to us, we often talk about how lucky we were that we had the experience that we had together, and how amazing it was compared with people who had more difficult birth stories or stories where it's been very intervention-heavy. A's always delighted that he was the first person to hold A and pass him to me. We look back at it in a really positive way. Apart from the midwifery bit afterwards, there's nothing about it that we would have changed. We're really pleased. Often I know that some women choose to freebirth after they've had their first, maybe negative, experience, so we're really pleased that this will probably be the only baby I have and I'm really pleased that my experience of birth has been one that was so positive. I hate the word 'empowering' but it was an empowering experience for me, as a woman, to do that at home unassisted. As I said before, it's weird because when I look back, I think wow, that was bloody amazing that I did that. But I think also really normal and dull – I was just another woman giving birth. But yes, it was one of those weird experiences that you can describe in two different ways. When I told people about it, I didn't think that I'd done anything special. A lot of people said, "oh, that's really brave." But I didn't feel it was a brave choice; I just felt it was the right choice for us. I just felt intuitively that I didn't want anybody that I didn't know around. I didn't want to be in an unfamiliar place. I wanted to be able to move around. I wanted my dog to be there. I wanted to be able to eat what I wanted. I wanted no-one to be interfering with me or needing to check me at certain points. I just wanted to do it. I just felt really confident that that was the right thing to do. I didn't feel frightened. I didn't, during my labour, have any fear about giving birth. I just wanted to give birth that way. It wasn't like I had anything against going into hospital or midwives or anything like that. It wasn't about not wanting to engage in services. It was just about wanting what I felt was intuitively right for me. I'm not someone who goes against the system as a general rule. I have a very boring teaching job, and I was quite a run of the mill, normal sort of person. I'm not a crazy hippy or anything. I'm just like a normal woman and I just knew that the way I wanted to give birth was to do it ourselves and without anybody about. I just felt that was right – and it was. **Lindsay**

Many saw the freebirth as having a long term impact upon them.

… the most wonderful birthing experience. I is our last baby and we ended on a lovely birth but I know in my heart that if I could do it all again I would freebirth. It's the most, most empowering spiritual experience. **Sarah M**

I am a different person now after that birth, the depths of myself that I found and what I now know, how much more deeply I'm able to believe in myself now is different. It's really interesting, because my first birth changed me as a person. But, I'm different. In a good way. **Beth**

So when I had the freedom, with O, I really was, it was really happening as I thought and it was really magical and special and… And it was real… it was very good, yes. And you really feel powerful and it really makes you high. And it was even something like… you will really feel like in connection with all the universe. And is something that goes higher… Yes. I really thought that it was going to be the closest I'm going to be of any god, if god is there, no. It's that kind of feeling. Yeah. **Bea**

Oh, it was amazing! You can never go back unless there is a real medical issue. It was very nice to have the experience of the unassisted pregnancy as well, I have to say. That was a completely different experience. We always knew what to do and I could really tune into my body during the pregnancy because I didn't have pictures of baby from scans and I didn't have people tell me where she is and how she is, so I really knew everything. The whole experience was really amazing, even for my husband. He's still taken by it and he said it was really incredible. You can see how the baby… she is very focused and really happy and different… she behaves differently, even as a baby, when she was born, she didn't cry, she just looked. It was a very beautiful experience. I could feel my placenta detach from my uterus… I could feel everything. There was such a concentration and tune-in to my body that I felt really little things. I knew how she was there, and I knew when she slid into the birth canal and I knew how she was rotating. I didn't have any tears. She was 3.8kg, quite a big baby. I could feel my placenta detach, so I just stood up, I pulled on the cord and it came out… Yes, it was a very interesting experience, and I could understand how women can tune into themselves. **Michaela**

After I gave birth, I was just like [makes loud growling noise]. I stood up with her and I brought her to my breast, and I was like, "F – get towels! C do this!" And I just started telling everyone what to do. C was like, oh my God – look at you! Like totally went into primal warrior woman stage. **Lacey**

And I hear so many stories of transfers in and I think my birth would have been an easy one to kind of high-jack, and I really, really feel really lucky… I've torn all three times. So I have a bad back from the scar tissue, but that can happen. So, and I have this tilted, twisted uterus. So that's why I struggle to get them out in the second stage. But I think I could easily be somebody that's had traumatic births. I could easily have been somebody that's been taken in and had one birth that was traumatic, and then maybe a second. And then just thought, "I'm not going to have any more children." So I feel so lucky to have had the experiences like an antenatal teacher and as a doula and then having an independent midwife. And that birth, and then being able to have two freebirths of my own. So I just feel tremendously blessed to have got to this point really. **Cathy S**

It was amazing. I would never, ever, ever consider doing it any other way; it was perfect. It was the perfect birth, it was exactly what we wanted. Everything was amazing. The midwife who we'd had towards the end of the process who was helpful in a way, she came a couple of days later. So she said, "Oh we're switching to whatever, continuous care model. So next time, if you want, you could just ask for me and we could work together. I don't have to do anything but you could just call me and I can just sit in the corner." And I just thought to myself, "Why would I ever downgrade this experience to that? Why do you… you don't need to be here." It was amazing and the whole thing just felt like this is how it should be. There was zero stress, there was zero concern, there were zero interruptions. I was able to completely focus on what I needed to do and listening to my body the entire time. I never had a distraction of anyone else trying to interject with something they needed to do for their tick list. It was brilliant. And I wish, I wish more women knew about it as an option, if they want to do it. Because it is such, it is such an incredible experience. Oh, it's amazing. I mean, it hurt like hell, don't get me wrong – it hurt. But you know that it's over. **ME**

Several women spoke of being healed by their freebirth.

I just felt really healed by the process I went through and really supported by the water and the two women who I know who were really in tune with me, and I knew they were in tune with me, because they knew things I was feeling and thinking. That was a real blessing and I wanted to have an intuitive process and if it wasn't going to be with midwives then I trusted in the women who had experienced home births and know about the process, that it is an intuitive process and that is what I wanted ultimately and just to be able to touch that. **Polly**

I did it [VBAC freebirth] actually, for my own healing and journey. It's really, really helped. **Katie H**

What's amazing with this second birth is it almost rebalanced in itself, that whole process, just rebalanced everything in my body again. It was an incredibly healing thing, and I wasn't drained, and I wasn't exhausted... I was forty-one when I had my second child, they give you these warnings about age, and I never believe any of that stuff because I think we're all different. **Katuš**

Many spoke of how their experience of freebirth strengthened and sustained them for the future as mothers.

Afterwards I was like, "God, if I can do that, I can do anything." And again, second time around, just feeling an immense sense of empowerment. **Rachel**

I actually got what I wanted and this is what I really did want and nobody stopped that from me, and so I think it has made me think right okay, just build on that, build on it. Yes definitely, and I would be much more assertive and I'm learning to be much more assertive and asking for what I want. **Polly**

I feel it has given me confidence to make the choices that I want to make as a mother. Yes, like the choice I made to breastfeed for longer like a lot of women do. I felt quite empowered to do that because I felt that after the birth I could make the choices that I wanted to. I could follow my instincts. I guess I felt that it was okay to do that and it would be okay if it wasn't what everybody else was doing. **Sarah-Anne**

I'm obviously so pleased that I did it, and it's an amazing story to have in my life, and amazing for R [baby] as well, a great start because it's just set us off on this really positive journey. **Rosalie**

… they've made me feel stronger because every time I went with my intuitions about something it turned out to be the right things to do, you know, **every** decision where I went against my intuitions it turned out to be the wrong thing to do so, yes, it's such a tremendous experience that it's very empowering to go through it your own way, and to trust that, it's great. **Charlie**

In the days following Z's birth, a profound elation lifted me beyond the physical ache which endured. I unravelled a deep admiration for my body and its capabilities, honouring every twinge, every bruise. As my memory recalled specific events, each word, each feeling was experienced again through my body – tensing, releasing, holding, flowing. Each element imprinted within my muscles, my bones, my very structure. From these foundations a story is born, meaning and value attributed, significance reflected in the learning.

The physical and the mental, the metaphysical; in a harmony of acceptance for the temporary truth of what the experience needed to be in those exact moments which are now history, non-existent. It brought forth words that allow me to conceptualise a meaning within the context of my life; an understanding in my mind that reflects the physical knowledge I hold within my body.

I feel strength, I feel power - these features have been absorbed, shaping the way forward. Each of my birth experiences, a trio of differing occurrences etched within, have offered thresholds for self-exploration. Z's birth brought deep intimate challenges yet simultaneously invited the innermost sincere insight, underpinning a replenished longevity and knowledge for my identity as a mother. **Melissa**

I sit holding on in the space she was born and feel so grateful that the birth before arrival on the previous year gave me the strength, courage, belief that I could, regardless of my health problems and premature babies, have the most wonderful birthing experience. **Sarah M**

It feels like an amazing start for my three children… I don't get a lot of things right parenting, but I think, "Well I got your birth right. Yes, I did everything I could to make sure that your very start to life was as kind of peaceful and as positive as it could be." And it was, so I comfort myself with that and a glass of wine on an evening when I've had a bad parenting day. **Cathy S**

For some women, their experience of freebirthing led them to suggest this could be an option for others.

At the appointment we had with the team of independent midwives at the end of my postnatal care, they asked if there was anything I thought they should tell clients. I suggested they mention to clients that it is okay to not call them and it is okay to freebirth. I had felt awkward about bringing this up with them before, as if they would be hurt or not understand someone booking independent midwives and also wanting to freebirth. But they did understand and said making clients aware of the option to freebirth would show how much they themselves trusted birth. **Virginia**

Some felt inspired to work to improve maternity services for others.

… just feeling immense sense of empowerment. And I think, for me, I mean I feel really passionate about birth and it's something that I feel like later in life, when I've got more time, I would love to sort of do some doula work and work with women. Because it makes such a difference having an empowered birth. **Rachel**

Now I feel, now I've had A, I feel much more confident in speaking that and saying that and supporting other people. And I'll continue to support other people in their choices, but also to know and be okay to say… I feel women are so disparaged, discouraged, unsupported in society as a whole, that no wonder we don't believe that our bodies work. We're told every day when we look at the media, "You're too fat. You're too thin." You know, the gaze that is upon us all the time is a critical one. And so when it comes to something like growing a healthy baby and giving birth in a way that is both positive in mind and body to baby and mother – it's no wonder people doubt themselves even subconsciously. So I feel like a lot of the work that I've done throughout my pregnancies has been trying to clear a lot of that away. Which is why the idea of having another baby appeals, because I just want to keep doing this work. I can keep doing it and supporting other people, and that's wonderful. And that's really wonderful. I'm glad I can do that. But, oh, it feels like there's so much work to do. And that can feel a bit exhausting and relentless, that we're in this situation within our culture and our society, that we've grown this belief of the lack in women's abilities to grow and birth babies. And... within that it's messed up. **Katy B**

I'm quite a baby in my career, but I'm in the middle of writing a course at the minute to help women who are considering freebirth, who might be mostly in the system, but aware that there might be something different. So, working on the margins of people who are choosing alternative care. Even if they might have, like I did, the appointments or they might still opt for the midwife there, but just thinking about a different way… Yes, I just talk about birth a lot (laughs). **Leonie**

I do wish that all women could have a birth like this, even with midwives there… In fact, all of the friends who've had freebirths who I know of, and where I've been at, have been just similarly exhilarating and transformative and empowering. I mean, there is a bit of an element of "fuck you" in there too. As in, this is my body, and if you're not going to respect it, then you're not coming near me, sorry. And I'm not saying that against midwives, because I work with midwives and I see so much good. **ST**, herself a midwife

I'm really interested to work with people. So it's really through my own experience, because of that I'd like to really try and help others to have such a positive experience as well. And help women to connect with their bodies, because I think so much of this is related to really trusting your own body. And trusting yourself, giving yourself that power, instead of giving it away to the professionals basically. **Gauri**

I think it's really extra-amazing because it was a VBAC. I had some midwifery attention before my labour even started and then after that, nothing. My local hospital, their VBAC success rate is only twenty percent. It's criminal really, because they make you all go to the labour ward, they have time moments, they have continuous monitoring, they have all of these things, which are just not conducive to giving birth. No wonder that they only have a twenty percent success rate. So I mean, I really, really try to advocate for women having home births for their VBACs, because I think it really gives them the best chance. Again, it's all about different things from the medical establishment…

It's interesting that my background is quite medical, but then I've stopped doing vet work and do the doula thing full time. **Katie H**

Actually one thing I'm really glad about is that after my complaint, I started attending the MSLC in Leeds and I met the midwife who dealt with our complaint and who was at the hospital on the day that we went in. I met her quite frequently and it does seem that because of what happened to us, lots of things have changed in Leeds for freebirthing women. So in some way I'm glad that I had that negative experience, because I feel like it's helped other women have a more positive experience. And while I wish I hadn't had to do that, I'm glad that something good has come out of it and that it hasn't just been something that happened to us and has happened to other people since. I feel happy in some way that my complaint and that my determination to make sure that other women weren't told, "what you've done is illegal, what you've done is wrong"… that doesn't happen anymore, I hope, because there is now something in place, some protocol in place for how to deal with freebirth in that area now. So you know, just try and look at the positive of what happened there and hope that other women… and I know that other women in Leeds have freebirthed since me, and have had more kindness shown to them and respect and their wishes being respected. So fingers crossed – it's been a positive outcome and not just… That midwife who came to me obviously had never experienced that before and was just totally out of her depth, and I think she was horrified but she also probably couldn't believe that we'd done it. I don't know. It was very bizarre, looking back. But you can't choose who gets sent out to you, unfortunately. **Lindsay**

Continuity of care, the NHS needs to value women's health in and of itself. And I just think if blokes were the ones that gave birth, we'd have continuity of care from day one. The system would have money pouring into it and that we need to, we need to fight for it. And it's not… I think with freebirth sometimes it can feel a bit, or it can be posed as a bit of an us and them against the NHS. And it might be against the system, but it's not the midwives, like the midwives are doing the best they can, they go into midwifery because they love women and they love babies and sometimes the system can just break them and they're still people who need to pay a mortgage, and they need a pay cheque at the end of every month, and they need to play that game because they still need to live their life. And so for the few midwives, like I wrote a big email to the Head of Midwifery and, because I found out from the midwife who came to our birth that she's getting to retirement… It's like now in these last few years, kick up a stink, become the loud one at the start, not, it's not even whistle-blowing but just being like, "Why aren't we moving to continuity of care? What is our plan to get more funding?" Now is the time to be that dissenting voice. **Jocelyn**

Doulas were very aware of the positive impact of freebirth on mothers and the importance of support towards that positive state.

The confidence in the women who birthed without the medical support or the medical interventions or disturbances was incredible. These women are, they're walking so tall and really feeling like they trusted themselves, they birthed on their own terms, nobody messed with them, nobody weighed the baby, nobody did anything, nobody talked really. That's phenomenal. I wish we could get midwifery in line with that.

I know you've been looking at this for years. But it's really just becoming clear to me now after what, twelve, thirteen years of being with women, that what they're needing is people who can sit and be with birth, people who they know, people who they can trust, people they can look forward to it with, and reflect back on it with. Because they see them in their community in the future.

And when I started this, I saw myself as a doula that could fill a gap, that doulas were a stopgap until they got maternity services sorted out. And now in some ways I feel like doulas are the last threads of midwifery. Kind of holding on to some of the knowledge, some of the wisdom, some of the tools that midwifery is no longer allowed to use or they don't have time to use. Like sitting patiently, like knitting, like not asking questions and just being there. **D**, doula

Our reflections

All those who contributed their stories to this book wanted their birth to be peaceful and uninterrupted. They wanted to tune into their bodies and their babies, and they wanted to feel safe. Everything we know of the physiology of birth suggests that these are wise choices. The tragedy is that they could only achieve this outside NHS maternity services.

These stories, unsurprisingly, are strikingly similar to stories from people all over the world wherever they plan to have their babies. Accounts from those planning to birth straightforwardly outside mainstream maternity services in high income countries particularly resonate with the stories in this book (Dahlen et al 2020, Gillan et al 2023, Hall et al 2022, Shorey et al 2023). Like all those giving birth, these women want to feel safe, respected, supported, and treated as capable and equal adults. In addition, those who birth outside maternity care systems and norms value being supported to make the decisions that they feel are right for them and their babies and families. They want to be cared for by people who see childbearing broadly in the same way that they do: a physiological process that usually goes well when women can birth unhindered in calm, quiet, non-medicalised surroundings with no routine time limits and no interference unless it is absolutely essential. While a few found support within the services from outstanding, courageous practitioners, overall they experienced their knowledge about birth, their babies, their bodies and aspirations as anathema to the mainstream medicalised, impersonal services they encountered. This made maternity units feel unsafe places for them to give birth.

Midwives have written eloquently about the need for women to feel "safe enough to let go" in labour (e.g. Anderson 2010). One of us (MK) has been concerned throughout her career with the importance of attention, and the need for the midwife to give her full attention to the individual in her care and hold safe space for her and her particular needs (Kirkham 1986 and 2010). Yet the midwifery service, now based on an industrial, rule driven model, has reached a point where women feel torn between attending to the midwife's requirements or attending to their own needs. Many no longer feel safe in the hands of midwives. This is heartbreaking. So many midwives leave midwifery (Ball et al 2002, Royal College of Midwives 2016) because they cannot practise as they would wish to practise, leaving the service even more short staffed, a tragically vicious circle. Or they give up trying to attend to individuals as this makes them vulnerable to pressure from management to ensure compliance with policies and guidelines. As many women are aware, midwives are often bullied and fearful, and some go on in their turn to bully women in their care. Nevertheless, it is unacceptable that so many women reported feeling "violated" by previous NHS care.

The intersection of safe and unsafe which we have written about previously (Edwards 2005, 2008) remains at the very heart of the tensions between the women who freebirth and those who believe (or who feel unable to challenge the belief) that birth in hospital supervised by health practitioners is not only desirable but essential to safe birth. This belief is usually accompanied by a further assumption, that the mother and baby are completely separate entities and that the baby must be prioritised during pregnancy and birth. This makes the definition of safety seem obvious, untouchable and therefore unchallengeable. These beliefs can portray freebirth, home birth and decisions outside usual medical protocols and policies as risky. Thus women who make these decisions are seen as deliberately and knowingly putting their babies at greater risk of harm than the women who acquiesce to the mainstream medical care on offer. While babies can and do die or be harmed during birth in any setting, these beliefs pose deeply moral obligations on mothers to conform to a system that is not based on evidence. Despite this, the heavy moral obligations on what it means to be a good mother currently pressing down on pregnant women are not shed lightly. These freebirthing women often thought about every possible aspect of pregnancy, labour and birth and came to carefully considered decisions about how best to proceed. Some had been so traumatised in previous births that they felt unable to consider using maternity services except in an emergency, because these services would have negative effects, including undermining their abilities to mother their babies well.

These women were aware that conformity can be imposed by drawing on coercive mechanisms and structures that can be threatened or used. The biggest threat identified by many of the women who contributed to this book was that of being referred to Social Services with their power to remove their children. Whilst a few midwives spoke up in defence of mothers referred to Social Services, most of the referrals were made by midwives. Two of the mothers who contributed their stories fled from their home area when referred to Social Services in fear of losing their children, and one family still feels unable to return. Both their babies are healthy and flourishing. One baby whose birth is described here has recently been taken into "care."

Despite coercive social norms and the ways in which they are enacted by health professionals, these women knew that conformity had already posed or would pose a risk to them and their babies, and that social and population norms are not necessarily positive or applicable to individuals. They described themselves and their babies as both inseparable and two beings. They believed that their immediate and long-term health and wellbeing would significantly impact on their babies' ongoing health and wellbeing, (as well as on their families). This makes for a much more complex definition of safety, which includes the physical, emotional, cultural and for many women spiritual safety of the mother baby dyad throughout the childbearing process (Edwards 2005, 2008).

A straightforward birth can thus be seen as a desirable and positive aspiration that protects the mother's and baby's health and wellbeing, potentially throughout life, and we now have overwhelming evidence that institutionalised obstetric units with their routine time limits and interventions mitigate against physiological birth rather than enhancing its likelihood (Olsen and Clausen 2023). And while the women could live with the uncertainties of life and birth, they *could not accept the uncertainties of the maternity services. The accounts in this book of the positive impact of their freebirths on these women speak for themselves.*

The women in this book emphasised the importance of preparation for labour and birth. They took responsibility for this preparation, as they did for the birth, and worked hard to prepare themselves. The doulas who supported many of them also emphasised the importance of their role in helping women to prepare for birth rather than the importance of their attendance at the birth. Independent midwives place similar emphasis, (often offered as preparation in case the woman gives birth before her midwife arrives) which women find empowering. The NHS has moved in the opposite direction, reducing or even removing antenatal classes especially for women who have already had babies, despite the fact that these women sometimes feel just as great a need for antenatal preparation, in particular if their first birth was difficult. These classes are now often focused on ensuring women's compliance with hospital policies, though there are a few innovative exceptions e.g. (Wiseman et al 2022).

An important part of preparing for a freebirth was seen as working through and moving away from fear and building trust and self confidence. This included surrounding themselves during pregnancy with people who trusted their ability to birth their babies. Fear is contagious, as is trust, so trusted supporters improve birth outcomes (Sandall et al 2016). The women felt this viscerally and tried to avoid having people around them, including midwives, who they experienced as fearful or negative. Traditionally midwives' main job was to support women, build their confidence and instil the belief that they could cope with labour and birth, which the vast majority of them did. Continuity of midwifery carer makes this possible and usually results in more women giving birth in Birth Centres and at home, better survival rates for babies, fewer preterm births, greater agency for women, fewer interventions in labour and birth, and increased breastfeeding rates (Sandall et al 2016). So many of the women in this book avoided NHS health professionals because of their negativity and fear, but were happy to consult supportive professionals such as hypnobirthing teachers, homoeopaths and independent midwives. NHS maternity care, with its emphasis on risk, prepared women for things going wrong, but did not prepare them for things going right. Indeed, by undermining women's self-confidence, the emphasis on risk is a negative self-fulfilling prophecy with many concerning implications: something that is recognised as negative in most other areas of life. Adjunct Professor of Midwifery, Nicky Leap, in her introduction to Birthing Outside the System: The Canary in the Coal Mine quoted from an interview she heard with an athlete, 'If only there was just a bit more positivity around health and well-being. [With our athletes] we don't sit down and quote stats at them, and quote how many times we've lost. We sit down and look at how we can win. [The doctors] go down the route of: 'Well, we're preparing you for the fail.' I don't prepare my team for the fail. Why is pregnancy not targeted like that? Why is it not given that positivity?' (Leap 2020 pxxii).

All the women stressed the need for a calm, quiet environment in which they could focus and listen to their bodies and babies without interference or intervention, but for many of the women, this did not mean being alone. Many chose to have people with them during labour and birth. Most had partners, some had their children, and many had doulas and/or friends and relatives. It is clear from their accounts that a professional presence with its monitoring gaze was often experienced as a negative intervention in the process of labour and birth. A presence that the woman perceives as negative undermines the mother's confidence when she needs it most. A presence that is trusted and seen to be wise holds safe space for the mother and baby. D had thought about this a lot as a doula. She emphasised the importance of watching and seeing how labour and birth unfolds and, crucially, focusing deeply on the women and whether or not she is giving any cues that anything needs to happen:

If the woman needs somebody, she'll let you know that she needs somebody, she'll ask for the somebody or she'll in some way struggle and look like she's needing something else, and then we might suggest something. But if we're suggesting something when she's not asking for it, what are we doing? We're interfering with her now… it's very emotional to see a woman birth undisturbed, kind of choking up thinking about it. It's really, really a sacred, beautiful and massive event that's very understated and whispery and precious and I very rarely see that when there are two strangers in the room. **D**, doula

This quietly encouraging, sensitive, "unobtrusive presence", described by women was exactly what they wanted. We know that a trusted relationship with a known doula or midwife improves birth outcomes (Sandall et al 2016). It is sad and immoral that we have reached a point where a supportive continuing midwife/mother relationship is very rare in the NHS, when the evidence shows so many benefits to the health and wellbeing of mothers, babies and families. Some women would have liked a midwife to support them during labour and birth but decided to freebirth because such a relationship was not possible.

It is also sad that the motivation which originally took MK into midwifery now leads midwives such as E (see chapter 15) to leave midwifery to become doulas. There is now a new kind of birth worker: doulas, birthkeepers and other birth supporters, whose aim is to be with women, the very meaning of the word midwife. They understand that birth is about relationships, helping women to feel safe in a web of support as they birth their babies and new family relationships are born. It is perhaps shocking but not surprising that some of the most experienced, holistic and woman-focused midwives in the UK have given up their midwifery registration with the Nursing and Midwifery Council in order to work as doulas.

People differ, and not all of the women wanted support from others during labour. Some women found solitude to be essential for them to be able to labour and give birth, even if they hadn't planned this. They needed privacy and did not want a doula or anyone else at their birth. Indeed a few said that excellent care for a previous birth had helped their confidence to a point where they wanted their next birth to be in private. The need for privacy could change during labour, even when being observed did not carry the monitoring implications of the medical gaze.

The structure and ideology of NHS maternity services held together by overworked midwives does not generally support women who want a peaceful birth with trusted supporters. In the past a Supervisor of Midwives might have been able to help these women. One of the roles of the statutory position of Supervisor of Midwives was as a senior midwife apart from NHS management to whom a mother could appeal when she felt her needs were not being met. That position was abolished in 2017 and not replaced. Some women found NHS midwifery managers were supportive, but this depended on the individual and was not part of their job.

The women who entrusted us with their stories are all UK residents. They were eligible for free NHS maternity care. They could accept all or part of maternity services offered by the NHS or opt out in the knowledge that NHS services would still be available for them and their babies in an emergency, and that they could opt into that service at any point during pregnancy, labour, birth or after the birth. The one woman who moved away from the safety net of NHS emergency services suffered a tragic outcome after she moved overseas to avoid Social Services to whom she had been referred by a midwife. The safety net of NHS emergency services was part of the planning of freebirths and was used when needed. This makes these women's stories particular to the UK where that service is available.

The women who contributed their stories spoke passionately about their experiences of lack of care from midwives and other practitioners, but were still able to access maternity services if they chose to, and could still sometimes find practitioners who could and would support them. As worrying beliefs and practices undermine our public services, (including our National Health Service), maternity services will look very different in the future. The almost universal safety net will decrease, especially for vulnerable women, and the way in which women make decisions about where and how to birth their babies will change, unless maternity services can be reshaped and resourced to embody genuine care for all pregnant women irrespective of their circumstances.

While these women were passionate about the importance of healthy, positive births, it was not always easy for them to speak out and they found that their visibility was often depicted in negative ways, because of the moral context in which they freebirthed. But they were abundantly clear and developed themes that women have been voicing for many decades in many different parts of the world. In this book we have sought to do justice to the women who entrusted us with their stories. Many of these women reported being "nourished" and "inspired" by other women's birth stories, which enabled them to move beyond their fears. We have shared their stories because we "believe in the transformative power of stories to bring people together, expand our cognitive horizons, and gently unlock our true potential for empathy and wisdom" (Shafak 2020 p88).

These stories opened our minds, taught, humbled and changed us. We hope that they will challenge certainty, inspire, and provoke deeper and more nuanced understanding and empathy towards pregnant women, the decisions they make and the support they need to grow, birth and nurture their babies and families in the most positive and healthy ways possible.

References

Alexievich S (2017) The Unwomanly Face of War. Penguin.

Alexievich S (2017) Boys in Zinc. Penguin.

Anderson T (2010) Feeling safe enough to let go: the relationship between a woman and her midwife during the second stage of labour. In Kirkham M Ed. The Midwife-Mother Relationship. Second Edition. Basingstoke, Macmillan.

de Bairacli Levy J (1991) The Complete Herbal Handbook for Farm and Stable. Farrar, Straus and Giroux.

Ball L, Curtis P, Kirkham M (2002) Why Do Midwives Leave? Royal College of Midwives, London.

Brink A (1996) Imaginings of Sand. London, Secker and Warburg.

Cohen Shabot S (2020) Why "Normal" Feels So Bad: violence and vaginal examinations during labour - a (feminist) phenomenology. Feminist Theory 22(3): 443–463.

Dahlen H, Kumar-Hazard B, Schmied V (eds) (2020) Birthing Outside the System: The Canary in the Coal Mine. Oxon, Routledge.

Davis E, Pascali-Bonaro D, Jolson A (2016) Orgasmic Birth. Audible Studios.

Dick-Read G (2004) Childbirth Without Fear. London, Pinter & Martin.

Edwards NP (2005) Birthing Autonomy: Women's experiences of planning home births. Oxon, Routledge.

Edwards NP (2008) Safety in birth: the contextual conundrums faced by women in a 'risk society', driven by neoliberal policies. MIDIRS Midwifery Digest 18:4: 463-70.

Gaskin IM (1977) Spiritual Midwifery. The Farm, Summertown, Tennessee.

Gillan P, Bamidele O, Healy M (2023) Systematic review of women's experience of planning home birth in consultation with maternity care providers in middle to high-income countries. Midwifery 124:103733. doi:10.1016/j.midw.2023.103733.

Greenfield M, Payne-Gifford S, McKenzie G (2021) Between a Rock and a Hard Place: Considering "Freebirth" During Covid 19. Frontiers in Global Women's Health. 2:603744. doi:3389/fgwh.2021.603744.

Gribble KD, Bewley S, Bartick MC *et al* (2022) Effective Communication about Pregnancy, Birth, Lactation, Breastfeeding and Newborn Care: the Importance of Sexed Language. Frontiers in Global Women's Health. 3:818856. doi:10.3389/fgwh.2022.818856.

Hall H, Fooladi E, Kloester J *et al* (2022) Factors that Promote a Positive Childbearing Experience: A Qualitative Study. Journal of Midwifery and Women's Health. 68(1): 44-51.

Kirkham M (1986) Basic, Supportive Care in Labour. PhD thesis, University of Manchester.

Kirkham M (1997) Stories and Childbirth in Kirkham M, Perkins E (eds) Reflections on

Midwifery. London, Bailliere Tindal.

Kirkham M (2010) The Midwife-Mother Relationship. Second Edition. Basingstoke, Macmillan.

Kirkham M (2018) Standardisation of care: a contradiction in terms. Midwifery Matters 157: 4-7.

Leap N (2020) Foreword. In Dahlen H, Kumar-Hazard B, Schmied V (eds) Birthing Outside the System: The Canary in the Coal Mine. Oxon, Routledge: xiv-xxiii.

McKenzie-Mohr S, Lafrance MN eds. (2014) Women Voicing Resistance. London, Routledge.

Olsen O, Clausen J (2023). Planned hospital birth compared with planned home birth for pregnant women at low risk of complications. Cochrane Database of Systematic Reviews, 3, CD000352. DOI: 10.1002/14651858.CD000352.pub3.

Owen A (2016) A Year in the Life of the Yorkshire Shepherdess. London, Pan Books.

Ray RA (1994) Buddhist Saints in India: a study in Buddhist values and orientations. New York, Oxford University Press.

Reed B (2016) Birth in Focus. London, Pinter & Martin.

Reed B, Edwards N (2023). Closure: How the flagship Albany Midwifery Practice, at the heart of its South London community, was demonised and dismantled. London: Pinter & Martin.

Robinson VS (2008) The Birthkeepers. Star Flower Press.

Royal College of Midwives (2016) Why Midwives Leave – revisited. London, RCM.

Sandall J, Soltani H, Gates S *et al* (2016) Midwife-led continuity models versus other models of care for women during pregnancy, birth and early parenting. Cochrane Database of Systematic Reviews, 9, CDOO4667. doi: 10.1002/14651858.CD004667.pub5

Shafak E (2020) How to stay sane in an age of division. London, Profile Books/Welcome Collection.

Shanley LK (1994) Unassisted Childbirth. Westport, Connecticut and London, Bergin& Garvey.

Shorey S, Jarašiūnaitė Fedosejeva G, Akik BK *et al* (2023) Trends and motivations for freebirth: A scoping review. Birth 50(1):16-31.

Schmid S translated by Neiger D (2015) Freebirth. Self-Directed Pregnancy and Birth. Edition Riedenburg.

Summers H (2020) There's no place like home. The Guardian Weekend, Dec 5, 34-37.

Wickham S (2022) What's right for me: making decisions in pregnancy and childbirth. Birthmoon Creations.

Wiseman O, Emmett L, Hickford G *et al* (2022) The challenges and opportunities of implementing group antenatal care ('Pregnancy Circles') as part of standard NHS maternity care: a co-designed qualitative study. Midwifery 109:103333. doi: 10.1016/j.midw.2022.103333.

Printed in Dunstable, United Kingdom